T0257984

Advances in Gastroenterology

Advances in Gastroenterology

Edited by **Sandra McLeish**

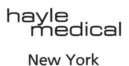

New York

Published by Hayle Medical,
30 West, 37th Street, Suite 612,
New York, NY 10018, USA
www.haylemedical.com

Advances in Gastroenterology
Edited by Sandra McLeish

International Standard Book Number: 978-1-63241-026-9 (Hardback)

Printed in the United States of America.

Contents

Preface   VII

Section 1   Pathophysiology and Treatment of
Pancreatic and Intestinal Disorders   1

Chapter 1   Pharmacology of Traditional Herbal
Medicines and Their Active Principles
Used in the Treatment of Peptic Ulcer,
Diarrhoea and Inflammatory Bowel Disease   3
Bhavani Prasad Kota, Aik Wei Teoh and Basil D. Roufogalis

Chapter 2   Emerging Approaches for the
Treatment of Fat Malabsorption
Due to Exocrine Pancreatic Insufficiency   17
Saoussen Turki and Héla Kallel

Chapter 3   Evaluating Lymphoma Risk in
Inflammatory Bowel Disease   45
Neeraj Prasad

Chapter 4   Development, Optimization and
Absorption Mechanism of DHP107, Oral Paclitaxel
Formulation for Single-Agent Anticancer Therapy   91
In-Hyun Lee, Jung Wan Hong, Yura Jang,
Yeong Taek Park and Hesson Chung

Chapter 5   Differences in the Development of the Small Intestine
Between Gnotobiotic and Conventionally Bred Piglets   109
Soňa Gancarčíková

Chapter 6   Superior Mesenteric Artery Syndrome   149
Rani Sophia and Waseem Ahmad Bashir

Chapter 7   The Surgical Management of Chronic Pancreatitis   153
S. Burmeister, P.C. Bornman, J.E.J. Krige and S.R. Thomson

Chapter 8   **Appendiceal MALT Lymphoma in
Childhood – Presentation and Evolution**   173
Antonio Marte, Gianpaolo Marte,
Lucia Pintozzi and Pio Parmeggiani

Chapter 9   **The Influence of Colonic Irrigation
on Human Intestinal Microbiota**   183
Yoko Uchiyama-Tanaka

Section 2   **Diseases of the Liver and Biliary Tract**   193

Chapter 10   **Pancreato-Biliary Cancers –
Diagnosis and Management**   195
Nam Q. Nguyen

Chapter 11   **Hepatic Encephalopathy**   211
Om Parkash, Adil Aub and Saeed Hamid

Chapter 12   **Adverse Reactions and Gastrointestinal Tract**   227
A. Lorenzo Hernández, E. Ramirez
and Jf. Sánchez Muñoz-Torrero

Chapter 13   **Recontructive Biliary Surgery in the
Treatment of Iatrogenic Bile Duct Injuries**   245
Beata Jabłońska and Paweł Lampe

Chapter 14   **Selected Algorithms of Computational
Intelligence in Gastric Cancer Decision Making**   263
Elisabeth Rakus-Andersson

             Permissions

             List of Contributors

Preface

The aim of this book is to describe complete clinical approaches based on current advancements in the field of gastroenterology. The most significant developments in the treatment of gastrointestinal disorders and pathophysiology are elucidated in this book including pancreatitis and irritable bowel disease (IBD). Special emphasis is laid on the disease of the liver and biliary tract. This book will provide important novel information which will be useful for clinicians, basic scientists and medical students.

This book is a result of research of several months to collate the most relevant data in the field.

When I was approached with the idea of this book and the proposal to edit it, I was overwhelmed. It gave me an opportunity to reach out to all those who share a common interest with me in this field. I had 3 main parameters for editing this text:

1. Accuracy – The data and information provided in this book should be up-to-date and valuable to the readers.

2. Structure – The data must be presented in a structured format for easy understanding and better grasping of the readers.

3. Universal Approach – This book not only targets students but also experts and innovators in the field, thus my aim was to present topics which are of use to all.

Thus, it took me a couple of months to finish the editing of this book.

I would like to make a special mention of my publisher who considered me worthy of this opportunity and also supported me throughout the editing process. I would also like to thank the editing team at the back-end who extended their help whenever required.

Editor

Section 1

Pathophysiology and Treatment of Pancreatic and Intestinal Disorders

Pharmacology of Traditional Herbal Medicines and Their Active Principles Used in the Treatment of Peptic Ulcer, Diarrhoea and Inflammatory Bowel Disease

Bhavani Prasad Kota[1], Aik Wei Teoh[2] and Basil D. Roufogalis[1]
[1]University of Sydney
[2]Ferngrove Pharmaceuticals
Australia

1. Introduction

The endocrine, exocrine and paracrine secretions of the gastrointestinal (GI) tract play a pivotal role in the digestion and absorption of food and orally administered drugs. The secretion of mucus by mucus-secreting cells protects the erosion of the gastric mucosa from the highly acidic gastric juice. The secretion of hydrochloric acid from parietal cells is regulated by acetylcholine, histamine and gastrin. Disturbances in secretory functions of the gastrointestinal tract can lead to several GI complications. Conventional therapies employ a range of drugs that have been pharmacologically well characterised. While these drug molecules are proven to be beneficial, the adverse effects and drug-drug interactions highlight the need for better treatment modalities for GI tract disorders.

Since ancient times, herbal medicines have been traditionally used to treat several diseases. The gastroprotective properties of these herbs and their active constituents have been experimentally demonstrated (Al Mofleh, 2010). Asian traditional medicine systems have identified several herbs and spices to treat GI tract disorders (Langmead & Rampton, 2006; Sengupta et al., 2004). In support of these traditional claims, several preclinical and clinical studies have provided the scientific basis for the effectiveness of herbal extracts (e.g. *Glycyrrhiza glabra*) and their active constituents (e.g. flavonoids) in treating GI tract disorders (Borrelli & Izzo, 2000). The discovery and development of anti-ulcer agents such as carbenoxolone from *Glycyrrhiza glabra* and gefarnate from cabbage further highlight the presence of pharmacologically active components in herbal extracts and suggests their use as an alternative therapy to treat GI tract disorders.

The effectiveness and the mechanisms of action of crude herbal extracts vary according the composition of their chemical constituents. Herbal medicine seems to fill this gap, especially when employing high manufacturing standardised forms of herbal medicine with regard to the quality and quantity of ingredients (Suzuki et al., 2009). In addition, well characterised herbal formulations may lead to the production of reliable clinical data on efficacy and safety. As several studies have shown that herbal medicines may produce adverse reactions and herb-drug interactions, the common assumption that 'herbal products are natural, they are safe' is no longer valid. Safety and quality data of herbal medicines should be made available to medical practitioners and other healthcare professionals to avoid these unwanted effects.

Several plants have been used by traditional healers around the world to treat various gastrointestinal tract diseases. Centuries ago the reliance on nature to cure human ailments was developed by great efforts of dedicated professionals by keen observation and trial and error method. This important knowledge is updated constantly and passed from generations to generations. Today traditional healing systems play important roles in several parts of the world, especially where modern pharmaceuticals are less accessible. Modern scientific research methods are invaluable to support traditional claims and also to develop traditional remedies as a viable alternative to mainstream pharmaceuticals. In recent years, a number of research papers have been published on herbal medicines to provide the experimental evidence for their traditional claims. Given the multitude of these research publications, it is not possible to cover all of them. In this chapter, we only attempted to provide the experimental (animal and human studies) evidence for the plants that have been traditionally used to treat most notable gastrointestinal diseases, namely, peptic ulcer, diarrhoea and inflammatory bowel syndrome.

2. Peptic ulcer

2.1 Animal models of gastric ulcer

Rats are commonly used animals to induce ulcers that resemble the human condition by various noxious chemical agents. NSAIDs (eg. Indomethacin and Aspirin) cause gastrointestinal ulceration, due to their ability to suppress cytoprotective prostaglandin synthesis (Wallace, 2001). The NSAIDS-induced ulcer model is important to identify mechanisms of action of plants that maintain the gastric mucosa integrity by balancing the toxic effects of NSAIDs. The widely used ethanol-induced gastric ulcer model is suitable to study gastric protective and free radical scavenging properties of plants. Stress induced gastric lesions in rats are useful to study gastric mucosal barrier strengthening properties (eg. increased mucus production) of potential plant extracts and their actives. Pylorus ligation in rats helps to screen plants for their antisecretory properties.

2.2 Plants used in the treatment of peptic ulcer

- *Diodia sarmentosa* (Rubiaceae), *Cassia nigricans* (Celsapinaceae), *Ficus exasperate* (Moraceae) and *Synclisia scabrida* (Menispermaceae) are the most popularly used antiulcer recipes in Nigeria. In vivo studies in mice and rats revealed their anti-ulcer activities by decreasing the ulcer index in aspirin-induced ulcerogenesis, delayed intestinal transit, increased pH, and decreased volume and acidity of gastric secretion (Akah et al., 1998).
- *Eruca sativa*, commonly known as Rocket, *is* a commonly used leaf vegetable in Unani, Ayurveda and Arab traditional medicine systems. Rocket is shown to possess significant anti-secretory, anti-ulcer and cytoprotective properties in rats (Alqasoumi et al., 2009). Pretreatment with ethanolic extract of Rocket attenuated gastric ulceration induced by ethanol, indomethacin and hypothermic stress. In pylorus ligated rats, Rocket dose-dependently reduced gastric acid secretion. In addition, the extract

Pharmacology of Traditional Herbal Medicines and Their Active Principles Used in the Treatment of Peptic Ulcer, Diarrhoea and Inflammatory Bowel Disease

5

significantly replenished gut wall mucous and reduced malondialdehyde (an indicator of lipid peroxidation) levels in ethanol treated rats. Gastroprotective effects of Rocket are attributed to the presence of flavonoids, sterols and triterpines.

- *Turnera ulmifolia* or 'chanana' (Turneraceae) is a small herb with wide geographical distribution ranging from Guyana to the North Eastern region of Brazil. It is a widely used folk medicine for its anti-inflammatory properties. The hydroalcoholic extract of *T. ulmifolia* inhibited gastric lesions induced by pylorus ligature, by indomethacin and by ethanol, but stress mediated lesions remained unaffected. As histamine plays a role in ulcerogenesis in pylorus ligation, it was postulated by the study authors that *T. ulmifolia* exerts gastroprotective actions by inhibiting histamine. The inhibition of gastric ulcers induced by indomethacin and ethanol indicate that gastroprotective effects of *T. ulmifolia* could be due to an enhancement of mucosal defensive factors such as gastric mucus (Antônio & Souza Brito, 1998).

- *Dodonaea viscosa* is a stiff bushy plant. Tribes who reside in the forest regions of South India (Kerala) use leaves of this plant for headaches and backaches. The hexane extract of *Dodonaea viscosa* dose dependently inhibited ethanol and indomethacin induced gastric lesions. Gastric secretion studies showed significant decrease of total acid in gastric juice (Arun & Asha, 2008). Furthermore, it decreased total acid content and increased gastric glutathione levels in ethanol and indomethacin treated rats.

- *Azadirachta indica* is a native tree to the Indian subcontinent. To the Indian it is commonly known as Neem and regarded as a 'village dispensary' due its multiple therapeutic properties. It has been extensively used in Ayurveda, Siddha, Unani and other local Indian folklore medicine systems (Brahmachari, 2004). Standardized aqueous extract of Neem exhibited remarkable anti-ulcer activity in restraint-cold stress and indomethacin induced gastric ulcers in rats. Animal studies suggest that the major gastroprotective effect of Neem bark extract against ulcer is mediated through inhibition of acid secretion by H+-K+-ATPase and prevention of oxidative damage (Bandyopadhyay et al., 2002).

- The aqueous extract of Neem bark when administered for 10 days at 30 mg dose twice daily significantly inhibited gastric acid secretion in patients with chronic gastric acid problem. The bark extract completely healed the duodenal ulcers at the dose of 30-60 mg twice daily for 10 weeks (Bandyopadhyay et al., 2004). Some important blood parameters for organ toxicity such as sugar, urea, creatinine, serum glutamate oxaloacetate transaminase, serum glutamate pyruvate transaminase, albumin, globulin, hemoglobin levels and erythrocyte sedimentation rate remained unaffected upon Neem exposure.

- *Pteleopsis suberosa* is traditionally used in Mali for the treatment of gastric ulcers. The aqueous extract of *P. suberosa* exhibited protective effects on gastric mucosa in ethanol and indomethacin treated rats (De Pasquale et al., 1995). It has also been shown that *Pteleopsis suberosa* decoction containing triterpenoid saponins and tannins is effective against *Helicobacter pylori* (Germano` et al., 1998).

- *Calligonum comosum* is a shrub distributed throughout Arabia and growing in sandy deserts. It is used by the local healers to treat stomach ailments. Pre-treatment with the 10% ethanolic extract displayed a significant and dose-dependent inhibition of acute gastric ulcers induced by NSAIDs (phenylbutazone and indomethacin) and necrotic agents (0.2 N NaOH and 80% ethanol) (Liu et al., 2001).

- *Solanum torvum*, a small tree, is widely used in African folk medicine to treat various diseases including gastric ulcer (Noumi et al., 2000). Aqueous and methanolic extracts from leaves of Solanum torvum produced significant anti-ulcer activity in HCl/ethanol, indomethacin, pylorus ligation and cold-restraint stress induced gastric ulcers in rats. The authors proposed that the cytoprotective activity of extracts could be due to strengthening of the mucosal barrier through the increase of mucus production (Nguelefack et al., 2008).

- *Tetrapleura tetraptera* and *Guibourtia ehie* Leonard are native trees to Ghana. The Ghanaian ethnomedical system employs these plant extracts in the management of stomach ulcers. In support of their traditional use, aqueous extracts of the barks of *Tet. Tetraprera* and *G. ethie* dose dependently inhibited HCl/ethanol induced gastric ulcers (Noamesi et al., 1994).

- *Glycyrrhiza glabra* is a legume native to southern Europe and parts of Asia. It is a well-known folk medicine for gastric ulcer (Aly et al., 2004). Gastric mucosal damage induced by NSAIDs is markedly reduced by *G. glabra* (Aly et al., 2004). Clinical data on *Gycrrhiza glabra* is inconsistent. In a double-blind clinical trial, administration of deglycyrrhizinized liquorice thrice daily at the dose of 760 mg for four weeks significantly accelerated the healing of gastric ulcer. In contrast, a cross over study at the same dose and treatment time reported no improvement in ulcer healing (Engqvist et al., 1973). A similar result was shown in a double-blind placebo- control study with administration of deglycyrrhizinized liquorice for one month at the dose of 380 mg thrice daily (Feldman et al., 1971). No side effects are reported in subjects who received deglycyrrhizinized liquorice extract in these studies.

Plant	Scientific Evidence	Active Constituent(s)	Reference
Diodia sarmentosa	Pre-clinical	Unknown	Akah et al
Cassia nigricans	Pre-clinical	Flavonoids	Akah et al
Ficus exasperate	Pre-clinical	Gallic acid & ellagic acid	Akah et al ; Sirisha et al
Synclisia scabrida	Pre-clinical	Alkaloids & flavonoids	Akah et al ; Orisakwe et al ; Obi et al
Eruca sativa	Pre-clinical	Flavonoids, sterols & triterpines	Alqasoumi et al
Turnera ulmifolia	Pre-clinical	Flavonoids	Antônio et al
Dodonaea viscosa	Pre-clinical	Flavonoids, saponins, bitter principles & phenols	Arun et al
Azadirachta indica	Pre-clinical & clinical	Phenolic glycoside	Bandyopadhyay et al
Pteleopsis suberosa	Pre-clinical	Triterpenoid saponins & tannins	De Pasquale et al ; Germanò et al
Calligonum comosum	Pre-clinical	Unknown	Liu et al
Solanum torvum		Flavonoids, sterols & triterpenes	Nguelefack et al
Tetrapleura tetraptera	Pre-clinical	Unknown	Noamesi et al
Guibourtia ehie	Pre-clinical	Unknown	Noamesi et al
Glycyrrhiza glabra	Pre-clinical & clinical	Unknown	Aly et al, Rees et al ; Engqvist et al; Feldman et al

Table 1. Plants and their active constituents with anti-ulcer activity

Pharmacology of Traditional Herbal Medicines and Their Active Principles Used in the Treatment of Peptic Ulcer, Diarrhoea and Inflammatory Bowel Disease

7

3. Diarrhoea

3.1 Experimental models

Rodents are commonly used to induce experimental diarrhea and to study mechanisms of action of plants and their active principles. Castor oil, Prostaglandin E2 (PG-E2) and heat-labile enterotoxin are commonly used agents to induce diarrhea in animals. The diarrhoeal effect of castor oil is mediated through ricinoleic acid which causes irritation and inflammation of intestinal mucosa, and consequesntly leads to the stimulation of intestinal motility and increased secretion of fluid and electrolytes. This model is ideal to study the antisecretory and antimotility potential of medicinal plants. Prostaglandin E2 causes enteropooling by stimulating fluid secretion and increasing propulsive activity in the colon (Pierre et al., 1991). Heat-labile enterotoxin (LT) is the virulent factor of *Escherichia coli* and diarrhea by accumulation of salt and water in the intestinal lumen (Spangler., 1992). Therefore, the LT-induced diarroheal model is suitable to study inhibitory effects of plant extracts on bacterial toxins. In addition, the charcoal meal test and charcoal-gum acacia-induced hyperperistalsis in animals are helpful to identity the effect of potential medicinal plants on intestinal motility.

3.2 Plants tested for antidiarrheal activity in animal models of diarrhoea

- *Ficus bengalensis, Eugenia jambolana, Ficus racemosa* and *Leucas lavandulaefolia* are commonly used folk medicine to treat diarrhoea by the people who live in Khatra region of West Bengal, India. Ethanolic exracts of *Ficus bengalensis* (hanging roots), *Eugenia jambolana* (bark), *Ficus racemosa* (bark) and *Leucas lavandulaefolia* (aerial parts) significantly inhibited castor oil induced diarrhoea and PGE2 induced enteropooling in rats. In addition, these extracts also showed a significant reduction in gastrointestinal motility in charcoal meal tests in rats (Mukherjee et al., 1997).
- *Geranium mexicanum* plant is a commonly used medicinal plant in Traditional Mexican Medicine for the treatment of diarrhoea. Methanolic extract of *Geranium mexicanum* (roots) remarkably inhibited charcoal–gum acacia-induced hyperperistalsis in rats. However the authors suggested that this medicinal plant should be used with care to avoid toxic effects (Clazada et al., 2009).
- *Galla chinensis and Chaenomeles speciosa* have been traditionally used in China to treat gastrointestinal disorders. These plant extracts significantly inhibited heat-labile enterotoxin-induced diarrhoea in the mouse (Chen et al., 2006, Chen et al., 2007).
- *Satureja hortensis* is an annual herb that is traditionally used in Iran for treating stomach and intestinal disorders. Essential oil isolated from *S. hortensis* exhibited antispasmodic activity in isolated rat ileum. In addition, it also inhibited castor oil-induced diarrhea in mice (Hajhashemi et al., 1999).
- *Thespesia populnea,* a large tree found in tropical regions and coastal forests of India, is traditionally used in India to treat several disorders including diarrhea and dysentery. Residue fraction of aqueous extract of *T. populnea* significantly inhibited castor oil and prostaglandin E2 (PGE$_2$)-induced diarrhea induced diarrhea in rats. In addition, it also inhibited intestinal motility in the charcoal meal test (Viswanatha et al., 2011).
- *Mitragyna speciosa* is an indigenous tree to Thailand, where it is commonly called kratom. In folk medicine, it is often used to treat diarrhea. Methanolic extract of *M. speciosa* dose dependently inhibited castor oil-induced diarrhea and intestinal transit in rats (Chittrakarn et al., 2008).

- *Punica granatum* is a deciduous shrub or small tree that is native to the Himalayas in north Pakistan and Northern India. Bark, rind of the fruit and seeds of this plant are used in folk medicine to treat diarrhea. Methanol extract of seeds of *P. granatum* dose dependently reduced castor oil induced diarrhea. It also significantly inhibited gastrointestinal motility and PGE$_2$ mediated enteropooling in rats (Das et al., 1999).

Plant	Scientific Evidence	Active Constituent(s)	Reference
Ficus bengalensis	Pre-clinical	Tannin	Mukherjee et al
Eugenia jambolana	Pre-clinical	Tannin	Mukherjee et al
Ficus racemosa	Pre-clinical	Tannin	Mukherjee et al
Leucas lavandulaefolia	Pre-clinical	Tannin	Mukherjee et al
Geranium mexicanum	Pre-clinical	(-)-epicatechin, tyramine	Calzada et al
Galla chinensis	Pre-clinical	Gallic acid	Chen et al
Chaenomeles speciosa	Pre-clinical	Oleanolic acid, ursolic acid & betulinic acid	Chen et al
Satureja hortensis	Pre-clinical	Carvacrol	Hajhashemi et al
Thespesia populnea	Pre-clinical	Unknown	Viswanatha et al
Mitragyna speciosa	Pre-clinical	Mitragynine & other alkaloids	Chittrakarn et al
Punica granatum	Pre-clinical	Tannin	Das et al

Table 2. Plants and their active constituent(s) with anti-diarrheal activity

4. Inflammatory Bowel Diseases (IBD)

4.1 Animal models of IBD

In IBD oxidative stress mediates disease progression by disrupting epithelial cell integrity. Acetic acid-induced colitis is helpful to screen herbs which can inhibit cytotoxic effects of reactive oxygen species (ROS). Dextran sulphate sodium (DSS)-induced colitis is also a frequently used animal colitis model in ethnopharmacological studies. This model is useful to test the effect of herbs on inflammatory cytokines mediated cellular injury (Dieleman et al., 1998). The transgenic rat model (HLA-B27) with overt chronic gastrointestinal tract inflammation also serves to screen medicinal herbs to treat IBD.

- *Zingiber officinale* is traditionally used to treat inflammatory gastrointestinal disorders. Ethanolic extract of dried rhizomes of ginger displayed protective effects against acetic acid-induced ulcerative colitis in rats (El-Abhar et al., 2008).
- *Cordia dichotoma* is a deciduous tree with many medicinal uses in Ayurveda. Traditionally bark of the plant is reported for the treatment of ulcerative colitis. Methanolic extract of C. Dichotoma improved lesions and reduced colonic myeloperoxidase (MPO) and malondialdehyde (MDA) in acetic acid induced UC in male swiss mice (Ganjare et al., 2011).
- *Patrinia scabiosaefolia* is a commonly used herbal medicine in Korea. It is used traditionally to treat colonic inflammations. Methanolic extract of P. Scabiosaefolia significantly attenuated dextran sulfate sodium induced colitis in mice. In addition, it

Pharmacology of Traditional Herbal Medicines and Their Active Principles Used in the Treatment of Peptic Ulcer, Diarrhoea and Inflammatory Bowel Disease

9

also suppressed colonic MPO accumulation and pro-inflammatory mediators (TNFα, IL-1, IL-6 and nitric oxide) (Cho et al., 2011).

- *Vitex negundo* is a shrub that grows in Southeast Asia. Traditionally its roots are used in the treatment of ulcerative colitis in India. Ethanolic extract of *V. negrundo* significantly inhibited acetic acid ulcerative colitis and reduced colonic MPO and MDA levels in mice (Zaware et al., 2011).
- *Pistacia lentiscus* is a dioecious shrub that grows in the Mediterranean region. Oleogum resin from *P. Lentiscus* is used in traditional Iranian medicine to treat IBD. Treatment with oleogum resin from *P. Lentiscus* improved the symptoms of dextran sulfate sodium (DSS) induced colitis in mice (Kim & Neophytou, 2009). A pilot study conducted in mild to moderate Crohn's disease patients demonstrated that mastic (resin) from *P. Lentiscus* significantly reduced disease activity index, plasma IL-6 and C-reactive protein (Kaliora et al., 2007a) and TNFα in peripheral blood mononuclear cells (Kaliora et al., 2007b). In addition, total antioxidant potential was significantly increased. No side effects are observed in mastic treated patients (Kaliora et al., 2007a). A double-blind clinical trial in patients with duodenal ulcers exhibited symptomatic relief in 80% patients on mastic and 50% patients on placebo, while endoscopically proven healing occurred in 70% patients on mastic (Al-Habbal et al., 1984).
- *Plantago ovata* is a well-known medicinal plant in the treatment of IBD. *P. ovate* seeds ameliorated the development of colonic inflammation in transgenic rats as evidenced by an improvement of intestinal cytoarchitecture, significant decrease in some of the pro-inflammatory mediators and higher production of short-chain fatty acids (Rodríguez-Cabezas et al., 2003). An open label, parallel-group, multicenter, randomized clinical trial in patients with ulcerative colitis concluded that *Plantago ovata* seeds (dietary fiber) might be as effective as mesalamine to maintain remission in ulcerative colitis (Ferna'ndez-Ban~ ares et al., 1999).
- *Boswellia serrata*, a tree which grows in the hilly areas of India, is an efficacious remedy for IBD in traditional Iranian medicine and also it has been used in the Ayurvedic medicine for the treatment of inflammatory diseases. Despite its traditional claims, *Boswellia* extracts are ineffective in ameliorating colitis in DSS-induced colitis in mice (Kiela et al., 2004). In contrast to animal studies, a double-blind, randomized, placebo-controlled, multicenter trial in colitis patients showed higher remission in Boswellia serrata extract treated group than in the pacebo group (Madisch et al., 2007). However, a recent double-blind, placebo-controlled, randomized, parallel study in patients with Crohn's disease has shown no difference between the Boswellia treated group and control group in disease remission (Holtmeier et al., 2011).

5. Quality, efficacy and safety of herbal medicines

5.1 Quality

The quality of herbal medicines is important to ensure their safe use and efficacy. In contrast to well characterized conventional medicine, assurance of the quality of herbal medicine is a major concern. The problems associated with the herbal products include deliberate or accidental inclusion of prohibited or restricted ingredients, substitution or adulteration of herbal materials, contamination with toxic substances and differences between labelled and actual contents (Barnes et al., 2nd ed). However, increased consumer awareness and

Plant	Scientific Evidence	Chemical Constituents	Reference
Zingiber officinale	Pre-clinical	Gingerols	El-Abhar et al ; Minaiyan et al
Cordia dichotoma	Pre-clinical	Apigenin	Ganjare et al
Patrinia scabiosaefolia	Pre-clinical	Oleanonic acid, oleanolic acid & ursolic acid	Cho et al
Vitex negundo	Pre-clinical	Unknown	Zaware et al
Pistacia lentiscus	Pre-clinical & clinical	Oleanolic acid	Kim et al; Kaliora et al; Al-Habbal
Plantago ovata	Pre-clinical & clinical	Unknown	Rodriguez-Cabezas et al ; Fernandez-Banares et al
Boswellia serrata	Pre-clinical & clinical	Boswellia acids	Kiela et al ; Madisch et al ; Holtmeier et al

Table 3. Plants and their active constituents for treatment of ulcerative colitis/IBD

regulatory agencies' strict guidelines on the quality and stability of herbal products has led to significant improvements in the quality control of herbal medicines. Recently the herbal manufacturing industry has focused on improving its quality assurance and quality control mechanisms to guard against the frequent episodes of substandard quality and possible adulterations. Use of high-performance liquid chromatograms, thin-layer chromatography, atomic absorption spectroscopy, gas chromatography and where necessary more sophisticated techniques such as NMR and LC/MS has now become common in complementary medicines manufacturing industries to ensure the quality of plant materials and final product (Rosenbloom et al., 2011). The emphasis on good manufacturing practice has steadily increased over years. In addition, new regulatory laws are now in place on product stability to support its shelf life. With the steady progress on different herbal quality control fronts, it is now possible to apply almost the same set of quality standards as for conventional medicines. As most of the traditional herbs listed in this chapter are not commercially manufactured, the data on the quality of these plant medicines is scarce.

5.2 Efficacy

Herbal medicines have a long history of traditional use. However, from today's stand point, traditional claims need to be verified. A well-designed randomized controlled trial is essential to determine the efficacy and safety of herbal medicines. The use of standardized herbal extracts in clinical trials is important to obtain reproducible data on the efficacy and safety of herbal medicines. Standardization of herbal extracts has become a common practice in phytomedicines. It allows the establishment of reproducible pharmaceutical quality by comparing a product with established reference substances and by defining the

Pharmacology of Traditional Herbal Medicines and Their Active Principles Used in the Treatment of Peptic Ulcer, Diarrhoea and Inflammatory Bowel Disease

11

specific quantity of one or several compounds. As the herbs are of natural origin, their chemical composition is affected by several factors (climate, growing conditions, time of harvesting, storage conditions and processing). Therefore, the use of standardized herbal extracts in preclinical and clinical research is helpful to develop evidence based traditional therapies. Although rigorous clinical investigations are lacking at present for many herbs used in GIT disorders, there is a vast literature on the *in vitro* and *in vivo* pharmacological effects of medicinal plants. These pre-clinical observations provide a rationale for further investigation of such plants.

5.3 Safety

The positive attitude towards herbal medicines is based on the testimony that herbs have been used since antiquity and the belief that they have the advantage of being 'natural' rather than 'synthetic'. Traditional healing systems employed herbal medicines for the symptomatic management of diseases. However, these herbs are now being used extensively for health promotion and disease prevention not only in underdeveloped and developing nations, but also increasingly in developed nations. As little is known regarding adverse effects of herbal medicines and their frequencies, the chronic exposure of these herbal ingredients may pose health risks. In particular, when herbs are extracted and purified, their toxicity might be increased due to increased concentration of potential toxic compounds. Therefore, the common assumption that herbal medicines are by inference 'safe' may not be valid by today's health standards.

Generally, traditional herbal medicines lack the following pharmacological data in humans:

- pharmacologically active chemical constituents and their metabolites
- mechanisms of action of active constituents/whole extract
- pharmacokinetics
- toxicology
- adverse effects and their frequencies
- drug–herb and food–herb interactions
- use in vulnerable individuals: children, elderly, individuals with renal or hepatic disease, gender effects, individuals with a different genetic profile
- contraindications

Phytochemical and pharmacological (preclinical and clinical) studies are important to address the above issues. The majority of the herbs mentioned in this chapter are tested only in animals. The main focus of these studies has been determining the efficacy of herbal extracts to support their traditional claims. However, it is a common procedure in these animal studies to measure toxic dose of herbal extracts. These toxicological studies are important to provide in vivo data in a whole animal situation on the dose and adverse effects of herbal extracts which may be relevant when tested in humans. None of these studies have reported any major adverse events in the experimental models of various GI disorders.

6. Conclusion

The use of plants in treating diseases is a very old human tradition. This knowledge, derived from observations and experiences, has been handed over from generation to generation verbally and also in the form of ancient texts. Medicinal plants are the foundations for modern therapeutic agents. Herbal medicines are an important part of the health care system in many developing countries. The use of herbal medicines, as health promoting agents, in developed countries has also increased and this trend is continuing. Healthcare professionals need to be aware of the pharmacology of these herbal medicines in order to provide well informed advice to patients. The traditional herbal medicines field is very vast. In this chapter we attempted to provide scientific evidence for the herbs with historical use in three major GIT disorders namely: peptic ulcer, diarrhoea and IBD. Researchers successfully reproduced these human disorders in animals by employing a range of chemical agents and scientific procedures. In some cases, these models not only have supported the traditional claims, but also provided important information on the mechanism of action of the plant extracts and in some cases their components. The majority of these preclinical studies established the scientific evidence to traditional herbal medicines. Unfortunately, very few clinical trials are conducted to translate animal data into humans. As clinical trials are important to furnish efficacy and safety data, the lack of clinical data has become the main impediment in developing traditional herbal remedies into mainstream medicines. Recent progress in the quality control of herbal products is very promising in gaining consumer confidence and promoting consideration of herbal medicines as complementary and in some cases alternative approaches to conventional therapies. Medicinal plants listed in this chapter have the potential to treat peptic ulcer, diarrhoea and IBD. Additional studies on quality, efficacy and safety in animals and humans will be required to integrate them in mainstream medicine.

7. References

Al Mofleh, IA. (2010). Spices, herbal xenobiotics and the stomach: friends or foes. *World journal of gastroenterology*, Vol.16, No.22 (June 2010), pp. 2710-2719. ISSN 1007-9327

Al-Habbal, MJ.; Al-Habbal, Z. & Huwez, FU. (1984). A double-blind controlled clinical trial of mastic and placebo in the treatment of duodenal ulcer. *Clinical and experimental pharmacology & physiology*, Vol.11, No.5 (September 1984), pp. 541-544. ISSN 0305-1870

Akah, PA.; Orisakwe, OE.; Gamaniel, KS. & Shittu, A. (1998). Evaluation of Nigerian traditional medicines: II. Effects of some Nigerian folk remedies on peptic ulcer. *Journal of ethnopharmacology*, Vol. 62, No. 2 (September 1998), pp. 123-127. ISSN 0378-8741

Alqasoumi, S.; Al-Sohaibani, M.; Al-Howiriny, T.; Al-Yahya, M. & Rafatullah, S. (2009). Rocket "*Eruca sativa*": a salad herb with potential gastric anti-ulcer activity. *World journal of gastroenterology*, Vol.15, No.16 (April 2009), pp. 1958-1965. ISSN 1007-9327

Aly, AM.; Al-Alousi, L. & Salem, HA. (2005). Licorice: a possible anti-inflammatory and anti-ulcer drug. *AAPS PharmSciTech*, Vol.6, No.1 (September 2005), pp. E74-82. ISSN 1530-9932

Antônio, MA. & Souza Brito, AR. (1998). Oral anti-inflammatory and anti-ulcerogenic activities of a hydroalcoholic extract and partitioned fractions of *Turnera ulmifolia* (Turneraceae). *Journal of ethnopharmacology*, Vol. 61, No.3 (July 1998), pp. 215-228. ISSN 0378-8741

Pharmacology of Traditional Herbal Medicines and Their Active Principles Used in the Treatment of Peptic Ulcer, Diarrhoea and Inflammatory Bowel Disease

13

Arun, M. & Asha, VV. (2008). Gastroprotective effect of *Dodonaea viscosa* on various experimental ulcer models. *Journal of ethnopharmacology*, Vol.118, No.3 (August 2008), pp. 460-465. ISSN 0378-8741

Ayo, RG. (2010). Phytochemical constituents and bioactives of the extracts of *Cassia nigricans* Vahl: A review. *Journal of medicinal plants research*, Vol.4, No.14 (July 2010), pp. 1339-1348. ISSN 1996-0875

Bandyopadhyay, U.; Biswas, K.; Chatterjee, R.; Bandyopadhyay, D.; Chattopadhyay, I.; Ganguly, CK.; Chakraborty, T.; Bhattacharya, K. & Banerjee RK. (2002). Gastroprotective effect of Neem (*Azadirachta indica*) bark extract: possible involvement of H(+)-K(+)-ATPase inhibition and scavenging of hydroxyl radical. *Life sciences*, Vol.71, No.24 (November 2002), pp. 2845-2865. ISSN 0024-3205

Bandyopadhyay, U.; Biswas, K.; Sengupta, A.; Moitra, P.; Dutta, P.; Sarkar, D.; Debnath, P.; Ganguly, CK. & Banerjee, RK. (2004). Clinical studies on the effect of Neem (*Azadirachta indica*) bark extract on gastric secretion and gastroduodenal ulcer. *Life sciences*, Vol.75, No.24 (October 2004), pp. 2867-2878. ISSN 0024-3205

Barnes, J.; Anderson, LA. & Phillipson JD. (2002). *Herbal Medicines* (2nd edition), Pharmaceutical Press, ISBN 0853694745, Great Britain.

Borrelli, F. & Izzo, AA. (2000). The plant kingdom as a source of anti-ulcer remedies. *Phytotherapy research*, Vol.14, No.8 (December 2000), pp. 581-591. ISSN 0951-418X

Brahmachari, G. (2004). Neem--an omnipotent plant: a retrospection. *European journal of chemical biology*, Vol.5, No.4 (April 2004), pp. 408-421. ISSN 1439-4227

Calzada, F.; Arista, R. & Pérez, H. (2010). Effect of plants used in Mexico to treat gastrointestinal disorders on charcoal-gum acacia-induced hyperperistalsis in rats. *Journal of ethnopharmacology*, Vol.128, No.1 (March 2010), pp. 49-51. ISSN 0378-8741

Chen, JC.; Ho, TY.; Chang, YS.; Wu, SL. & Hsiang, CY. (2006). Anti-diarrheal effect of *Galla Chinensis* on the Escherichia coli heat-labile enterotoxin and ganglioside interaction. *Journal of ethnopharmacology*, Vol.103, No.3 (February 2006), pp. 385-391. ISSN 0378-8741

Chen, JC.; Chang, YS.; Wu, SL.; Chao, DC.; Chang, CS.; Li, CC.; Ho, TY. & Hsiang, CY. (2007). Inhibition of Escherichia coli heat-labile enterotoxin-induced diarrhea by *Chaenomeles speciosa*. *Journal of ethnopharmacology*, Vol.113, No.2 (September 2007), pp. 233-239. ISSN 0378-8741

Chittrakarn, S.; Sawangjaroen, K.; Prasettho, S.; Janchawee, B. & Keawpradub, N. (2008). Inhibitory effects of kratom leaf extract (*Mitragyna speciosa Korth.*) on the rat gastrointestinal tract. *Journal of ethnopharmacology*, Vol.116, No.1 (February 2008), pp. 173-178. ISSN 0378-8741

Cho, EJ.; Shin, JS.; Noh, YS.; Cho, YW.; Hong, SJ.; Park, JH.; Lee, JY.; Lee, JY. & Lee, KT. (2011). Anti-inflammatory effects of methanol extract of *Patrinia scabiosaefolia* in mice with ulcerative colitis. *Journal of ethnopharmacology*, Vol.136, No.3 (July 2011), pp. 428-435. ISSN 0378-8741

Das, AK.; Mandal, SC.; Banerjee, SK.; Sinha, S.; Das, J.; Saha, BP. & Pal, M. (1999). Studies on antidiarrhoeal activity of *Punica granatum* seed extract in rats. *Journal of ethnopharmacology*, Vol.68, No.1-3 (December 1999), pp. 205-208. ISSN 0378-8741

De Pasquale, R.; Germanò, MP.; Keita, A.; Sanogo, R. & Iauk, L. (1995). Antiulcer activity of *Pteleopsis suberosa*. *Journal of ethnopharmacology*, Vol.47, No.1 (June 1995), pp. 55-58. ISSN 0378-8741.

Dieleman, LA.; Palmen, MJ.; Akol, H.; Bloemena, E.; Peña, AS.; Meuwissen, SG. & Van Rees, EP. (1998). Chronic experimental colitis induced by dextran sulphate sodium (DSS) is characterized by Th1 and Th2 cytokines. *Clinical and experimental immunology*, Vol.114, No.3 (December 1998), pp. 385-391. ISSN 0009-9104

El-Abhar, HS.; Hammad, LN. & Gawad, HS. (2008). Modulating effect of ginger extract on rats with ulcerative colitis. *Journal of ethnopharmacology*, Vol.118, No.3 (August 2008), pp. 367-372. ISSN 0378-8741

Engqvist, A.; Von Feilitzen, F.; Pyk, E. & Reichard, H. (1973). Double-blind trial of deglycyrrhizinated liquorice in gastric ulcer. *Gut*, Vol.14, No.9 (September 1973), pp. 711-715. ISSN 0017-5749

Feldman, H. & Gilat, T. (1971). A trial of deglycyrrhizinated liquorice in the treatment of duodenal ulcer. *Gut*, Vol.12, No.6 (June 1971), pp. 449-451. ISSN 0017-5749

Fernández-Bañares, F.; Hinojosa, J.; Sánchez-Lombraña, JL.; Navarro, E.; Martínez-Salmerón, JF.; García-Pugés, A.; González-Huix, F.; Riera, J.; González-Lara, V.; Domínguez-Abascal, F.; Giné, JJ.; Moles, J.; Gomollón, F. & Gassull, MA. (1999). Randomized clinical trial of *Plantago ovata* seeds (dietary fiber) as compared with mesalamine in maintaining remission in ulcerative colitis. Spanish Group for the Study of Crohn's Disease and Ulcerative Colitis (GETECCU). *The American journal of gastroenterology*, Vol.94, No.2 (February 1999), pp. 427-433. ISSN 0002-9270

Ganjare, AB.; Nirmal, SA.; Rub, RA.; Patil, AN. & Pattan, SR. (2011). Use of *Cordia dichotoma* bark in the treatment of ulcerative colitis. *Pharmaceutical biology*, Vol.49, No.8 (August 2011), pp. 850-855. ISSN 1388-0209

Germanò, MP.; Sanogo, R.; Guglielmo, M.; De Pasquale, R.; Crisafi, G. & Bisignano, G. (1998). Effects of *Pteleopsis suberosa* extracts on experimental gastric ulcers and Helicobacter pylori growth. *Journal of ethnopharmacology*, Vol.59, No.3 (January 1998), pp. 167-172. ISSN 0378-8741

Hajhashemi, V.; Sadraei, H.; Ghannadi, AR. & Mohseni, M. (2000). Antispasmodic and anti-diarrhoeal effect of *Satureja hortensis L.* essential oil. *Journal of ethnopharmacology*, Vol.71, No.1-2 (July 2000), pp. 187-192. ISSN 0378-8741

Holtmeier, W.; Zeuzem, S.; Preiss, J.; Kruis, W.; Böhm, S.; Maaser, C.; Raedler, A.; Schmidt, C.; Schnitker, J.; Schwarz, J.; Zeitz, M. & Caspary, W. (2011). Randomized, placebo-controlled, double-blind trial of *Boswellia serrata* in maintaining remission of Crohn's disease: good safety profile but lack of efficacy. *Inflammatory bowel diseases*, Vol. 17, No.2 (February 2011), pp. 573-582. ISSN 1078-0998

Kaliora, AC.; Stathopoulou, MG.; Triantafillidis, JK.; Dedoussis, GV. & Andrikopoulos, NK. (2007). Chios mastic treatment of patients with active Crohn's disease. *World journal of gastroenterology*, Vol.13, No.5 (February 2007), pp.748-753. ISSN 1007-9327

Kaliora, AC.; Stathopoulou, MG.; Triantafillidis, JK.; Dedoussis, GV. & Andrikopoulos NK. (2007). Alterations in the function of circulating mononuclear cells derived from patients with Crohn's disease treated with mastic. *World journal of gastroenterology*, Vol.13, No.45 (December 2007), pp. 6031-6036. ISSN 1007-9327

Kiela, PR.; Midura, AJ.; Kuscuoglu, N.; Jolad, SD.; Sólyom, AM.; Besselsen, DG.; Timmermann, BN. & Ghishan, FK. (2005). Effects of *Boswellia serrata* in mouse models of chemically induced colitis. *American journal of physiology. Gastrointestinal and liver physiology*, Vol. 288, No.4 (April 2005), pp. G798-808. ISSN 0193-1857

Pharmacology of Traditional Herbal Medicines and Their Active Principles Used in the Treatment of Peptic Ulcer, Diarrhoea and Inflammatory Bowel Disease

15

Kim, HJ. & Neophytou, C. (2009). Natural anti-inflammatory compounds for the management and adjuvant therapy of inflammatory bowel disease and its drug delivery system. *Archives of pharmacal research*, Vol.32, No.7 (July 2009), pp. 997-1004. ISSN 0253-6269

Langmead, L. & Rampton, DS. (2006). Review article: complementary and alternative therapies for inflammatory bowel disease. *Alimentary pharmacology & therapeutics*, Vol.23, No.3 (February 2006), pp. 341-349, ISSN 0269-2813

Liu, XM.; Zakaria, MN.; Islam, MW.; Radhakrishnan, R.; Ismail, A.; Chen, HB.; Chan, K. & Al-Attas, A. (2001). Anti-inflammatory and anti-ulcer activity of *Calligonum comosum* in rats. *Fitoterapia*, Vol.72, No.5 (June 2001), pp. 487-491. ISSN 0367-326X

Madisch, A.; Miehlke, S.; Eichele, O.; Mrwa, J.; Bethke, B.; Kuhlisch, E.; Bästlein, E.; Wilhelms, G.; Morgner, A.; Wigginghaus, B. & Stolte, M. (2007). *Boswellia serrata* extract for the treatment of collagenous colitis. A double-blind, randomized, placebo-controlled, multicenter trial. *International journal of colorectal disease*, Vol.22, No.12 (December 2007), pp.1445-14451. ISSN 0179-1958

Minaiyan, M.; Ghannadi, A.; Mahzouni, M. & Nabi-Meibodi, M. (2008). Anti-ulcerogenic effect of ginger (rhizome of *Zingiber officinale* Roscoe) hydroalcoholic extract on acetic acid-induced acute colitis in rats. *Research in pharmaceutical sciences*, Vol.3, No.2 (October 2008), pp. 15-22. ISSN 1735-5362

Mukherjee, PK.; Saha, K.; Murugesan, T.; Mandal, SC.; Pal, M. & Saha BP. (1998). Screening of anti-diarrhoeal profile of some plant extracts of a specific region of West Bengal, India. *Journal of ethnopharmacology*, Vol.60, No.1 (February 1998), pp. 85-89. ISSN 0378-8741

Nguelefack, TB.; Feumebo, CB.; Ateufack, G.; Watcho, P.; Tatsimo, S.; Atsamo, AD.; Tane, P. & Kamanyi, A. (2008). Anti-ulcerogenic properties of the aqueous and methanol extracts from the leaves of *Solanum torvum* Swartz (Solanaceae) in rats. *Journal of ethnopharmacology*, Vol.119, No.1 (September 2008), pp. 135-140. ISSN 0378-8741

Noamesi, BK.; Mensah, JF.; Bogale, M.; Dagne, E. & Adotey, J. (1994). Antiulcerative properties and acute toxicity profile of some African medicinal plant extracts. *Journal of ethnopharmacology*, Vol.42, No.1 (March 1994), pp. 13-18. ISSN 0378-8741

Obi, E.; Emeh, JK.; Orisakwe, OE.; Afonne, OJ.; Ilondu, NA. & Agbasi, PU. (2000). Investigation of the biochemical evidence for the antiulcerogenic activity of *Synclisia scabrida*. *Indian Journal of Pharmacology*, Vol.32, No.6 (September 2000), pp. 381-383. ISSN: 0253-7613

Orisakwe, OE.; Afonne, OJ.; Dioka, CE.; Ufearo, CS.; Okpogba, AN. & Ofoefule, SI. (1996). Some pharmacological properties of *Synclisia scabrida* II. *Indian journal of medical research*, Vol.103 (May 1996), pp. 282-284. ISSN 0971-5916

Rees, WD.; Rhodes, J.; Wright, JE.; Stamford, LF. & Bennett, A. (1979). Effect of deglycyrrhizinated liquorice on gastric mucosal damage by aspirin. *Scandinavian journal of gastroenterology*, Vol.14, No.5, (1979), pp. 605-607. ISSN 0036-5521

Rodríguez-Cabezas, ME.; Gálvez, J.; Camuesco, D.; Lorente, MD.; Concha A,; Martinez-Augustin, O.; Redondo, L. & Zarzuelo, A. (2003). Intestinal anti-inflammatory activity of dietary fiber (*Plantago ovata* seeds) in HLA-B27 transgenic rats. *Clinical nutrition*, Vol.22, No. 5 (October 2003), pp. 463-471. ISSN 0261-5614

Rivière, PJ.; Farmer, SC.; Burks, TF. & Porreca, F. (1991). Prostaglandin E2-induced diarrhea in mice: importance of colonic secretion. *The Journal of pharmacology and experimental therapeutics*, Vol.256, No.2 (February 1991), pp. 547-552. ISSN 0022-3565

Rosenbloom, RA.; Chaudhary, J. & Castro-Eschenbach, D. (2011). Traditional botanical medicine: an introduction. *American journal of therapeutics*, Vol.18, No.2 (March 2011), pp. 158-161. ISSN 1075-2765

Sengupta, A.; Ghosh, S.; Bhattacharjee, S. & Das, S. (2004). Indian food ingredients and cancer prevention - an experimental evaluation of anticarcinogenic effects of garlic in rat colon. *Asian Pacific journal of cancer prevention*, Vol.5, No.2 (April 2004), pp. 126-132. ISSN 1513-7368

Sirisha, N.; Sreenivasulu, M.; Sangeeta, K. & Madhusudhana Chetty C. (2010). Antioxidant properties of Ficus species- A review. *International journal of pharmtech research*, Vol.2, No.4 (October 2010), pp. 2174-2182. ISSN 0974-4304

Spangler, BD. (1992). Structure and function of cholera toxin and the related Escherichia coli heat-labile enterotoxin. *Microbiological reviews*, Vol.56, No.4 (December 1992), pp. 622-647. ISSN 0146-0749

Suzuki, H.; Inadomi, JM. & Hibi, T. (2009). Japanese herbal medicine in functional gastrointestinal disorders. *Neurogastroenterology and motility*, Vol.21, No.7 (Jul 2009), pp. 688-696. ISSN 1350-1925

Viswanatha, GL.; Hanumanthappa, S.; Krishnadas, N. & Rangappa, S. (2011). Antidiarrheal effect of fractions from stem bark of *Thespesia populnea* in rodents: Possible antimotility and antisecretory mechanisms. *Asian Pacific journal of tropical medicine*, Vol.4, No.6 (June 2011), pp. 451-456. ISSN 1995-7645

Wallace, JL. (2001). Pathogenesis of NSAID-induced gastroduodenal mucosal injury. *Best practice & research. Clinical gastroenterology*, Vol.15, No.5 (October 2001), pp. 691-703. ISSN 1521-6918

Zaware, BB.; Nirmal, SA.; Baheti, DG.; Patil, AN. & Mandal, SC. (2011). Potential of *Vitex negundo* roots in the treatment of ulcerative colitis in mice. *Pharmaceutical biology*, Vol.49, No.8 (August 2011), pp. 874-878. ISSN 1388-0209

2

Emerging Approaches for the Treatment of Fat Malabsorption Due to Exocrine Pancreatic Insufficiency

Saoussen Turki and Héla Kallel
Unité de Biofermentation, Institut Pasteur de Tunis
Tunisia

1. Introduction

The main purpose of the gastrointestinal tract is to digest and absorb nutrients (fat, carbohydrates, and proteins), micronutrients (vitamins and trace minerals), water, and electrolytes. Digestion involves both mechanical and enzymatic breakdown of food. Mechanical processes include chewing, gastric churning, and the to-and-fro mixing in the small intestine. Enzymatic hydrolysis is initiated by intraluminal processes requiring gastric, pancreatic, and biliary secretions. The final products of digestion are absorbed through the intestinal epithelial cells.

Malabsorption is a state arising from abnormality in absorption of food nutrients across the gastrointestinal (GI) tract. Depending on the abnormality, impairment can be of single or multiple nutrients leading to malnutrition and a variety of anaemias. Symptoms of malabsorption are varied because the disorder affects so many systems. General symptoms may include loss of appetite (anorexia), weight loss, fatigue, shortness of breath, dehydration, low blood pressure, and swelling (edema). Nutritional disorders may cause anemia (lack of iron, folate and vitamin B12), bleeding tendency (lack of vitamin K), or bone disease (lack of vitamin D). Gastrointestinal symptoms include flatulence, stomach distention, borborygmi (rumbling in the bowels), discomfort, diarrhea, steatorrhea (excessive fat in stool) and frequent bowel movements (Bai, 1998). Intestinal malabsorption can be due to : mucosal damage (enteropathy), congenital or acquired reduction in absorptive surface, defects of specific hydrolysis, defects of ion transport, impaired enterohepatic circulation or pancreatic insufficiency (Walker-Smith & al.,2002). This chapter will particularly focus on fat malabsorption, the overriding problem caused by severe pancreatic insufficiency.

Pancreatic insufficiency is a condition commonly associated with diseases such as pancreatitis or cystic fibrosis. Patients suffering from these pathologies show a shortage of the digestive enzymes necessary to break down food. Hence, a common feature of these diseases is a severe dietary malabsorption due to the poor hydrolysis of lipid in the lumen of small intestine. Digestive lipases are the key enzymes of fat digestion. The most common example of these enzymes is human pancreatic lipase. Nevertheless, the human lipases include the pre-duodenal lingual and gastric lipase, the extra-duodenal pancreatic, hepatic, lipoprotein and the recently described endothelial lipase. In this chapter, a short basic overview of these fat-digesting enzymes and their physiological contribution to fat digestion is first presented. Thereafter, pathophysiology of fat malabsorption resulting from exocrine pancreatic insufficiency, clinical symptoms, incidence and diagnosis of the pathology are described as well.

Standard strategies for exocrine pancreatic insufficiency management are based on oral administration of porcine derived pancreatic extracts. Unfortunately, this approach is being unsatisfactory for many reasons. Greater attention has been paid over the last decade to optimize correction of fat malabsorption and essential fatty acid deficiency in order to improve the quality of life and extend the life span of patients with severe pancreatic insufficiency. Hence, we interestingly discuss herein drawbacks of therapeutic use of currently available lipase preparations before focusing mainly on research forces joined for the development of new oral enzyme substitution approaches and future promising opportunities to treat intestinal fat malabsorption caused by exocrine pancreatic insufficiency.

2. Human digestive lipases

Lipases are key enzymes responsible for digesting lipids in the digestive system. In humans, gastrointestinal lipases include pre-duodenal lipases (gastric lipase and lingual lipase) and the other members of the lipase gene family: pancreatic, hepatic, lipoprotein and endothelial lipases. The chromosomal localization of genes encoding these lipases and their tissue of origin has been described (Table 1).

Lipase	Chromosomal localization of gene	Tissue of origin	References
Lingual lipase	-*	Serous glands of the tongue	Hamosh, 1990
Gastric lipase	10q23.2	Fundic mucosa of the stomach	Bodmer & al., 1987
Pancreatic lipase	10q26.1	Pancreas	Sims & al., 1993
Hepatic lipase	15q21–q23	Liver	Ameis & al., 1990
Lipoprotein lipase	8p22	Adipose, heart, skeletal muscle	Wion et al., 1987
Endothelial lipase	18q21.1	Endothelial cells, liver, lung, kidney, placenta	Hirata et al., 1999

* Unknown data

Table 1. Human digestive lipases

2.1 Lingual lipase

The serous von Ebner glands of the tongue secrete lingual lipase in the saliva. Unlike rodents, lingual lipase is present in trace amounts in humans (Hamosh, 1990). Human lipase purified from lingual serous glands or gastric juice has a MW of 45 kDa to 51 kDa but tends to aggregate (MW 270-300 kDa and 500 kDa) and is highly hydrophobic (Hamosh, 1990). Lingual lipase has unique characteristics including an optimum activity at pH 4,5 – 5,4 and ability to catalyze reactions without bile salts (Hamosh & Scow, 1973). Lingual lipase breaks down short and medium chain saturated fatty acids and helps in their digestion. It has been stated that 10 to 30% of dietary fat is hydrolyzed in the stomach by lingual lipase. The enzyme uses a catalytic triad consisting of Aspartatic Acid-203 (Asp), Histidine-257 (His), and Serine-144 (Ser), to initiate the hydrolysis of a triglyceride into a diacyglyceride and a free fatty acid (Hamosh & Scow, 1973). Secreted in the buccal cavity, lingual lipase is one of the key components that make the digestion of milk fat in newborns possible. In humans lipolytic activity is present in gastric aspirates as early as 26 weeks of gestational age which is evidence enough for the fact that lingual lipase is present at birth (Hamosh, 1979). New born infants indeed secrete only low amounts of pancreatic lipase and bile salts and it has been demonstrated that pancreatic lipase alone does not readily hydrolyze a lipid emulsion as well as native milk fat globules (Miled & al., 2000).

2.2 Gastric lipase

Gastric lipase (EC 3.1.1.3) is the predominant pre-duodenal lipase in humans. The enzyme is secreted in the gastric juice by the chief cells of fundic mucosa in the stomach (Moreau & al., 1988). The pre-duodenal enzyme was purified from human gastric aspirates and its N-terminal amino-acid sequence was determined. The amino-acid sequence from the isolated protein and the DNA sequence obtained from the cloned gene indicated that human gastric lipase consists of a 379 amino acid unglycosylated polypeptide with a molecular weight of 43 162 Da (Bodmer & al., 1987). However, native human gastric lipase (HGL) (molecular weight 50 kDa) is a highly glycosylated protein with four potential glycosylation sites (Bodmer & al., 1987). Human gastric and rat lingual lipase share a high degree of sequence homology and have identical gene organizations (Lohse & al., 1997). Gastric lipase belongs to the α/β-hydrolase-fold family. It possesses a classical catalytic triad (Ser-153, His-353, Asp-324) and an oxyanion hole (backbone NH groups of Gln-154 and Leu-67) analogous to serine proteases (Roussel & al., 1999). It has an optimum pH activity around 5.4, hydrolyzes long-, medium- and short-chain triacylglycerols and do not require bile acid or colipase for optimum enzymatic activity (Denigris et al., 1985). For many years, the exact physiological contribution of gastric lipase to the overall process of lipolysis was unknown. Carrière et al. (1993a) established, for the first time, that most of the HGL secreted in the stomach was still active in the duodenum. They estimated that the gastric lipase contribution in the hydrolysis of triglycerides is about 25 %. The stereoselectivity of HGL toward triglycerides was also investigated. It was clearly demonstrated that HGL shows a stereopreference for the sn-3 position of the triglyceride (Rogalska & al., 1990).

Hence, gastric lipase, together with lingual lipase, make up 30% of lipid hydrolysis occurring during digestion in the human adult, with gastric lipase contributing the most of the two acidic lipases. In neonates, these acidic pre-duodenal lipases are much more important, they have the unique ability to initiate the degradation of maternal milk fat globules.

2.3 Pancreatic lipases

A limitation of acidic lipases is that they remove only one fatty acid from each triacylglycerol. The free fatty acid can readily cross the epithelial membrane lining the gastrointestinal tract, but the diacylglycerol cannot be transported across. Hence, hydrolysis of dietary triacylglycerols by both gastric and pancreatic lipase is essential for their absorption by enterocytes. Human pancreatic lipase (HPL) (EC 3.1.1.3) is produced by the pancreatic acinar cells. The lipase is located into the zymogen granules, together with many other enzymes and secreted into the intestinal lumen together with the bile (Miled & al., 2000). Contrary to most of the pancreatic enzymes which are secreted as proenzymes and further activated by proteolytic cleavage in the small intestines, HPL is directly secreted as an active enzyme. Purified from pancreatic juice, the protein showed to have a molecular weight of 48 kDa (De Caro & al., 1977) and has been characterized as a glycoprotein consisting of 449 amino acid polypeptide (Lowe & al., 1989). The resolution of the HPL 3D structure (Fig.1) revealed the presence of a catalytic triad (Ser[152]-Asp[176] –His[263]) similar to that found in other serine hydrolases, Ser [152] being part of the G-X-S-X-G consensus sequence (Lowe & al., 1989). Pancreatic lipase acts maximally around pH 8-9 (Winkler et al., 1990) and was found to be poorly stereoselective (Rogalska & al., 1990). Unlike pre-duodenal lipases, pancreatic lipase requires colipase−a pancreatic protein−as cofactor for its enzymatic activity (Fig.1). Colipase relieves phosphatidyl choline-mediated inhibition of the interfacial lipase–substrate complex, helps anchor the lipase to the surface and stabilizes it in the 'open', active conformation (Brockman, 2000; Lowe, 1997).

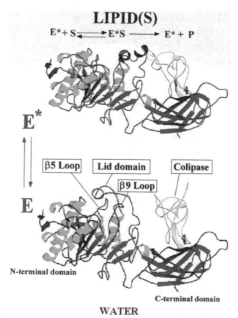

Fig. 1. 3-D Structure of the HPL-procolipase complex in the closed conformation (E) and in the open conformation (E*). These two diagrams show the conformational changes in the lid, the β-5 loop and the colipase during interfacial activation (Adapted from Miled et al., 2000 as cited in van Tilbeurgh et al., 1992; 1993).

The lipase gene family includes also two other pancreatic proteins: pancreatic lipase related proteins 1 and 2, with strong nucleotide and amino acid sequence homology to pancreatic triglyceride lipase. All three proteins have virtually identical three-dimensional structures (Lowe, 2000). Of the pancreatic triglyceride lipase homologues, only pancreatic lipase related protein 2 has lipase activity (Table 2).

Enzyme Name	Substrate specificity	References
Pancreatic lipase	Triglycerides (lipid-droplet)	Thirstrup & al., 1994
Pancreatic lipase related protein 1 (PLRP1)	Unknown Inhibitory effect of HPL (regulatory effect of TG digestion in the duodenum?)	Crenon & al., 1998 Berton & al., 2009
Pancreatic lipase related protein 2 (PLRP2)	Broad range of substrate specificity Triglycerides (milk lipid-droplet) Synergistic effect of HPL (regulatory effect of TG digestion in the duodenum?) Phospholipids Galactolipids Esters of vitamin A	Berton & al., 2009 Thirstrup & al., 1994 Sias & al., 2004 Reboul & al., 2006
Carboxyl ester lipase	Nonspecific enzyme Esters of lipid-soluble vitamins Esters of cholesterol Triglycerides, diglycerides, monoglycerides Phospholipids Ceramides	Hui & Howles , 2002
Phospholipase A2	Phospholipids	Verheij & al., 1983

Abbreviations: HPL, human pancreatic lipase; TG, triglycerides

Table 2. Human pancreatic enzymes involved in lipid digestion

It should be stressed that adult pancreas also produces an enzyme equivalent to the colipase-dependant pancreatic lipase (CDL) called bile-salt-stimulated lipase (BSSL) or carboxyl ester lipase (EC 3.1.1.1) (Hui & Howles, 2002). Originally discovered in milk of humans and various other primates (Swan & al., 1992), BSSL participates to the intestinal digestion of dietary lipids (Table 2). While colipase-dependent pancreatic lipase facilitates the uptake of fatty acids, bile-salt-stimulated lipase facilitates the uptake of free cholesterol from the intestinal lumen (Sahasrabudhe & al., 1998). A distinguishing feature of this 722 - amino acid native protein is that it requires primary bile salts for the hydrolysis of emulsified long chain triacylglycerols (Sahasrabudhe & al., 1998).

The exocrine pancreas secretes another group of phospholipid-hydrolyzing enzymes including phospholipase A1 (EC 3.1.1.32), and phospholipase A2 (EC 3.1.1.4). These enzymes are secreted in their zymogen form and activated by trypsin on entering the duodenum (Nouri-Sorkhabi & al., 2000).

PLA1 catalyzes the hydrolysis of fatty acids exclusively at the sn-1 position of phospholipids. A free fatty acid (FFA) and a lysophospholipid (lysoPL) are the products of this reaction. However, this class of phospholipase is not well understood, and no crystal structures exist. The assignment of a function for this pancreatic enzyme has yet to be firmly established (Richmond & Smith, 2011).

In intraluminal digestion, phospholipase A2 is primarily responsible for hydrolyzing phosphatidyl-choline to 2-lysophophatidyl-choline. This reaction is important in triglyceride digestion as the amphipathic phosphatidyl-choline, in a manner similar to bile salts, will adsorb to the surface of the lipid droplets, preventing contact between the lipase-colipase complex and its lipid substrate. Hydrolysis of phosphatidyl-choline by phospholipase 2 will allow desorption of lysophosphatidyl-choline, which is water soluble. The subsequent mucosal absorption of lysophosphatidyl-choline is important in the generation of enterocyte phospholipids and lipoproteins and, thus, chylomicron formation (Nouri-Sorkhabi & al., 2000).

2.4 Hepatic lipase

As the name suggests, hepatic lipase (EC 3.1.1.3) is synthesized mostly by hepatocytes in the liver and found localized at the surface of liver sinusoidal capillaries (Perret & al., 2002). The human hepatic lipase presents four glycosylation sites, which are localized at positions 20, 56, 340, and 375, and a molecular mass around 65 kDa (Ben-Zeev & al., 1994 ; Wolle & al., 1993). Together with lipoprotein lipase (LPL), hepatic lipase (HL) could be considered as a lipase of the vascular compartment (Perret & al., 2002). Unlike pancreatic lipase, hepatic lipase does not require a cofactor for its activity; is stable at high salt concentrations and is inactivated by sodium dodecyl sulfate (Mukherjee, 2003). HL exerts both triglyceride lipase and phospholipase A1 activities, and is involved at different steps of lipoprotein metabolism (Santamarina-Fojo & al., 2004). The preferred physiological substrate of hepatic lipase is triglyceride of intermediate density lipoprotein (IDL) particle, which it hydrolyses to form triglyceride-poor and cholesterol-rich low-density lipoprotein (LDL). Hepatic lipase also converts post-prandial triglyceride rich high-density lipoprotein (HDL) particle (i.e.HDL2) to post-absorptive triglyceride poor HDL (i.e. HDL3) (Mukherjee, 2003).

2.5 Lipoprotein lipase

Lipoprotein lipase (EC 3.1.1.34) (LPL) is a non-covalent homodimeric protein produced mainly by the adipose, heart and muscle tissue and to some extent by macrophages (Camp & al., 1990). LPL is secreted from parenchymal cells as a glycosylated homodimer, after which it is translocated through the extracellular matrix and across endothelial cells to the capillary lumen. After secretion, however, the mechanism by which LPL travels across endothelial cells is still unknown (Braun & Severeson 1992; Mead & al., 2002). The glycosylation sites of LPL are Asn-43, Asn-257, and Asn-359 (Mead & al., 2002). Lipoprotein lipase has multiple functional domains including lipid-binding, the dimer formation, heparin binding, cofactor interaction and fatty acid-binding domains (Santamarina-Fojo & Dugi, 1994). Interaction of the enzyme with the lipoprotein substrate takes place in the lipid-binding domain. This results in a conformational change that leads to the movement of a short helical segment or 'lid' to expose the active site containing the Ser-Asp-His catalytic triad, where hydrolysis of triacylglycerol takes place (Emmerich & al., 1992). As a homodimer, LPL has the dual function of triglyceride hydrolase and ligand/bridging factor for receptor-mediated lipoprotein uptake. Through catalysis, triacylglycerol present in very low-density lipoprotein (VLDL) and chylomicron particles is converted to triglyceride-poor intermediate-density lipoprotein (IDL) and chylomicron remnants, respectively (Mukherjee, 2003). Apolipoprotein CII (ApoCII) present on VLDL particles is the co-factor required for activating the enzyme (Mukherjee, 2003).

2.6 Endothelial lipase

Endothelial lipase (EC 3.1.1.3) which was firstly characterized in 1999 was also added to the lipase gene family (Jaye & al., 1999). Mature endothelial lipase is a 68 kDa glycoprotein with five potential N-linked glycosylation sites (Yasuda & al., 2010). It has 44% primary sequence homology with lipoprotein lipase, 41% with hepatic lipase and 27% with pancreatic lipase (Choi & al., 2002). The enzyme is secreted by endothelial cells from various tissues like lung, liver, kidney and placenta. However, heart and skeletal muscles do not express endothelial lipase (Jaye & al., 1999). Endothelial lipase differs from the other enzymes of the lipase gene family in the sequence of the 'lid' domain. Its 19-residue 'lid' region is 3 residues shorter and less amphipathic than 'lid' region of lipoprotein or hepatic lipase indicating a different enzymatic function (Jaye & al., 1999). Indeed, unlike lipoprotein or hepatic lipases that have triacylglycerol lipase activity, endothelial lipase has primarily a phospholipase A1 activity. It was suggested that endothelial lipase plays a physiologic role in HDL metabolism probably by catalyzing hydrolysis of HDL phospholipids thereby facilitating a direct HDL receptor-mediated uptake (Cohen, 2003). Endothelial lipase may also facilitate the uptake of apolipoprotein B-containing remnant lipoprotein. As the placental tissue abundantly expresses endothelial lipase, it may also have a role in the development of fetus (Choi & al., 2002).

3. Human dietary lipid digestion process and regulation of pancreatic fluid in healthy state

Protein digestion begins in the stomach with the concomitant action of hydrochloric acid and pepsin, continues with pancreatic proteases in the duodenum, and finishes with numerous brush border peptidases located all over the small intestine (Fieker & al., 2011 as cited in Alpers, 1994). Starch digestion begins in the mouth with salivary amylase, continues with pancreatic amylase, and ends with several intestinal brush border oligosaccharidases (Fieker & al., 2011 as cited in Alpers, 1994). In contrast, the majority of lipid digestion and absorption occurs between the pylorus and the ligament of Treitz. Prior to this step, 5% to 40% of the dietary triglyceride acyl chains are released in the stomach by gastric lipase (Armand & al., 1994, 1996, 1999; Carrière & al., 1993b ; Hamosh, 1990) which continues its action in the duodenum together with pancreatic lipase until these enzymes are degraded by pancreatic proteases. Although a pH of 8 to 9 appears to be optimal for pancreatic lipase activity *in vitro*, bile salts allow the enzyme to work efficiently at a pH of 6 to 6.5 *in vivo* (Borgstrom, 1964; Carrière & al., 2005). HPL is responsible for the hydrolysis of 40% to 70% of triglycerides (Fig.2).

The pancreatic lipase-related 2 protein (hPLRP2), with a broader substrate specificity, hydrolyzes milk triglycerides (Berton & al., 2009) phospholipids (Jayne & al., 2002; Lowe, 2002; Thirstrup & al., 1994) galactolipids (Sias & al., 2004) and esters of lipid-soluble vitamins (Reboul & al., 2006). Carboxyl ester lipase (also called bile salt-stimulated lipase,

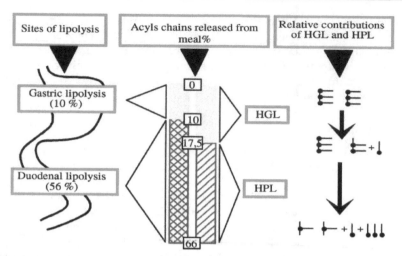

Fig. 2. Schematic representation of the relative contributions of HGL and HPL to the overall digestion of dietary triacylglycerides. On a weight basis, the ratio of pancreatic lipase to gastric lipase total secretory outputs was found to be around four after 3 hours of digestion. The level of gastric hydrolysis was calculated to be 10% of the acyl chains released from the meal triglycerides. Gastric lipase remained active in the duodenum where it might still hydrolyze 7.5% of the triglyceride acyl chains. Hence, globally, during the whole digestion period, gastric lipase hydrolyzes 17.5% of all the triglyceride acyl chains. (Reproduced from Carrière & al., 1993b).

(BSSL)) will hydrolyze triglycerides, diglycerides, phospholipids, and esters of lipid-soluble vitamins and of cholesterol (Hui & Howles, 2002). Phospholipase A2 hydrolyzes phospholipids to lysophospholipids20 which is essential for an optimal absorption of lipid nutrients (Fieker & al., 2011, as cited in Tso, 1994).

Products generated during lipolysis are solubilized in bile salts–mixed micelles and liposomes (vesicles) which allow absorption across the intestinal villi. Once absorbed, the digested lipids are converted back to triglycerides, phospholipids, and esters of cholesterol and of lipid-soluble vitamins, then packaged as chylomicrons and transported through the thoracic duct into the systemic circulation for delivery to various sites throughout the body (Fieker & al., 2011, as cited in Tso, 1994).

To execute this digestive function, postprandial pancreatic juice secretion can increase up to 1 to 2 L per day in response to physiologic stimuli, mainly secretin and vagal output (Lee & Muallem, 2009). Appropriate enzyme delivery in the duodenum is allowed through a specific orchestration of the pancreatic fluid secretion during the fed state. In fact, during the gastric phase, digestion of proteins by pepsin and of triglycerides by gastric lipase generates amino acids and free fatty acids, respectively (Fieker & al., 2011, as cited in Alpers, 1994). When delivered through the pylorus, they become powerful stimulants of the cholecystokinin hormone (CCK) produced by the duodenal endocrine cells which stimulates pancreatic enzymes secretion and controls the gastric emptying rate. The acidic pH of the chyme entering the duodenum stimulates the release of secretin, which increases the secretion of water and bicarbonate ions from the pancreas (Fieker & al., 2011 as cited in

Solomon, 1994). This gastric phase of digestion represents an important aspect in the overall postprandial regulation of pancreatic secretion. During the intestinal phase, enterohormones, such as CCK, together with neurotransmitters and neuropeptides further stimulate pancreatic secretion (Chey & Chang, 2001). Thus, digestive pancreatic enzyme response to a meal follows a specific pattern in which the degree and duration depend on nutrient composition, caloric content and physical properties of the meal. Enzyme secretion into the duodenum increases quickly reaching peak output within the first 20 to 60 minutes postprandially, then decreasing to a stable level before reaching an interdigestive level at the end of the digestive period, ie, about 4 hours after meal intake (Keller & Layer, 2005).

4. Exocrine pancreatic insufficiency & fat malabsorption

As previously described, the pancreas functions as the main factory for the digestive enzymes. The gland produces pancreatic juice that consists of a mixture of more than two dozen digestive enzymes in the pre-activated form, called zymogens. Zymogens are produced by acinar cells and mixed with a bicarbonate rich fluid that is produced by pancreatic ducts cells (Whitcomb & Lowe, 2007). Trypsin, chymotrypsin, amylase and lipase are responsible for the majority of the enzyme activity derived from the pancreas (Whitcomb & Lowe, 2007). Lipase is one of the most important enzymes because it plays a leading role in the digestion of fat, which is the highest dietary source of calories.

Pancreatic exocrine insufficiency, partial or complete loss of digestive enzyme synthesis, occurs primarily in disorders directly affecting pancreatic tissue integrity (Table 3).

Pancreatic parenchymal disease
Chronic pancreatitis Post-necrotizing acute pancreatitis Cystic fibrosis Pancreatic cancers/tumors Autoimmune pancreatitis
Extrapancreatic disease
Celiac disease Inflammatory bowel disease Diabetes mellitus Zollinger-Ellison syndrome
Postsurgical states
Gastric resection Whipple's pancreaticoduodenectomy Short bowel syndrome Bariatric surgeries (eg, gastric bypass)

Table 3. Conditions Causing EPI (adapted from Keller et al., 2009).

It is most frequently due to chronic pancreatitis (in adults) or cystic fibrosis (in children) (Keller & al., 2009). Other pancreatic causes include acute pancreatitis, pancreatic tumors and pancreatic surgery (Table 3).

While protein and starch digestion are usually maintained at a normal physiological level even in severe cases of pancreatic insufficiency, lipid malabsorption becomes the overriding problem and causes many of the clinical symptoms and nutritional deficiencies.

4.1 Pathophysiology

Clinically evident EPI occurs only when 90% of the function is lost and the secretion of pancreatic enzymes is less than 10% of normal (Lankisch & al., 1986; Layer & al., 1986). In chronic pancreatitis, an earlier decrease of lipase secretion is observed in comparison with amylase and protease. This is due to higher susceptibility of lipase to acidic pH caused by concomitant impairment of bicarbonate secretion, higher susceptibility of lipase to proteolytic destruction during small intestinal transit, additional acidic denaturation of bile acids and marked inhibition of bile acid secretion in malabsorptive states (Keller & Layer, 2005). Hence, in case of EPI, fat malabsorption precedes malabsorption of proteins and carbohydrates and is clinically more apparent. Additionally, due to the low bicarbonate secretion, the intraduodenal pH may drop below 4 late postprandially, bile salts may precipitate which leads to a decrease in post- prandial duodenal lipid solubilisation and contribute to impaired lipolysis (Zentler-Munro & al., 1984). The increased presence of lipids and other nutrients in the distal small bowel causes significant alterations in gut motility leading to accelerated gastric emptying and intestinal transit. This results in a marked decrease in the time available for digestion and absorption of nutrients, which also contributes to the malabsorption (Layer & al. 1997). However, more than 80% of carbohydrates can be digested and absorbed in the absence of pancreatic amylase activity and the colonic flora can further metabolizes malabsorbed carbohydrates (Layer & al., 1986). By contrast, gastric lipase, the only extrapancreatic source of lipolytic activity in humans, does not compensate efficiently for pancreatic lipase deficiency although it may be elevated in patients with chronic pancreatitis compared to healthy individuals (Carrière & al., 1993b). That's why fat malabsorption remains the first problem to be considered when treating EPI.

4.2 Clinical symptoms and complications

Maldigestion of fat results in steatorrhoea. In western countries steatorrhoea is diagnosed when daily stool fat content exceeds 7 g during ingestion of a diet containing 100 g fat per day. This corresponds to a decrease of the enteral absorption rate to less than 93% (Dimagno & al., 1973). Steatorrhoea causes symptoms such as foul-smelling, voluminous, greyish, fatty stools, abdominal cramps, bloating and chronic abdominal pain (Pasquali & al., 1996). It may also cause weight loss due to the loss of the highest dietary source of calories (fat contains 38 kJ/g, carbohydrates and protein contain 17 kJ/g) (Rosenlund & al., 1974). Steatorrhoea and weight loss are the overt clinical symptoms of EPI. They usually only occur if pancreatic enzyme secretion falls below 5–10% of normal levels (Keller & al., 2009).

Due to fat malabsorption fat-soluble vitamins (A, D, E and K), magnesium, calcium and essential fatty and amino–acids are insufficiently resorbed (Dutta & al., 1982; Keller & al., 2009) which results in a variety of associated complications. Deficiencies in these vitamins and nutrients may lead to tetany, glossitis, cheilosis, and in a more progressive stage, to peripheral neuropathy (Dimagno , 1993). Patients with PEI may exhibit low vitamin D levels and develop osteopathy, i.e. osteopenia, osteoporosis and osteomalacia. There are reports on vitamin A deficiency causing night-blindness, visual impairment and other ocular affections. As a consequence of vitamin E and K deficiencies neurologic symptoms or coagulopathy can occur (Keller & al., 2009). There seems also to be an increased risk for cardiovascular events in PEI, independent of life style factors (Gullo & al., 1996).

4.3 Incidence and diagnosis

The prevalence of EPI is increasing with the higher proportion of patients with cystic fibrosis who survive into adult life and the incidence of chronic pancreatitis, which rises in parallel with alcohol consumption. In fact, the incidence of cystic fibrosis is approximately 1 in 2500 live births. The lack of chloride secretion in the pancreatic duct is responsible for severe exocrine pancreatic insufficiency in approximately 85% of CF newborns (Levy, 2011). In case of chronic pancreatitis, an incidence of 8.2 per 100 000 population per year and a prevalence of 26.4 cases per 100 000 along with a 3.6-fold increase in mortality in patients with alcohol-induced chronic pancreatitis compared with a population without chronic pancreatitis has been signaled (Keller & al., 2009). Hence, to avoid malnutrition related morbidity and mortality, it is pivotal to start treatment as soon as EPI is diagnosed.

Several direct and indirect function tests are available for assessment of pancreatic function. Direct invasive function tests like the secretin-caerulein test are still the gold standard with highest sensitivity and specificity. However, their availability is limited to specialized centers, they are costly, time consuming and uncomfortable for the patient (Keller & al., 2009). Determination of fecal elastase is convenient and widely available but its sensitivity is low in mild to moderate cases. Moreover, due to low specificity, it is of limited value for differential diagnosis in patients with diarrhea (Dominguez-Munoz & al., 1995; Stein & al., 1996). Other non-invasive tests such as 13C-breath tests are becoming more important but are not widely established, yet (Dominguez-Munoz & al., 2007).

5. Standard approaches for the treatment of fat malabsorption due to exocrine pancreatic insufficiency

The main focus in the management of EPI is to prevent weight loss, EPI related symptoms, vitamin deficiencies, and to improve the patient's nutritional status. Whatever the aetiology, oral pancreatic enzyme supplements are widely used as the first-line approach to treat malabsorption secondary to exocrine pancreatic insufficiency (Breithaupt & al., 2007).

5.1 Formulations and galenic properties

Pancreatic enzyme preparations (PEPs) are typically a mixture of porcine-derived pancreatic enzymes. These preparations, also called pancreatin, contain a variable mixture of protease, lipase and amylase depending on the brand. Various preparations are commercially available. The main formulations are immediate-release, enteric-coated microspheres and minimicrospheres, enteric-coated microtablets and enteric-coated microspheres with a bicarbonate buffer (Table 4). A Comprehensive table of these preparations has been summarized in other reviews (Krishnamurty & al., 2009, Ferrone & al., 2007).

Formulation	Number of available products	Product example (manufacturer)
Immediate–release formulations	6	Pancrelipase tablets (various manufacturers) Vikokase powder (Axcan Scandipharm)
Enteric-coated microspheres	24	Lipram capsules (Global Pharmaceuticals) Pangestym (Ethex) Pancrelipase capsules (various manufacturers)
Enteric-coated microtablets	7	Pancrease (McNeil) Ultrase (Axcan Scandipharm)
Enteric-coated minimicrospheres	3	Creon capsules (Solvay Pharmaceuticals)
Enteric-coated microsphere with bicarbonate buffer	3	Pancrecarb (Digestive Care)

Table 4. Commercially available pancreatic enzyme formulations (adapted from Krishnamurty et al., 2009)

The uncoated formulations are susceptible to acidic inactivation in the stomach and are currently used largely in clinical practice to treat the pain of chronic pancreatitis and not malabsorption (Chauhan & Forsmark, 2010). The enteric-coated pancreatic enzyme formulations have been developed to solve problems associated with acid-mediated inactivation of pancreatic lipase, especially in patients with EPI who also show low pH values in the small intestine. First generation of these preparations was the enteric coated tablet with diameter of 11-20 mm. Due to their large size, these formulations did not empty into the duodenum as quickly as smaller food particles and did not show any additional benefits over conventional preparations (Meyer & al., 1988; Meyer & Lake, 1997). Next generation of enteric-coated preparations consist of capsules (over 2 mm in size) coated with acid resistant agents designed to release the enzyme between pH 5.0-5.5. No therapeutic benefit of these preparations was seen. Studies of labeled capsules suggest that even with varying sizes of microspheres, the ingested lipid may enter the duodenum in advance of the pancreatic enzyme (Meyer & Lake, 1997). Hence, newer formulations consisting of capsules containing mini-microspheres, pellets or micro-tablets of less than 2 mm in size were designed to promote an adequate intragastric mixture of exogenous enzymes with chyme. Whether the use of these enteric coated mini-microsphere preparations adds any special advantage over the existing treatment options remains, however, subject to great discussion (Halm & al., 1999; Stern & al, 2000).

The most recent innovation in the formulation of pancreatic enzymes supplements has been the development of enteric-coated "buffered" micro-sphere preparations which have 1.5-2.5 mEq of bicarbonate per capsule. Clinical trials conducted to compare these formulations to standard enteric coated microspheres showed controversy results (Brady & al., 2006; Kalnins & al., 2006).

In Europe, availability of preparations varies by country and they are regulated nationally and not by the European Medicines Agency. In products in which the enzyme content has been standardized, marked variability in particle size, enzyme release, and for some, acid stability has been noted and may result in differences in clinical effect (Walters & Littlewood, 1996; Aloulou & al., 2008; Löhr & al., 2009). In the United States, marked variation in the enzyme content of the various formulations especially with generic products has been attributed to a lack of stringent regulation (Fieker & al., 2011).

5.2 Dosage recommendation and schedule of administration

Some general guidelines are given in spite of the absence of an easy applicable and objective method to establish the adequate dose of oral pancreatic enzymes to treat exocrine pancreatic insufficiency.

In general, the recommended dosage of Pancreatic enzyme supplements (PES) for a main meal (breakfast, lunch, or dinner) ranges from 25,000 to 75,000 units of lipase and from 10,000 to 25,000 units of lipase for snacks, depending on the fat content of the meal (Sikkens et al., 2010). Initial dose must ensure supplementation of 60 UI/min of lipase activity in postparandial chyme throughout the digestive period; hence, dosing is adjusted considering this recommendation and the amount of lipase in the supplement (Krishnamurty et al., 2009) but it is not recommended to exceed 10,000 units of lipase per kg of body weight per meal (Fieker et al., 2011).

The timing of ingestion of the capsules is important to optimize therapeutic efficacy. A recent study compared three different administration schedules using enzyme replacement before, during or after meals. Better lipid digestion was found when giving enzymes during or after meals (Dominguez-Munoz & al., 2005).

5.3 Efficacy assessment of the treatment with pancreatic enzyme supplements

Numerous randomized placebo controlled trials have shown that treatment with pancreatic enzyme supplements improves steatorrhea, as measured by increased fat absorption, reduced fecal fat excretion, decreased stool weight and frequency, improved stool consistency and improved symptom scores (Guarner et al., 1993; O'keefe et al., 2001; Dominguez-Munoz et al., 2005; Safdi et al., 2006, Trapnell et al., 2009; Wooldridge et al., 2009; Whitcomb et al., 2010). Enzyme supplements have been found to improve lipid malabsorption in children even those who are younger than 7 years old (Graff et al., 2010a, 2010b). In yet other studies, increased cholesterol absorption and improved enterohepatic cycling of bile salts have been reported (Dutta et al., 1986; Vuoristo et al., 1992). Moreover, it has been demonstrated that improvement of lipid digestion contributes to effective correction of motility disorders (Mizushima et al., 2004). Altered levels of gastro-intestinal hormones were normalized (Nustede et al., 1991); accelerated gastric emptying and abnormal antroduodenal motility were corrected (Layer et al., 1997).

Even though, randomized controlled trials have suggested, years ago, that non-enteric coated pancreatic enzyme supplements reduce pain in chronic pancreatitis (Isaksson et al., 1983; Slaff et al., 1984), a more recent study did not support the use of these preparations for the relief of pain in all patients (Brown et al., 1997). Unfortunately, pancreatic enzyme supplements were reported to be not sufficient for correcting fat soluble vitamin deficiencies or B12 deficiency without simultaneous vitamin supplementation (Dutta et al., 1982; Bang et al., 1991).

The most surprising fact regarding efficacy assessment of this therapy is that few investigations are made considering nutritional status and quality of life improvements as well as weight gain (Czako et al., 2003; Trolli et al., 2001; Dominguez-Munoz, 2007). Reduction in stool fat achieved by pancreatic enzyme replacement therapy has not been proven by robust research to be correlated with a complete correction of nutritional deficiency in patients with pancreatic insufficiency. Accordingly, an overall assessment of this therapy efficacy is yet dependent on future demonstration of long-term interesting outcomes.

5.4 Safety concerns, side effect and treatment failure

Enzyme replacement therapy using pancrelipase (pancreatin) delayed-release capsules (i.e. Creon®, Solvay Pharmaceuticals, Inc., Marietta, GA, USA) have been available in the United States of America for more than 20 years with very few observed side effects (Krishnamurty et al., 2009). Meanwhile, allergic reactions to the porcine proteins and some others side effects may occur: Pancreatin extracts are prone to form insoluble complexes with folic acid resulting in folate deficiency (Russell & al., 1980). One serious adverse effect has been reported by Smyth et al. (1994, 1995). The authors described five children with cystic fibrosis in which a colonic obstruction developed due to fibrosing colonopathy (FC) after using very high doses of the enteric-coated micro- minisphere preparations (i.e. more than 20000 lipase units/capsule). Fortunately, the cases of reported FC have decreased considerably since the Medicine Control Agency (MCA) recommended in 1994 that the dose of pancreatic enzymes should not exceed 10,000 IU lipase/kg/day in patients with CF (Taylor , 2002 as cited in Medicine Control Agency, 1994).

Recently, Axcan Pharma Inc. and its subsidiaries received safety update reports describing a total of 46 adverse events observed in a clinical study carried out between 01 November 2008 and 31 May 2009 and involving three pancreatic enzyme preparations: ULTRASE®, VIOKASE® and PANZYTRAT® (Table 5). Fifty-three patients were enrolled, 40 of these patients completed the study.

In most cases, adverse effects were single occurrences. Drug ineffectiveness was the most frequently reported adverse effect for ULTRASE® (Table 5). A lack of therapeutic effect was also reported for some other preparations (Kraisinger et al., 1994). In fact, among marketed PEPs, great variability in the amount of enzymes included in each capsule has been noted (Case & al., 2005; US Food and Drug Administration, 2006; Wooldridge & al., 2009) due in part to the manufacturer practice of overfilling capsules to account for enzyme degradation that occurs over the course of the product's shelf life (US Food and Drug Administration, 2004). While instability of the enzymes results in delivery medications that contain less than the packaged amount of enzyme, the practice of "overfilling" in an effort to address enzyme degradation may result in excess enzyme content, resulting in formulations that deliver inadequate or excess amounts of enzyme.

The possible safety risk posed by high-dose enzyme therapy, particularly fibrosing colonopathy , in combination with the issue of enzyme overfill, recently prompted the FDA to require the manufacturers of PEPs to demonstrate drug efficacy and safety in randomized, placebo-controlled trials before approval (Trapnell & al., 2009). The FDA ruled that manufacturers of pancreatic enzyme supplements must file new drug applications

SOC / Preferred Term	ULTRASE®	VIOKASE®	PANZYTRAT®	Total
Cardiac disorders				
Cardio-respiratory arrest	0	1	0	1
Gastrointestinal disorders				
Abdominal pain	0	2	0	2
Abdominal pain upper	1	1	1	3
Abnormal faeces	0	1	0	1
Diarrhoea	1	3	1	5
Dyspepsia	0	1	0	1
Faecal volume increased	1	0	0	1
Frequent bowel movements	1	0	0	1
Gastritis	0	1	0	1
Glossodynia	0	1	0	1
Groin pain	0	1	0	1
Lip swelling	0	1	0	1
Nausea	0	1	1	2
Oral discomfort	0	1	0	1
Steatorrhoea	1	0	0	1
Swollen tongue	0	1	0	1
Tongue ulceration	0	1	0	1
Vomiting	0	0	1	1
General disorders and administration site conditions				
Asthenia	0	1	0	1
Drug effect decreased	1	0	0	1
Drug ineffective	4	0	0	4
Feeling abnormal	0	1	0	1
Product commingling	0	1	0	1
Therapeutic response decreased	0	1	0	1
Injury, poisoning and procedural complications				
Incorrect dose administered	0	1	0	1
Investigations				
Blood glucose increased	1	0	0	1
Blood sodium decreased	0	1	0	1
Blood sugar level fluctuation	0	1	0	1
Drug screen positive	0	1	0	1
Weight decreased	1	0	0	1
Metabolism and nutrition disorders				
Diabetes mellitus	1	0	0	1
Nervous system disorders				
Loss of consciousness	0	1	0	1
Respiratory, thoracic and mediastinal disorders				
Throat irritation	0	1	0	1
Skin and subcutaneous tissue disorders				
Rash macular	0	1	0	1
Urticaria	0	1	0	1

Coded with MedDRA dictionary

Table 5. Adverse Events (Preferred Term) Recorded for Pancreatic Enzyme Preparations in the Axcan Pharma Safety Database Classified by System Organ Class from November 1, 2008, to May 31, 2009 (Reproduced from Page 8 of the Safety Update for NDA 22-222 dated August 4, 2009).

(NDA) to ensure consistent efficacy, safety, and quality of these agents (US Food and Drug Administration, 2006). Therefore, in order to comply with the FDA 2004 mandate, several studies have been recently conducted to ensure safety and effectiveness of some new reformulated pancreatic enzyme supplements such as Creon® 24,000 and EUR-1008 (Zenpep™) (Wooldridge & al., 2009; Trapnell & al., 2009). Nevertheless, these products of animal origin present yet a risk of viral transmission. Accordingly, there remains a need for new alternatives to treat correctly exocrine pancreatic insufficiency.

6. Enzyme replacement therapy: What's in the pipeline?

6.1 Bovine enzymes

Even though bovine enzymes have been suggested as a potential alternative for individuals who refuse to consume porcine products for religious or other cultural reasons; there remain some safety concerns about transmittable pathogens such as Foot and mouth disease and Bovine spongiform encephalopathy from these preparations. Additionally, lipase activity is approximately 75% lower than the porcine preparations (Layer and Keller, 2003)

6.2 Recombinant mammalian/human lipases

Owing to rapid development of plant biotechnology in recent times, Merispase a recombinant mammalian gastric lipase was produced in transgenic corn by Meristem Therapeutics and proposed as new oral substitute for the treatment of pancreatic insufficiency. Dog gastric lipase was selected because it is naturally resistant to inactivation by stomach acids and maintains a high enzymatic activity after passage through the stomach. Enzyme expression was stable over 11 generations with an approximate level of 1,000 mg kg-1 kernel (Shama & Peterson, 2008). According to Fieker et al. (2011), this approach could be problematic for several reasons: gastric lipase specific activity is about 10 times lower than that of pancreatic lipase (measured on tributyrin), it is highly sensitive to trypsin proteolysis, and endogenous secretion of gastric lipase can be increased in patients with pancreatic insufficiency because of possible nutritional adaptation. Meanwhile, clinical trials showed that the recombinant gastric lipase is well tolerated and efficient when administered either alone or combined with porcine pancreatic extract to patients with cystic fibrosis (Fieker & al., 2011, as cited by Lenoir et al., 2006, 2008). The highest efficiency is obtained when 250 mg of recombinant gastric lipase is associated with low dose of pancreatic extract (Fieker & al., 2011, as cited by Lenoir et al., 2008). Despite these encouraging results, Mersitem therapeutics went out of business in September 2008 while the product was blocked in clinical phase II trial.

Expected to offer superior safety by decreasing the risk of allergic reactions, recombinant human bile salt- stimulated lipase was suggested as promising candidate for the treatment of lipid malabsorption in pancreatic insufficiency. Human bile salt-stimulated lipase is naturally acid resistant and able to: (i) hydrolyze triglycerides and phospholipids (Lindquist & Hernell, 2010) (ii) generate lysophospholipids necessary for an efficient lipid absorption rate by the small intestine (Fieker & al., as cited by Tso, 1994) (iii) participate in chylomicron assembly and secretion through its ceramidase activity (Hui and Howles, 2002). For these reasons, Swedish Orphan Biovitrum - a leading company focused on treatment of rare diseases developed two preparations of recombinant bile salt-stimulated lipase: Kiobrina for preterm infants and

Exinalda for cystic fibrosis patients. A phase I clinical trial showed that addition of recombinant bile salt-stimulated lipase to standard pancrelipase (Creon) enabled a dose reduction of pancrelipase. The treatment had the advantage of restoring a normal level and pattern of plasma chylomicron secretion (Fieker & al., 2011, as cited by Strandvik et al., 2004). The combined results from two Phase II studies evaluating Kiobrina in preterm infants demonstrated an increase in growth velocity and uptake of long chain polyunsaturated fatty acids such as docosahexanoic acid and arachidonic acid. The safety and tolerability profile of rhBSSL added to formula was similar compared to placebo (Maggio et al., 2010). Based on these encouraging results, Swedish Orphan Biovitrum enrolls in August 2011 the first patient in Kiorbina phase III clinical trial. An open-label exploratory phase II study on Exinalda (rhBSSL) in patients with cystic fibrosis and pancreatic insufficiency has been completed. The aim was to study the effect of Exinalda on fat absorption as well as safety in this patient population. The results showed that Exinalda is safe and tolerable at a dose level of 170 mg three times a day. In terms of efficacy (coefficient of fat absorption CFA) the primary endpoint was not met. Swedish Orphan Biovitrum is now assessing options to continue the development (Swedish Orphan Biovitrum website www. sobi.com).

6.3 Microbial and plant derived lipases

With the aim of developing porcine-free enzyme supplements and in order to avoid the short-life of lipolytic enzymes of pancreatic origin, microbial lipases of fungal or bacterial origin were suggested for replacement therapy. Therefore, potential efficacy of many fungal Lipases derived from *Aspergillus niger* (Griffin & al., 1989), *Rhizopus arrhizus* (Iliano & Lodewijk, 1990), *Rhizopus delemar* (Galle & al., 2004), *Candida cylindracea* (Schuler & Schuler, 2008) and *Yarrowia lipolytica* (Turki & al., 2010a) was investigated. The *Yarrowia lipolytica* lipase seemed to be of potential interest because of its acid and protease-stable properties and its resistance to the detergent action of bile salts as shown *in vitro* (Turki & al., 2010a). Supporting its use as a pharmaceutical, safety assessment of the enzyme in rats showed that there were no toxicologically severe changes in clinical signs, growth, hematology, clinical chemistry, organ weight and pathology related to oral administration of *Yarrowia lipolytica* lipase in animals (Turki & al., 2010b). Actually, a substitute for EPI treatment based on Lip2p is under investigation by Laboratoire Mayoly Spindler, a French pharmaceutical company specialized in gastroenterology therapeutics (Fickers & al., 2011, as cited in http://www.mayoly-spindler.com/). The process development in cGMP conditions for the production of the *Yarrowia lipolytica* MS1819 lipase was completed in 2009 with the Swiss biotech company DSM Nutritional Product Ltd (Fickers & al., 2011, as cited in http://www.dsm.com, press release, December 22th, 2009). In 2010, a drug development partnership was established with Protea Biosciences to initiate phase I/IIA clinical trials in France with the aim of demonstrating safety and proof-of-concept of the therapeutic use of this recombinant lipase (Fickers & al., 2011).

A pipeline preparation Liprotamase (formerly known as ALTU 135 and Trizytek) containing bacterial lipase, fungal protease and amylase was developed by Eli Lilly company (Eli Lilly, IN, USA, www. Lilly.com). An open-label Phase III safety study was carried out in order to evaluate 214 patients, of which 145 CF patients, ages 7 and above, completed 12 months of treatment with Liprotamase. Investigators found that 96 percent of all CF patients who received liprotamase for 12 months maintained or gained weight. Based on key nutritional parameters, the study showed that patients who completed 12 months of treatment with liprotamase demonstrated that they maintained their nutritional status; and survival in people living with cystic fibrosis was maintained too (Borowitz & al., 2011). Subsequent to the completion of the stage III clinical study on liprotamase, the drug's manufacturer submitted a New Drug Application to the U.S. Food and Drug Administration (FDA) for approval. However, on January 13th of this year, the FDA panel stated that he was not convinced that Liprotamase was any better than the current pancreatic enzyme products available now. The manufacturer disclosed that another clinical trial must be conducted before the FDA will consider the approval of this drug (Eli Lilly, IN, USA, www. Lilly.com).

In yet other approaches, plant acid-stable lipases were suggested as good alternatives to porcine preparations. Hence, considerable attention has focused in these enzymes and suitable techniques for isolating and purifying them have been well documented. A lipase sourced from *Carica papaya* latex has been recently proposed as suitable candidate for use as a therapeutic tool in patients with pancreatic exocrine insufficiency (Abdelkafi et al., 2009). The enzyme showed several biochemical properties enabling it to act in the gastro-intestinal tract like mammalian digestive lipases (Abdelkafi et al., 2009): (i) its activity on long-chain Triacylglycerols reaches an optimum at pH 6.0 in the presence of bile, (ii) it is only weakly inhibited by bile salts, (iii) it shows a similar pattern of regioselectivity to that of human pancreatic lipase, generating 2-Mono acylglycerol and free fatty acids (FFA), the lipolysis products absorbed at the intestinal level, and (iv) it shows significant levels of stability and activity at low pH values at a temperature of 37 °C. Therefore, *Carica papaya* lipase seems to be tailored to act optimally under the physiological conditions pertaining in the gastro-intestinal tract. However, its sensitivity to digestive proteases still needs to be tested.

6.4 Future therapies and new research areas

Development of non-porcine enzyme replacement therapies is currently extended to new research areas including design, by direct molecular evolution, of human pancreatic lipase variants that display lipolytic activity at acidic pH higher than that of the native enzyme. Colin et al. (2008) investigated, first, the feasibility of altering the pH optimum of pancreatic lipase to improve its performances in the intestinal conditions of cystic fibrosis by site-directed mutagenesis. Later, they demonstrated that directed molecular evolution approach combined to a sensitive screening strategy could be useful to improve pancreatic lipase activity at acidic pH. The authors showed that a single round of random mutagenesis was successful in identifying lipase variant with approximately 1.5-fold increased activity at low pH (Colin et al., 2010).

Future therapies may also include structuring food emulsions and creation of functional dietary lipids that are more effectively digested. This new area of research could substantially help patient suffering from pancreatic insufficiency with the design of specific more digestible or absorbable lipid sources. Hence, the addition of specific phospholipids able to enhance lipase activity in enzyme supplements or in formula would both increase lipase activity and, in parallel, enhance lipid nutrient absorption (Fieker et al., 2011).

7. Conclusion

Pancreatic exocrine insufficiency is a condition commonly associated with diseases such as pancreatitis or cystic fibrosis. When pancreatic insufficiency is severe, impaired absorption of nutrients by the intestines may result, leading to deficiencies of essential nutrients and the occurrence of loose stools containing unabsorbed fat (steatorrhea). A shortage of the digestive enzymes necessary to break down food is the main cause of this dietary malabsorption. Unlike protein and starch digestion, lipid malabsorption is the overriding problem and the main cause of clinical symptoms and nutritional deficiencies. Until recently, approaches used to address problem of fat malabsorption due to pancreatic insufficiency have been focusing primarily on oral administration of exogenous pancreatic enzymes extracted from porcine source. Standard clinical practices dictate administration of lipase 25,000-75,000 units/meal by using pH-sensitive pancrelipase microspheres, along with dosage increases, compliance checks, and differential diagnosis in cases of treatment failure. Various pancreatin preparations are available, however, differences in galenic properties and release kinetics and other factors such as early acid inactivation, under dosage and patient incompliance may decrease clinical efficacy of the treatment. The FDA decreed that all manufacturers of pancreatic enzyme supplements must file new drug applications (NDA) to ensure consistent efficacy, safety, and quality of these agents. Accordingly, improved approaches to treat efficiently problem of fat malabsorption secondary to pancreatic insufficiency are investigated. New alternatives of enzyme substitution therapy are being developed. Emerging therapeutic landscape includes use of porcine free - lipase preparations. Enzyme supplements either from human, mammalian, microbial or plant origins are wisely suggested. Interestingly, newest approaches state the design of acid -stable variants of human pancreatic lipase as well as creation of functional dietary food with specific more digestible/absorbable lipid sources. However, how these pipeline therapies may help meet the ongoing challenges in treating lipid malabsorption in patients with pancreatic insufficiency and improve the long-term outcomes of these patients remains yet to be assessed.

8. References

Abdelkafi, S.; Fouquet, B. ; Barouh, N. ; Durner, S. ; Pina, M. ; Scheirlinckx, F. ; Villeneuve, P. & Carrière F. (2009). In vitro comparisons between Carica papaya and pancreatic lipases during test meal lipolysis: Potential use of CPL in enzyme replacement therapy. *Food Chemistry*, Vol.115, No. 2, pp. 488–494

Aloulou, A. ; Puccinelli, D. ; Sarles, J. ; Laugier, R. ; Leblond, Y. & Carrière, F. (2008). In vitro comparative study of three pancreatic enzyme preparations: dissolution profiles, active enzyme release and acid stability. *Alimentary Pharmacology and Therapeutics*. Vol. 27, No. 3, pp. 283-392.

Ameis, D.; Stahnke, G.; Kobayashi, J.; McLean, J.; Lee, G.; Buscher, M.; Schotz, M.C. & Will, H. (1990). Isolation and characterization of the human hepatic lipase gene. *Journal of Biological Chemistry*. Vol. 265, pp. 6552–6555.

Armand, M.; Borel, P.; Dubois, C.; Senft, M.; Peyrot, J.; Salducci, J.; Lafont, H. & Lairon, D. (1994).Characterization of emulsions and lipolysis of dietary lipids in the human stomach. *American Journal of Physiology Gastrointestinal and Liver Physiology*, Vol., 266, No. 3, pp. 372-381.

Armand, M.; Hamosh, M.; Mehta, N.R.; Angelus, P.A.; Philpott, J.R.; Henderson, T.R.; Dwyer, N.K.; Lairon, D. & Hamosh, P. (1996). Effect of human milk or formula on gastric function and fat digestion in the premature infant. *Pediatric Research.* Vol. 40, No. 3, pp.429–437.

Armand, M. ; Pasquier, B.; Andre, M.; Borel, P. ; Senft, M.; Peyrot, J.; Salducci, J. ; Portugal, H. ; Jaussan, V. & Lauron, D. (1999). Digestion and absorption of 2 fat emulsions with different droplet sizes in the human digestive tract. *The American Journal of Clinical Nutrition.* Vol. 70, No. 6, pp.1096–1106.

Bai, J. (1998).Malabsorption syndromes. *Digestion,* Vol. 59, No.5, pp 530–546.

Bang Jørgensen, B.; Thorsgaard Pedersen, N. & Worning, H. (1991). Short report: lipid and vitamin B12 malassimilation in pancreatic insufficiency. *Alimentary Pharmacology & Therapeutics,* Vol. 5, No. 2, pp. 207–210.

Ben-Zeev, O.; Stahnke, G.; Liu, R.; Davis, C. & Doolittle, M. H. (1994). Lipoprotein lipase and hepatic lipase: the role of asparagine linked glycosylation in the expression of a functional enzyme. *Journal of Lipid Research.* Vol. 35, pp. 1511–1523.

Berton, A.; Sebban-Kreuzer, C.; Rouvellac, S.; Lopez, C. & Crenon, I. (2009) Individual and combined action of pancreatic lipase and pancreatic lipase-related proteins 1 and 2 on native versus homogenized milk fat globules. *Molecular Nutrition & Food Research.* Vol.53, No.12. pp.1592–1602.

Breithaupt, D. E.; Alpmann, A. & Carrière, F. (2007). Xanthophyll esters are hydrolysed in the presence of recombinant human pancreatic lipase. *Food Chemistry,* 103, 651–656.

Bodmer, M.W.; Angal, S.; Yarranton, G.T.; Harris, T.J.R.; Lyons, A.; King, D.J.; Pieroni, G.; Riviere, C.; Verger R. & Lowe P.A. (1987).Molecular cloning of human gastric lipase and expression of the enzyme in yeast, *Biochimica and Biophysica Acta,* Vol. 909, pp. 237–244.

Borgstrom, B. (1964). Influence of bile salt, pH, and time on the action of pancreatic lipase. *Journal of Lipid Research.* Vol. 5, pp.522–531.

Borowitz, D.; Stevens, C.; Brettman, L.R.; Campion, M.; Chatfield, B. & Cipolli, M. & for the Liprotamase 726 Study Group (2011).. International phase III trial of liprotamase efficacy and safety in pancreatic-insufficient cystic fibrosis patients. *Journal of Cystic Fibrosis,* In press doi:10.1016/j.jcf.2011.07.001 |

Brady, M.S.; Garson, J.L.; Krug, S.K.; Kaul, A.; Rickard, K.A.; Caffrey, H.H.; Fineberg, N., Balistreri, W.F.; Stevens, J.C. (2006). An enteric-coated high-buffered pancrelipase reduces steatorrhea in patients with cystic fibrosis: a prospective, randomized study. *Journal of American Dietetic Association.* Vol. 106, No. 8, pp. 1181-1186.

Braun, J.E. & Severson, D.L. (1992). Regulation of the synthesis, processing and translocation of lipoprotein lipase. *Biochemistry Journal.* Vol. 287, No 2, pp. 337–347.

Brockman, H.L. (2000). Kinetic behaviour of the pancreatic lipase– colipase–lipid system. *Biochimie,* Vol. 82, pp. 987–995.

Brown, A.; Hughes, M.; Tenner, S. & Banks, P.A. (1997). Does pancreatic enzyme supplementation reduce pain in patients with chronic pancreatitis: a meta-analysis. *American Journal of Gastroenterology,* Vol.92, pp. 2032–2035.

Case, C.L.; Henniges, F. & Barkin, J.S. (2005). Enzyme content and acid stability of enteric-coated pancreatic enzyme products in vitro. *Pancreas,* Vol. 30, No. 2, pp.180–183.

Carrière, F.; Barrowman, J.A. ; Verger, R. & Laugier, R. (1993a). Secretion and contribution to lipolysis of gastric and pancreatic lipases during a test meal in humans, *Gastroenterology*, Vol.105, pp. 876–888.

Carriere, F.; Laugier, R.; Barrowman, J.A.; Douchet, I.; Priymenko, N. & Verger, R. (1993b) Gastric and pancreatic lipase levels during a test meal in dogs. *Scandinave Journal of Gastroenterology*. Vol. 28, pp. 443–454.

Carrière, F.; Grandval, P.; Renou, C. ; Palomba, A. ; Priéri, F. ; Giallo, J. ; Henniges, F. ; Sander-Struckmeier, S. & Laugier, R. (2005). Quantitative study of digestive enzyme secretion and gastrointestinal lipolysis in chronic pancreatitis. *Clinical Gastroenterology & Hepatology*.Vol. 3, No 1, pp. 28–38.

Camp, L.; Reina, M.; Llobera, M.; Vilaro, S. & Olivecrona, T. (1990). Lipoprotein lipase: cellular origin and functional distribution, *American Journal of Physiology*. Vol. 258, pp. 673 – 681.

Chauhan, S. & Forsmark, C.E. (2010). Pain management in chronic pancreatitis: A treatment algorithm. *Best Practice Research in Clinical Gastroenterology*. Vol. 24, No. 3, pp. 323–335.

Chey, W.Y. & Chang, T. (2001). Neural hormonal regulation of exocrine pancreatic secretion. *Pancreatology*. Vol.1, No. 4, pp.320–335.

Choi, S.Y.; Hirata, K.; Ishida, T.; Quertermous, T. & Cooper, A.D. (2002). Endothelial lipase: a new lipase on the block. *Journal of Lipid Research*. Vol. 43, pp. 1763–1769.

Czakó, L.; Takács, T.; Hegyi, P., Prónai, L.; Tulassay, Z.; Lakner, L.; Döbrönte, Z.; Boda, K. & Lonovics, J. (2003). Quality of life assessment after pancreatic enzyme replacement therapy in chronic pancreatitis. *Canadian Journal of Gastroenterology*, Vol. 17, No. 10, pp. 597–560.

Crenon, I.; Foglizzo, E.; Kerfelec, B.; Vérine, A.; Pignol, D.; Hermoso, J.; Bonicel, J. & Chapus C. (1998). Pancreatic lipase-related protein type I: a specialized lipase or an inactive enzyme. *Protein Engineering*. Vol. 11, No. 2, pp.135–142.

Cohen, J.C. (2003). Endothelial lipase: direct evidence for a role in HDL metabolism. *Journal of Clinical Investigation*. Vol. 111, pp. 318–321

Colin,D.Y. ; Deprez-Beauclair,P. ; Allouche,M. ; Brasseur,R. & Kerfelec,B. (2008). Exploring the active site cavity of human pancreatic lipase. *Biochemical and Biophysical Research Communication*, Vol. 370, No. 3, pp. 394–398.

Colin,D.Y. ; Deprez-Beauclair,P.; Silva, N.; Infantes, L. & Kerfelec, B. (2010). Modification of pancreatic lipase properties by directed molecular evolution. *Protein Engineering, Design & Selection*, Vol. 23, No. 5, pp. 365–373.

De Caro, A.; Figarella, C.; Amic, J.; Michel, R. & Guy, O. (1977). Human pancreatic lipase: A glycoprotein. *Biochimica and Biophysica Acta (BBA)-Protein Structure*, Vol. 490, No 2, pp. 411-419.

DeNigris, S.J.; Hamosh, M.; Kasbekar, D.K.; Fink, C.S.; Lee, T.C. & Hamosh, P. (1985). Secretion of human gastric lipase from dispersed gastric glands. *Biochimica & Biophysica Acta (BBA) -Lipids and Lipid Metabolism*. Vol. 836, No 1, pp. 67-72.

DiMagno, EP. (1993). A short eclectic history of exocrine pancreatic insufficiency and chronic pancreatitis. *Gastroenterology*, Vol. 104, No. 5, pp. 1255 - 1262.

DiMagno, E.P.; Go, V.L. & Summerskill, W.H (1973). Relations between pancreatic enzyme outputs and malabsorption in severe pancreatic insufficiency. *New England Journal of Medecine*, Vol. 288, pp. 813–815.

Dominguez-Munoz, J.E., Hieronymus, C., Sauerbruch, T., & Malfertheiner, P. (1995). Fecal elastase test: evaluation of a new noninvasive pancreatic function test. *American Journal of Gastroenterology*, Vol. 90, No. 10, pp.1834–1837.

Domínguez-Muñoz, J.E.; Iglesias-García, J.; Iglesias-Rey, M.; Figueiras, A. & Vilariño-Insua, M. (2005). Effect of the administration schedule on the therapeutic efficacy of oral pancreatic enzyme supplements in patients with exocrine pancreatic insufficiency: a randomized, three-way crossover study. *Alimentary Pharmacology and Therapeutics*. Vol. 21, pp. 993-1000.

Dominguez-Munoz, J.E.; Iglesias-Garcia, J.; Vilarino-Insua, M. & Iglesias-Rey M. (2007). 13C-mixed triglyceride breath test to assess oral enzyme substitution therapy in patients with chronic pancreatitis. *Clinical Gastroenterology and Hepatology*, Vol. 5, pp. 484–488.

Dutta, S.K.; Bustin, M.P., Russell, R.M. & Costa, B.S. (1982). Deficiency of fat-soluble vitamins in treated patients with pancreatic insufficiency. *Annals of Internal Medcine*, Vol. 97, pp. 549–552.

Duttan, S.K.; Anand, K. & Gadacz, T.R. (1986). Bile salt malabsorption in pancreatic insufficiency secondary to alcoholic pancreatitis. *Gastroenterology*, Vol. 91, pp.1243–1249.

Eli Lilly, IN, USA, Liprotamase Liprotamase Regulatory Review Bus (Liprotamase) is a biologic entity that combines three biotechnology-produced enzymes. *http://www.lilly.com/SiteCollectionDocuments/FlashFiles/PipeLine/Clinical Development Pipeline/14.html*.

Emmerich, J.; Beg, O.U.; Peterson, J.; Previato, L.; Brunzell, J.D.; Brewer, J.r.H.B. & Santamarina-Fojo, S. (1992). Human lipoprotein lipase. Analysis of catalytic triad by site-directed mutagenesis of Ser-132, Asp-156 and His-241, *Journal of Biological Chemistry*, Vol. 267, pp. 4161–4165

Ferrone, M., Raimondo, M., Scolapio, J.S.(2007). Pancreatic enzyme pharmacotherapy. *Pharmacotherapy*, Vol. 27, No.6, pp. 910-920.

Fickers, P.; Marty, A. & Nicaud, J.M (2011). The lipases from *Yarrowia lipolytica*: Genetics, production, regulation, biochemical characterization and biotechnological applications, *Biotechnology Advances*, doi: 10.1016/j.biotechadv.2011.04.005

Fieker, A.; Philpott, J. & Armand, M. (2011). Enzyme replacement therapy for pancreatic insufficiency: present and future. *Clinical and Experimental Gastroenterology*. Vol. 4, pp. 55-73.

Galle, M.; Gregory, P.C.; Potthoff, A. & Henniges, F. (2004). Microbial enzyme mixtures useful to treat digestive disorders. US Patent 20040057944

Graff, G.R.; Maguiness, K.; McNamara, J.; Morton, R.; Boyd, D.; Beckmann, K. & Bennett, D. (2010a). Efficacy and tolerability of a new formulation of pancrelipase delayed-release capsules in children aged 7 to 11 years with exocrine pancreatic insufficiency and cystic fibrosis: a multicenter, randomized, double-blind, placebo-controlled, two-period crossover, superiority study. *Clinical Therapeutics*, Vol. 32, No. 1, pp. 89-103.

Graff, G.R.; McNamara, J.; Royall, J.; Caras, S.; Forssmann, K. (2010b). Safety and tolerability of a new formulation of pancrelipase delayed-release capsules (CREON) in children under seven years of age with exocrine pancreatic insufficiency due to cystic fibrosis: an open-label, multicentre, single-treatment-arm study. *Clinical Drug Investigation*, Vol.30, No. 6, pp. 351- 364.

Griffin, S. M.; Alderson, D.; Farndon, J.R. (1989). Acid resistant lipase as replacement therapy in chronic pancreatic exocrine insufficiency: a study in dogs. *Gut*, Vol. 30, pp. 1012-1015

Guarner, L. ; Rodriguez, R. ; Guarner, F. ; Malagelada, J. R. (1993). Fate of oral enzymes in pancreatic insufficiency. *Gut*, Vol. 34, pp. 708–712.

Gullo, L.; Tassoni, U.; Mazzoni, G. ; Stefanini F. (1996). Increased prevalence of aortic calcification in chronic pancreatitis. *American Journal of Gastroenterology*, Vol. 91, No. 4, pp. 759-761.

Halm, U.; Löser, C.; Löhr, M.; Katschinski, M. & Mössner, J. (1999). A double-blind, randomized, multicentre, crossover study to prove equivalence of pancreatin minimicrospheres versus microspheres in exocrine pancreatic insufficiency. *Alimentary Pharmacology and Therapeutics*. Vol. 13, No. 7, pp. 951-957.

Hamosh, M. (1979). The role of lingual lipase in neonatal fat digestion. *Ciba Foundation Symposium*, Vol. 16-18, No. 70, pp. 69-98.

Hamosh, M. (1990). Lingual and gastric lipase. *Nutrition*, Vol. 6, pp. 421–428.

Hamosh, M. & Scow, R.O. (1973). Lingual lipase and its role in the digestion of dietary lipid. *Journal of Clinical Investigation*. Vol. 52, No. 1, pp. 88–95.

Hirata, K.-I.; Dichek, H.L.; Cioffi, J.A.; Choi, S.Y.; Leeper, N.J.; Quintana, L.; Kronmal, G.S.; Cooper, A.D. & Quertermous, T. (1999). Cloning of a unique lipase from endothelial cells extends the lipase gene family. *Journal of Biological Chemistry*. Vol. 274, pp.14170 -14175.

Hui, D.Y. & Howles, P.N. (2002). Carboxyl ester lipase: structure-function relationship and physiological role in lipoprotein metabolism and artherosclerosis. *Journal of Lipid Research*. Vol. 43, No. 12, pp.2017-2030.

Iliano, L.O. & Lodewijk, J.S. (1990). A composition for the treatment of exocrine insufficiency of the pancreas, and the use of said composition. European Pat. ES 2059986 (T3).

Isaksson, G.; Ihse, I. (1983). Pain reduction by an oral pancreatic enzyme preparation in chronic pancreatitis. *Digestive Disease Science*, Vol. 28, pp. 97–102.

Jaye, M.; Lynch, K.J.; Krawiec, J.; Marchadier, D.; Maugeais, C.; Doan, K.; South, V.; Amin, D.; Perrone, M. & Rader, D.J. (1999). A novel endothelial-derived lipase that modulates HDL metabolism. *Nature Genetics*. Vol. 21, pp. 424–428.

Jayne, S.; Kerfelec, B.; Foglizzo, E.; Chapus, C. & Crenon, I. (2002). High expression in adult horse of PLRP2 displaying a low phospholipase activity. *Biochimica & Biophysica Acta*. Vol.1594, No. 4, pp. 255–265.

Kalnins, D., Ellis, L.; Corey, M.; Pencharz, P.B., Stewart, C., Tullis, E., Durie, P.R. (2006). Enteric-coated pancreatic enzyme with bicarbonate is equal to standard enteric-coated enzyme in treating malabsorption in cystic fibrosis. *Journal of Pediatric Gastroenterology and Nutrition*. Vol. 42, No. 3, pp. 256-261.

Keller, J. & Layer P. (2005). Human pancreatic exocrine response to nutrients in health and disease. *Gut*. Vol. 54, No. 6, pp.1–28.

Keller, J.; Aghdassi, A.A.; Lerch, M.M.; Mayerle, J.V. & Layer, P. (2009). Tests of pancreatic exocrine function – Clinical significance in pancreatic and non-pancreatic disorders. *Best Practice & Research Clinical Gastroenterology*, Vol. 23, pp. 425–439.

Krishnamurty, D. M.; Rabiee, A.; Jagannath, S. B. & Andersen, D.K. (2009) Delayed release pancrelipase for treatment of pancreatic exocrine insufficiency associated with chronic pancreatitis. *Therapeutics and clinical risk management*, Vol. 5, pp. 507-520.

Kraisinger, M.; Hochhaus, G.; Stecenko, A.; Bowser, E. & Hendeles, L. (1994). Clinical pharmacology of pancreatic enzymes in patients with cystic fibrosis and *in vitro* performance of microencapsulated formulations. *Journal of Clinical Pharmacology*, Vol. 34, No. 2, pp.158–166.

Lankisch, P.G.; Lembcke, B.; Wemken, G. & Creutzfeldt, W. (1986). Functional reserve capacity of the exocrine pancreas. *Digestion*, Vol. 35, No. 3, pp. 175 - 181.

Layer, P.; Go, V.L. & DiMagno, E.P. (1986) Fate of pancreatic enzymes during small intestinal aboral transit in humans.*American Journal of Physiology*. Vol. 251, No. 4, pp. 475- 480.

Layer, P.; vonderOhe, M.R.; Holst, J.J.; Jansen, J.B.; Grandt, D.; Holtmann, J. & Goebell, H. (1997). Altered postprandial motility in chronic pancreatitis: role of malabsorption .*Gastroenterology*, Vol. 112, No.5, pp. 1624- 1634.

Layer, P. & Keller J. (2003). Lipase Supplementation Therapy: Standards, Alternatives, and Perspectives. *Pancreas*, Vol. 26, No. 1, pp. 1-7.

Lee, M.G. & Muallem, S. (2009). Physiology of duct cell secretion, *In : The Pancreas: An Integrated Textbook of Basic Science, Medicine, and Surgery, Second Edition*, (eds H. G. Beger, A. L. Warshaw, M. W. Büchler, R. A. Kozarek, M. M. Lerch, J. P. Neoptolemos, K. Shiratori, D. C. Whitcomb and B. M. Rau), pp.78-90, Blackwell Publishing Ltd., 9781444300123, Oxford, UK.

Levy, E. (2011). Nutrition-related derangements and managements in patients with cystic fibrosis: Robust challenges for preventing the development of co-morbidities. *Clinical Biochemistry*, Vol. 44, pp. 489–490

Löhr, JM, Hummel FM, Pirilis KT, Steinkamp G, Körner A, Henniges F. (2009). Properties of different pancreatin preparations used in pancreatic exocrine insufficiency. *European Journal of Gastroenterology and Hepatology*. Vol. 21, No. 9, pp. 1024-1031.

Lohse, P.; Chahrokh-Zadeh, S. & Seidel, D. (1997). The acid lipase gene family: three enzymes, one highly conserved gene structure. *Journal of Lipid Research*. Vol. 38, pp. 880–891

Lowe, M.E. (1997). Molecular mechanisms of rat and human pancreatic triglyceride lipases. *Journal of Nutrition*. Vol. 127, pp.549–557.

Lowe, M.E. (2000). Properties and function of pancreatic lipase related protein 2. *Biochimie*, Vol. 82, No 11, pp. 997-1004.

Lowe, M.E. (2002). The triglyceride lipases of the pancreas. *Journal of Lipid Research*, Vol. 43, No. 12, pp. 2007–2016.

Lowe, M.E , Rosemblum, J.L. & Strauss, A.W. (1989). Cloning and characterization of human pancreatic lipase cDNA. *Journal of Biological Chemistry*. Vol. 264, pp. 20042-20048.

Lindquist, S. & Hernell, O. (2010). Lipid digestion and absorption in early life: an update. *Current Opinion of Clinical Nutrition Metabolism Care*. Vol. 13, No. 3, pp. 314-320.

Maggio, L.; Bellagamba, M.; Costa, S.; Romagnoli, C.; Rodriguez, M.; Timdahl, K.; Vågerö, M.; Carnielli, V.P. A prospective, randomized, double-blind crossover study comparing rhBSSL (recombinant human Bile Salt Stimulated Lipase) and placebo added to infant formula during one week of treatment in preterm infants born before 32 weeks of gestational age. Abstract EAPS meeting.

Mead, J.R.; Irvine, S.A. & Ramji, D.P. (2002). Lipoprotein lipase: structure, function, regulation, and role in disease. *Journal of Molecular Medicine*. Vol. 80, No. 12, pp. 753- 769.

Meyer, J.H.; Elashoff, J.; Porter-Fink, V., Dressman, J. & Amidon, G.L. (1988). Human postprandial gastric emptying of 1-3-millimeter spheres. *Gastroenterology*, Vol. 94, pp. 1315-1325.

Meyer, J.H. & Lake, R. (1997). Mismatch of duodenal deliveries of dietary fat and pancreatin from enterically coated microspheres. *Pancreas*, Vol. 15, pp. 226-235.

Miled, N.; Canaan, S.; Dupuis, L.; Roussel, A.; Rivière, M.; Carrière, A.; Caro, A.; Cambillau, C. & Verger, R. (2000). Digestive lipases: From three-dimensional structure to physiology. *Biochimie*, Vol. 82, pp. 973-986.

Moreau, H.; Laugier, R.; Gargouri, Y.; Ferrato, F. & Verger, R. (1988). Human pre-duodenal lipase is entirely of gastric fundic origin. *Gastroenterology*, Vol. 95, pp.1221-1226.

Mukherjee, M. (2003).Human digestive and metabolic lipases—a brief review. *Journal of Molecular Catalysis B: Enzymatic*. Vol. 22, pp. 369-376.

Mizushima, M.; Ochi, K.; Ichimura, M.; Kiura K.; Harada, H. & Koide, N. (2004). Pancreatic enzyme supplement improves dysmotility in chronic pancreatitis patients. *Journal of Gastroenterology and Hepatology*, Vol. 19, No. 9, pp. 1005-1009.

Nouri-Sorkhabi, M.H.; Chapman, B.E.; Kuchel, P.W.; Gruca, M.A. & Gaskin, K.J. (2000). Parallel Secretion of Pancreatic Phospholipase A2, Phospholipase A1, Lipase, and Colipase in Children with Exocrine Pancreatic Dysfunction. *Pediatric Research*. Vol. 48, No. 6, pp. 735-740

Nustede, R.; Köhler, H.; Fölsch, U.R. & Schafmayer, A. (1991). Plasma concentrations of neurotensin and CCK in patients with chronic pancreatitis with and without enzyme substitution. *Pancreas*. Vol. 6, No. 3, pp. 260-265.

O'Keefe, S.J.; Cariem, A.K. & Levy, M. (2001).The exacerbation of pancreatic endocrine dysfunction by potent pancreatic exocrine supplements in patients with chronic pancreatitis. *Journal of Clinical Gastroenterology*, Vol. 32, pp. 319-323.

Pasquali, C.; Fogar, P.; Sperti, C.; Bassob, D.; De Paolib, M.; Plebanib, M. & Pedrazzoli, S. (1996). Efficacy of a pancreatic enzyme formulation in the treatment of steatorrhea in patients with chronic pancreatitis. *Current Therapeutic Research & Clinical Experimentation*, Vol. 57, No. 5, pp. 358-365.

Perret, B.; Mabile, L.; Martinez, L.; Tercé, F.; Barbaras, R. & Collet, X. (2002). Hepatic lipase: structure/function relationship, synthesis, and regulation. *Journal of Lipid Research*. Vol. 43, No. 8, pp. 1163-1169.

Reboul, E.; Berton, A.; Moussa, M.; Kreuzer, C.; Crenon, I. & Borel, P. (2006). Pancreatic lipase and pancreatic lipase-related protein 2, but not pancreatic lipase-related protein 1, hydrolyze retinyl palmitate in physiological conditions. *Biochimica & Biophysica Acta.* Vol. 1761, No. 1, pp. 4–10.

Richmond, G.S. & Smith, T.K. (2011). Phospholipases A1. *International Journal of Molecular Sciences.* Vol. 12, pp. 588- 612.

Rogalska, E.; Ransac, S. &Verger, R. (1990). Stereoselectivity of lipases. II. Stereoselective hydrolysis of triglycerides by gastric and pancreatic lipases. *Journal of Biology &. Chemistry.* Vol. 265, pp. 20271–20276

Rosenlund, M.L.; Kim, H.K. & Kritchevsky, D. (1974). Essential fatty acids in cystic fibrosis. *Nature.* Vol. 25, pp. 251(5477):719.

Roussel, A.; Canaan, S.; Egloff, M.P.; Rivière, M.; Dupuis, L.; Verger, R. & Cambillau, C. (1999). Crystal structure of human gastric lipase and model of lysosomal acid lipase, two lipolytic enzymes of medical interest. *Journal of Biology and Chemistry,* Vol. 274, No. 24, pp. 16995–7002

Russell, R.M.; Dutta, S.K.; Oaks, E.V.; Rosenberg, I.H. & Giovetti, A.C. (1980). Impairment of folic acid absorption by oral pancreatic extracts. *Digestive Diseases and Sciences,* Vol. 25, No. 5, pp. 369-373.

Sahasrabudhe, A.V.; Solapure, S.M.; Khurana, R.; Suryanarayan, V.; Ravishankar, S.; deSousa, S.M. & Das, G. (1998) Production of Recombinant Human Bile Salt Stimulated Lipase and Its Variant in *Pichia pastoris. Protein expression and purification,* Vol. 14, pp. 425–433.

Safdi, M.; Bekal, P.K.; Martin, S.; Saeed, Z.A.; Burton, F.; Toskes, P.P. (2006). The effects of oral pancreatic enzymes (Creon 10 capsule) on steatorrhea: a multicenter, placebo controlled, parallel group trial in subjects with chronic pancreatitis. *Pancreas,* Vol. 33, pp.156–162.

Santamarina-Fojo, S. & Dugi, K.A. (1994). Structure, function and role of lipoprotein lipase in lipoprotein metabolism. *Current Opinion in Lipidology.* Vol. 5, pp. 117–125.

Santamarina-Fojo, S.; Gonza´lez-Navarro, H.; Freeman, L.; Wagner, E. & Nong, Z. (2004). Hepatic Lipase, Lipoprotein Metabolism, and Atherogenesis. *Arteriosclerosis Thrombosis Vascular Biology.* Vol. 24, pp.1750-1754

Schuler, C. & Schuler, E.F. (2008). Composition With a Fungal (Yeast) Lipase and Method For Treating Lipid Malabsorption in Cystic Fibrous as Well as People Suffering From Pancreatic Lipase Insufficiency. *US Patent 20080279839.*

Shama, L.M. & Peterson, R.K.D. (2008).Assessing risk of plant-based pharmaceuticals: I. human dietary exposure. *Human and Ecological Risk Assessment,* Vol. 14, pp. 179-193.

Sias, B.; Ferrato, F.; Grandval, P.; Lafont, D.; Boullanger, P.; De Caro, A.; Leboeuf, B.; Verger, R. & Carriere, F. (2004). Human pancreatic lipase-related protein 2 is a galactolipase. *Biochemistry,* Vol. 43, pp. 10138–10148.

Sims, H.F.; Jennens, M.L. & Lowe, M.E. (1993). The human pancreatic lipase-encoding gene: structure and conservation of an Alu sequence in the lipase gene family. *Gene,* Vol. 131, pp. 281–285.

Sikkens, E.C.M.; Cahen, D.L.; Kuipers, E.J. & Bruno, M.J. (2010). Pancreatic enzyme replacement therapy in chronic pancreatitis. *Best practice research Clinical gastroenterology*,Vol. 24, No. 3, pp. 337-347.

Slaff, J.; Jacobson, D.; Tillman, C.R.; Curington, C. & Toskes, P. (1984). Protease-specific suppression of pancreatic exocrine secretion. *Gastroenterology*, Vol. 87, pp. 44–52.

Smyth, R.L.; Smyth, A.R.; Lloyd, D.A.; vanVelzen, D. & Heaf D.P. (1994). Strictures of a scending colon in cystic fibrosis and high-strength pancreatic enzymes. *The Lancet,* Vol. 343, No. 8889, pp. 85- 86.

Smyth, R.L.; O'Hea, U.; Burrows, E.; Ashby, D.; Lewis, P. & Dodge, J.A. (1995). Fibrosing colonopathy in cystic fibrosis: results of a case-control study. *The Lancet,* Vol. 346, No. 8985, pp.1247-1251.

Stein, J.; Jung, M.; Sziegoleit, A.; Zeuzem, S.; Caspary, W.F. & Lembcke, B. (1996). Immunoreactive elastase I: clinical evaluation of a new noninvasive test of pancreatic function. *Clinical Chemistry,* Vol. 42, pp. 222–226.

Stern, R.C.; Eisenberg, J.D.; Wagener, J.S.; Ahrens, R.; Rock, M.; doPico, G.; Orenstein, D.M. (2000). A comparison of the efficacy and tolerance of pancrelipase and placebo in the treatment of steatorrhea in cystic fibrosis patients with clinical exocrine pancreatic insufficiency. *The American Journal of Gastroenterology.* Vol. 95, No. 8, pp. 1932-1938.

Swan, J.S.; Hoffman, M.M.; Lord, M.K. & Poechmann, J.L. (1992).Two forms of human milk bile-salt-stimulated lipase. *Biochemistry Journal*, Vol. 283, No. 1, pp. 119 –122.

Swedish Orphan Biovitrum website www. sobi.com

Taylor, C.J. (2002). Fibrosing colonopathy unrelated to pancreatic enzyme supplementation. *Journal of Pediatric Gastroenterology and Nutrition*, Vol. 35, No. 3, pp. 268-269.

Thirstrup, K.; Verger, R. & Carrière, F. (1994). Evidence for a pancreatic lipase subfamily with new kinetic properties. *Biochemistry*, Vol. 33, No. 10, pp. 2748–2756.

Trapnell, B.C.; Maguiness, K.; Graff, G.R., Boyd, D.; Beckmann, K. & Caras, S. (2009). Efficacy and safety of Creon® 24,000 in subjects with exocrine pancreatic insufficiency due to cystic fibrosis. *Journal of Cystic Fibrosis,* doi:10.1016/j.jcf.2009.08.008.

Trolli, P.A.; Conwell, D.L.; Zuccaro, G. Jr (2001). Pancreatic enzyme therapy and nutritional status of outpatients with chronic pancreatitis. Gastroenterology Nursing, Vol. 24, No. 2, pp. 84 - 87.

Turki, S.; Mrabet, G.; Jabloun Z.; Destain, J.; Thonart, P. & Kallel, H. (2010a). A highly stable *Yarrowia lipolytica* lipase formulation for the treatment of pancreatic insufficiency. *Biotechnology and Applied Biochemistry*, Vol. 57, No. 4, 134 -149.

Turki, S.; Jabloun, Z.; Mrabet, G.; Marouani, A.; Thonart, P.; Diouani, M.F.; Ben Abdallah, F.; Amra A.; Rejeb, A. & Kallel, H. (2010 b). Preliminary safety assessment of Yarrowia lipolytica extracellular lipase: Results of acute and 28-day repeated dose oral toxicity studies in rats. *Food and Chemical Toxicology*, Vol. 48, pp. 2393-2400.

U.S. Food and Drug Administration. (2004). FDA requires pancreatic extract manufacturers to submit marketing applications. FDA News. *http://www. fda.gov/bbs/topics/news/2004/NEW01058.html.* Published April 27, 2004. Accessed 8 August 2008

U.S. Food and Drug Administration (2006). Center for Drug Evaluation and Research. Guidance for Industry: Exocrine Pancreatic Insufficiency Drug Products— Submitting NDAs. *http://www.fda.gov/cder/guidance/6275fnl.htm.* Published April 13, 2006. Accessed March 9 2009.

Verheij, M.H.; Westerman, J.; Sternby, B. & de Haas, G.H. (1983). The complete primary structure of phospholipase A2 from human pancreas. *Biochimica & Biophysica Acta.* Vol. 747, No. 1-2, pp. 93-99.

Vuoristo, M.; Vaananen, H.; Miettinen, T.A. (1992). Cholesterol malabsorption in pancreatic insufficiency: effects of enzyme substitution. *Gastroenterology.* Vol. 102, pp. 647-655.

Walker-Smith, J.; Barnard, J.; Bhutta, Z.; Heubi, J.; Reeves, Z. & Schmitz, J. (2002). Chronic Diarrhea and Malabsorption (Including Short Gut Syndrome): Working Group Report of the First World Congress of Pediatric Gastroenterology, Hepatology, and Nutrition. *Journal of Pediatric Gastroenterology and Nutrition,*Vol 35, No. 2, pp. 98-105.

Walters, M.P. & Littlewood, J.M. (1996). Pancreatin preparations used in the treatment of cystic fibrosis-lipase content and in vitro release. *Alimentary Pharmacology & Therapeutics.* Vol. 10, No. 3, pp. 433-440.

Whitcomb, D.C. & Lowe, M.E (2007).Human pancreatic digestive enzymes. *Digestive Diseases & Sciences,* Vol. 52, No. 1, pp. 1-17.

Winkler, F.K.; D'Arcy, A. & Hunziker, W. (1990). Structure of Human pancreatic lipase. *Nature,* Vol. 343, pp.771-774.

Wion, K.L.; Kirchgessner, T.G.; Lusis, A.J.; Schotz, M.C. & Lawn, R.M. (1987). Human lipoprotein lipase complementary DNA sequence. *Science,* Vol. 235, pp. 1638-1641.

Wolle, J.; Jansen, H.; Smith, L.C. & Chan, L. (1993). Functional role of N-linked glycosylation in human hepatic lipase: asparagine- 56 is important for both enzyme activity and secretion. *Journal of Lipid Research.* Vol. 34, pp. 2169-2176.

Wooldridge, J.L.; Heubi, J.E.; Amaro-Galvez, R.; Boas, S.R.; Blake, K.V.; Nasr, S.Z.; Chatfield, B.; McColley, S.A.; Woo, M.S.; Hardy, K.A.; Kravitz, R.M.; Straforini, C.; Anelli, M. & Lee, C. (2010). EUR-1008 pancreatic enzyme replacement is safe and effective in patients with cystic fibrosis and pancreatic insufficiency. *Journal of Cystic Fibrosis.* Vol. 8, No. -, pp. 405- 417.

Whitcomb, D.C.; Lehman, G.A.; Vasileva, G.; Malecka-Panas, E.; Gubergrits, N.; Shen, Y.; Sander-Struckmeier, S. & Caras S. (2009). Pancrelipase Delayed-Release Capsules (CREON) for Exocrine Pancreatic Insufficiency due to Chronic Pancreatitis or Pancreatic Surgery: A Double-Blind Randomized Trial. *The American Journal of Gastroenterology,* Vol. 105, pp. 2276-2286.

Whitcomb, D.C. & Lowe, M.E. (2007). Human pancreatic digestive enzymes. *Digestive diseases & Sciences.* Vol. 52, N°. 1, pp. 1-17

Yasuda, T.; Ishida, T. & Rader, D.J. (2010). Update on the Role of Endothelial Lipase in High-Density Lipoprotein Metabolism, Reverse Cholesterol Transport, and Atherosclerosis. *Circulation Journal,* Vol. 74, pp. 2263 - 2270.

Zentler-Munro, P.L.; Fitzpatrick, W.J.; Batten, J.C. & Northfield, T.C. (1984). Effect of intrajejunal acidity on aqueous phase bile acid and lipid concentrations in pancreatic steatorrhoea due to cystic fibrosis. *Gut.* Vol.25, No. 5, pp. 500- 507.

3

Evaluating Lymphoma Risk in Inflammatory Bowel Disease

Neeraj Prasad
Royal Albert Edward Infirmary, Wigan
University of Salford
United Kingdom

1. Introduction

The risk of lymphoma in inflammatory bowel disease (IBD) has been a topic of great interest for many years. In 1928, the first published series of colorectal malignancies in ulcerative colitis (UC) patients included a case of lymphosarcoma, the name given to an early classification of lymphoma (Bargen, 1928). Since then a huge number of case reports, case series, cohort studies, population-based studies and meta-analyses have been presented on the topic but the matter remains controversial with conflicting results based on poor quality evidence. Most recently, a type of non-Hodgkin's lymphoma (NHL) known as hepatosplenic T-cell lymphoma (HSTCL) has understandably drawn much attention despite its rarity. HSTCL has an invariably fatal outcome despite reports of early response to treatment, it almost exclusively affects young men with Crohn's disease (CD) and seems to be linked to commonly used drugs for the management of IBD, the thiopurines and tumour necrosis factor (TNF) antagonists (Kotlyar et al., 2011). A further source of concern stems from a trend by IBD physicians to use these drugs earlier in the course of disease and also in combination because recent studies suggest that these strategies may improve outcomes (Colombel et al., 2010, D'Haens, 2009).

Proving causality has been difficult because it is difficult to separate the multiple factors involved in lymphomagenesis using the evidence that is available (see Figure 1). It has long been suspected that the chronic inflammation seen in IBD itself may be the cause of lymphoma in this setting but there has been growing concern that it is in fact the drugs used in the treatment of IBD which confers this risk. One could also speculate that it is the combination of both these factors which results in the development of lymphoma.

The case of lymphosarcoma identified by Bargen in 1928 was in an era when immunomodulators were not available for the treatment of IBD suggesting that the disease itself may predispose to lymphoma development. There are other reports of lymphoma in drug-naïve IBD patients (Aydogan et al., 2010). There does appear to be an increased risk of lymphoma in other chronic inflammatory and autoimmune conditions as well including rheumatoid arthritis (RA), primary Sjögren's syndrome, systemic lupus erythematosus (SLE) and Hashimoto's thyroiditis (Smedby et al., 2006). There is some evidence that increased severity of the disease may increase the risk of lymphoma in these conditions (Baecklund et al., 2006, Theander et al., 2006, Lofstrom et al., 2007).

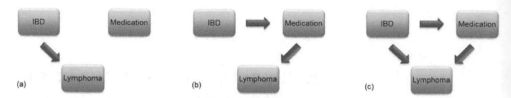

Fig. 1. Assessing the causality of lymphoma in IBD. IBD itself may be the cause of lymphoma (a), or lymphoma may be due to the medication used to treat it (b) or lymphoma may be due to a combination of the disease and the treatment (c).

Both primary and acquired immunodeficiency states have been associated with lymphoma which is important because many of the drugs used for the treatment of IBD have immunosuppressive effects. There is an increased risk of lymphoma with Human Immunodeficiency Virus (HIV) infection and in post-transplant patients treated with immunosuppressives (Serraino et al., 1992, Grulich et al., 2007b). The role of Epstein-Barr virus (EBV) is well established in lymphomagenesis in post-transplant patients and this also appears to be important in IBD patients (Dayharsh et al., 2002).

IBD is associated with significant morbidity and a small mortality (Rubin et al., 2004, Ghosh and Mitchell, 2007). It is important that IBD physicians are able to help patients weigh up the risk of lymphoma with the benefits of drugs used to treat IBD. A number of attempts have been made to quantify this risk. One of the largest population-based studies utilised a primary care database from the United Kingdom but did not find a statistically significant increased background risk of lymphoma in IBD patients (Lewis et al., 2001). A cohort study from Dublin found an alarmingly higher rate of lymphoma in their IBD patients with up to a 59-fold increase (Farrell et al., 2000). Kandiel et al performed a meta-analysis of 6 studies to evaluate the risk of lymphoma in IBD patients treated with thiopurines and found a 4-fold increased risk of lymphoma in these patients (Kandiel et al., 2005).

A number of more recent studies have been presented in the literature including large cohort studies from the United States (US) and Spain (Chiorean et al., 2010, Van Domselaar et al., 2010) as well as large population-based studies from the UK and the Netherlands (Armstrong et al., 2010, Vos et al., 2010). Most notably, the French CESAME study published in 2009 with almost 50,000 patient-years of follow up, set out to quantify the risk of lymphoma and made attempts to distinguish the background risk of lymphoma due to IBD itself from the risk conferred by its treatment (Beaugerie et al., 2009a).

This chapter aims to provide an up to date systematic review of the available literature regarding the risk of lymphoma in inflammatory bowel disease. Meta-analysis techniques have been used to pool data from multiple studies.

2. Inflammatory bowel disease

Inflammatory bowel disease (IBD) is a chronic, idiopathic, remitting and relapsing disorder of the gastrointestinal tract. It comprises of two main disease types, ulcerative colitis (UC) and Crohn's disease (CD), which have many similar but also certain distinct pathological and clinical characteristics.

2.1 Epidemiology

IBD affects 400 per 100,000 population in the United Kingdom but there is considerable variation worldwide with the highest prevalence in developed countries (Rubin et al., 2000). It most commonly presents in teenage or young adult life but it can affect any age and there is an approximate equal sex distribution.

2.2 Aetiology

The aetiology is unknown but evidence suggests an immune dysfunction which is triggered by an environmental factor in a genetically susceptible individual (Cho, 2008) leading to chronic inflammation and injury to the gastrointestinal tract. Many of the susceptibility genes identified in recent studies have been shown to have important roles in immune regulation but there is increasing evidence that these genes pertain to the innate immune system and are involved in the sensing or intracellular processing of bacteria (Packey and Sartor, 2008). Potential microbial triggers which have been studied include a form of enteroadherent *Escherichia coli* and *Mycobacterium paratuberculosis*, but more recent investigation suggests that a disturbance of normal enteric microflora may play a role in aetiology (Sartor, 2008). Additionally, a number of other potential environmental factors have also been studied including diet, smoking, appendiceal inflammation, certain drugs and stress but causality has remained difficult to establish (Bernstein, 2010). The particular combination of susceptible genes and environmental triggers probably varies between individuals with IBD and leads to different patterns and severity of disease.

Ulcerative colitis causes a continuous mucosal inflammation of the colorectum, whereas Crohn's disease can affect any part of the GI tract, characteristically with skip lesions and transmural inflammation. Additionally, chronic inflammation in Crohn's disease can lead to fistulising and stricturing disease behaviours (Satsangi et al., 2006).

2.3 Treatment

A curative treatment for inflammatory bowel disease is yet to be identified. Strategies for the management of IBD involve treatment of flares and maintenance of remission. Although a wide range of therapies including enteral nutrition (Zachos et al., 2007), antibiotics (Lal and Steinhart, 2006) and complementary medicines (Langmead and Rampton, 2006) are used in IBD, the mainstay of treatment has been with anti-inflammatory and immunomodulatory drugs. Corticosteroids, 5-aminosalicylates (5ASA), azathioprine (AZA), mercaptopurine (6MP), methotrexate (MTX) and cyclosporin A (CSA) have been the most commonly used drugs. In an attempt to reduce steroid exposure and maintain remission, immunomodulatory therapy is being used earlier, for prolonged periods and in combination. The concern is of an increased risk of side effects with this approach. Estimates suggest that up to 30% of patients may not respond to this treatment and may require more aggressive strategies. The increased understanding of the pathogenesis of IBD, has led to investigation in to a number of therapies targeted towards the abnormal cytokine expression seen in patients with IBD. Of these, only the monoclonal antibodies against tumour necrosis factor are currently in clinical use but other targets have been identified and are undergoing laboratory and clinical study. Infliximab (IXB) and adalimumab (ADA) are the two anti-tumour necrosis factor (anti-TNF) drugs available in the United Kingdom and a number of studies have proven their efficacy (Hanauer et al., 2006, Hanauer et al., 2002, Jarnerot et al., 2005). A third, pegylated anti-TNF drug, certolizumab has also been studied and appears to have equivalent clinical efficacy (Sandborn et al., 2007a). Despite medical therapy, up to 50-70% of patients with CD will undergo surgery within 5 years of diagnosis and UC patients have a 20-30% lifetime risk of colectomy (Cosnes et al., 2005).

2.4 Cancer risk in IBD

The increased risk of colonic adenocarcinoma in patients with ulcerative colitis and Crohn's colitis is well documented (Rutter et al., 2006, Jess et al., 2006). One study has suggested a protective role for thiopurines in this context (Beaugerie et al., 2009b) though these patients were not corrected for co-administration of 5ASA preparations which may also have a protective role in this setting.

There also appears to be an increased risk of certain non-colorectal malignancies amongst IBD patients. In the same cohort of patients from the CESAME study, prospective data suggested a 20-fold increased risk of small bowel adenocarcinoma and suggestion of an increased risk of skin and cervical malignancy (Beaugerie et al., 2009c). In a database of over 27,000 UC patients from Sweden, the standardised incidence ratio (SIR) for all cancers was 1.46 with increased risk of malignancy of the liver, small bowel (carcinoid), prostate and breast (Hemminki et al., 2008). In a recent review of malignancies associated with thiopurine therapy, Smith et al concluded that these drugs did not increase the risk of cervical dysplasia, colonic cancer or solid organ tumours in IBD patients (Smith et al., 2010). A retrospective cohort study of over 50,000 IBD patients from the US suggested an increased risk of non-melanomatous skin cancer and that this risk was highest in patients treated with thiopurines (Odds Ratio 4.27) and biological therapies (Odds Ratio 2.18) (Long et al., 2010).

Many of these studies have also shown an increased risk of lymphoma and this will be discussed further in this chapter.

3. Lymphoma

Lymphoma is a broad term used to describe a variety of neoplasms due to proliferation of lymphoid cells. Traditionally, lymphoid neoplasms that presented with bone marrow and blood involvement were referred to by the term *leukaemia* and those that presented with a mass would be called a *lymphoma*. However, it is now appreciated that any *lymphoma* can present with or evolve in to a leukaemic picture and occasionally, *leukaemia* can present with a mass lesion.

3.1 Classification of lymphoma

The earliest classifications of lymphoma were based entirely on the morphological features of the neoplastic cells involved. Historically, lymphomas represented by large cells were known as *reticulosarcomas* and those by small cells were *lymphosarcomas* (Diebold, 2001). Later, lymphomas began to be distinguished according to their origin from B or T lymphocytes. With the development of immunophenotyping and cytogenetics, as well as an appreciation of differences in prognosis and patient stratification, more complex classification systems have developed. The World Health Organisation (WHO)

Classification of Tumours of Haemopoietic and Lymphoid Tissues, updated in 2008 (see Table 1), is now widely accepted (Swerdlow et al., 2008) and categorises lymphoid neoplasms in to those derived from:

- B cell progenitors - bone marrow derived
- T cell progenitors - thymus derived
- Mature T lymphocytes - cytotoxic or killer T cells, helper T cells or T regulatory cells
- Mature B lymphocytes - B cells or plasma cells

Non-Hodgkin's Lymphoma	
Precursor B-cell lymphomas	**Precursor T-cell and NK-cell lymphomas**
Precursor B-cell lymphoblastic lymphoma	Precursor T-cell lymphoblastic lymphoma
	Blastic NK-cell lymphoma
Mature B-cell lymphomas	
	Mature T-cell and NK-cell lymphomas
Small lymphocytic lymphoma	
Lymphoplasmacytic lymphoma	T-cell prolymphocytic leukaemia
Splenic marginal zone lymphoma	T-cell large granular lymphocytic leukaemia
Hairy cell leukaemia	Aggressive NK-cell leukaemia
Plasma cell neoplasms	Adult T-cell lymphoma/leukaemia
Extranodal marginal zone B-cell MALT lymphoma	Extranodal NK-/T-cell lymphoma, nasal type
Nodal marginal zone B-cell lymphoma	Enteropathy-type T-cell lymphoma
Follicular lymphoma (grades 1, 2, 3a and 3b)	Hepatosplenic T-cell lymphoma
Diffuse follicle centre lymphoma	Subcutaneous panniculitis-like T-cell lymphoma
Mantle cell lymphoma	Mycosis fungoides
Diffuse large B-cell lymphoma	Peripheral T-cell lymphoma unspecified
Mediastinal (thymic) large B-cell lymphoma	Angioimmunoblastic T-cell lymphoma
Intravascular large B-cell lymphoma	Anaplastic large cell lymphoma
Primary effusion lymphoma	
Burkitt lymphoma	
B-cell proliferations of uncertain malignant potential	
Lymphomatoid granulomatosis	
Post-transplant lymphoproliferative disorder	

Hodgkin's Lymphoma
Classical Hodgkin's lymphoma
Nodular sclerosis classical HL
Mixed cellularity classical HL
Lymphocyte rich classical HL
Lymphocyte depleted classical HL
Nodular lymphocyte predominant HL

Table 1. WHO Classification of Non-Hodgkin's and Hodgkin's Lymphoma (Swerdlow et al, 2008). (MALT – mucosa-associated lymphoid tissue; HL – Hodgkin's Lymphoma; NK – Natural Killer).

Hodgkin's lymphoma (formerly known as Hodgkin's disease) arises from B-cells of germinal or post-germinal centres of peripheral lymph nodes. It is pathologically and clinically distinct from other lymphoid neoplasia and generally has a good prognosis. Hodgkin's lymphoma has a distinguishing cellular composition on biopsy of lymphomatous tissues with abundant inflammatory cells and only a minority of neoplastic cells, known as Reed-Sternberg cells. Reed-Sternberg cells are large, binucleated or multinucleated containing multiple eosinophilic nucleoli and have prominent cytoplasm. Hodgkin's lymphoma (HL) is classified in to *nodular lymphocyte predominant HL* and *classical HL*, which is further subdivided in to *nodular sclerosis, mixed cellularity, lymphocyte-rich* and *lymphocyte-depleted* types (see Table 1).

The term Non-Hodgkin's lymphoma encompasses all other types of lymphoma. Although the WHO classification does not distinguish NHL on the basis of disease activity, it has classically been divided in to two subtypes:

- High-grade NHL develops quickly and aggressively.
- Low-grade or indolent NHL develops slowly and there may be no symptoms for many years.

3.2 Non-Hodgkin's lymphoma

NHL can occur in children and adults but over two-thirds are diagnosed in people aged over 60 years. There is a male preponderance with a ratio of up to 1.5 in older age groups. NHL is the fifth most common cancer in the UK with over 10,000 people diagnosed with the condition in 2007 and an age-standardised rate of 14.2 per 100,000 population (Cancer-Research-UK, 2011) (see Figure 2A). In the United States, the Surveillance Epidemiology & End Results (SEER) registry provides an age-standardised rate of 19.6 per 100,000 between 2003 and 2007 (Altekruse et al., 2010). The incidence of NHL seems to be rising in the UK

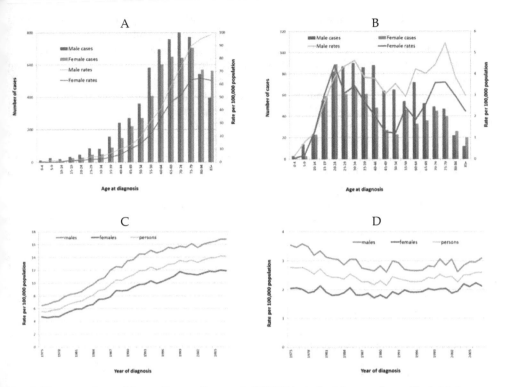

Fig. 2. Figures adapted from Cancer Research UK 2011. A: Incidence of non-Hodgkin's lymphoma by gender. B: Incidence of Hodgkin's lymphoma by gender. C: Age standardised incidence rates for non-Hodgkin's lymphoma. D: Age standardised incidence rates for Hodgkin's lymphoma.

with an increase of 35% during the 20 year interval between 1988 and 2007 (see Figure 2C). This trend seems to be reflected throughout the world. Mortality in the UK is estimated at 6.9 per 100,000 from NHL and with improvements in treatment, it is estimated that over half of patients now survive for at least 10 years following diagnosis. Up to 15% of all extra-nodal NHL presents in the GI tract (Newton et al., 1997).

A number of risk factors for the development of NHL have been studied:

- **Infectious agents** – It is thought that a proportion of the worldwide rise in incidence of NHL parallels, but is not completely explained by, the HIV epidemic. The risk of NHL in HIV and AIDS is well documented but only 3-5% of these patients will develop NHL (Serraino et al., 1992). Epstein-Barr virus has been linked to Burkitt's lymphoma and post-transplant lymphoma (Epstein et al., 1964). Other infections associated with an increased risk of NHL include *Helicobacter Pylori* (Xue et al., 2001), Hepatitis C (Dal Maso and Franceschi, 2006) and Human T-cell Lymphotropic Virus (HTLV-1) (Parkin, 2006).
- **Immunosuppression** – The use of immunosuppression following organ transplant has been shown to increase the risk of NHL and in a significant proportion of these, EBV

infection has been implicated (Kawashima et al., 1994). A recent meta-analysis suggests an 8-fold increased risk of NHL in post-transplant patients (Grulich et al., 2007b).

- **Autoimmune conditions** – Conditions such as autoimmune haemolytic anaemia, systemic lupus erythematosus and Sjögren's syndrome, where there is a longstanding stimulation of the immune system have been shown to carry an increased risk of NHL but the exact mechanisms remain poorly understood (Ekstrom Smedby et al., 2008). Coeliac disease is associated with T-cell lymphoma and less frequently, B-cell lymphoma (Chandesris et al., 2010, Oruc et al., 2010). This risk can be reduced by treatment with a gluten-free diet (Silano et al., 2008).
- **Genetic susceptibility** – The sibling or progeny of an affected individual has an approximate two-fold increased risk of developing NHL and there appears to be concordance in NHL subtype (Altieri et al., 2005).
- **Exposure to chemical carcinogens** – A number of studies and meta-analyses suggest an increased risk of NHL in individuals with occupational exposure to agricultural pesticides (Merhi et al., 2007), benzene (Steinmaus et al., 2008) and aromatic hydrocarbons (Miligi et al., 2006).
- **Diet and obesity** – Dietary factors and the risk of lymphoma are controversial. A recent study from Iowa found a 31% risk reduction for women with a higher intake of fruit and vegetables (Thompson et al., 2010). However, an earlier cohort study did not corroborate this finding (Zhang et al., 2000). NHL appears to be associated with obesity with one meta-analysis showing a relative risk of 1.4 for diffuse large B-cell NHL amongst individuals with a BMI $\geq$ 30 kg/m^2 (Larsson and Wolk, 2007).

3.3 Hodgkin's lymphoma

Hodgkin's lymphoma represents 15% of all lymphomas and accounts for only 0.6% of all cancers diagnosed in the United Kingdom (Cancer-Research-UK, 2011). The age standardised incidence in 2007 was 2.6 per 100,000 population in the UK and 2.8 per 100,000 in the USA (Altekruse et al., 2010) (see Figure 2B). In the UK, age-specific peaks in incidence occur in early adult life (for men at 30 to 34 years and women at 20 to 24 years old) and in later life (over 70 years). Unlike NHL, the incidence of Hodgkin's lymphoma seems to have fallen in the 1970s and has plateaued since the 1980s (see Figure 2D). This may be explained by changes in classification of different types of lymphoma. With treatment, prognosis for Hodgkin's lymphoma is good with around 78% of patients with HL diagnosed in 2007 in the UK predicted to survive for at least 10 years according to calculations by Cancer Research UK. The overall age-standardised survival rate for patients diagnosed with HL in England between 1996 and 1999 was 80% (Coleman, 1999). The Nodular Sclerosis subtype of classical HL is the commonest occurring in 60% of cases and is associated with younger age and more affluent populations.

Many of the risk factors for Hodgkin's lymphoma are similar to those of NHL but certain factors may be more important in the development of HL:

- **Genetic susceptibility** – a family history of Hodgkin's lymphoma appears to have a much more dramatic effect on risk when compared to NHL. Monozygotic twin studies suggest a 99-fold increased risk (Mack et al., 1995) and a first degree relative diagnosed with any haematological malignancy confers a two to three-fold increased risk (Chang et al., 2005, Goldin et al., 2004). Studies from the USA suggest racial differences in susceptibility with lower risk in blacks than whites (Glaser, 1991).

- **Epstein-Barr virus** – EBV infection has long been implicated in the development of Hodgkin's lymphoma. EBV DNA can be found in 40% of cases with higher rates of association found in the paediatric population (Jarrett et al., 1996). EBV positivity is more commonly found in the Mixed Cellularity than the Nodular Sclerosis subtypes of classical HL. A previous history of infectious mononucleosis confers an increased risk of HL with an SIR of 3.49 in patients aged 15 to 34 years (Hjalgrim et al., 2000).
- **Previous non-Hodgkin's lymphoma** – Studies suggest that patients who have previously been treated for NHL are at increased risk of subsequently developing HL with a magnitude in the order of four- to twelve-fold (Travis et al., 1991, Travis et al., 1993).

4. Pathogenesis of lymphoma in IBD

Lymphoma is a clonal expansion of B- and T- lymphocytes caused by the accumulation of a series of genetic mutations affecting proto-oncogenes and tumour suppressor genes. This results in dysregulated proliferation, evasion of immune surveillance mechanisms and inhibition of apoptosis (Jaffe et al., 2001). Significant progress has been made in to the understanding of these mechanisms at a molecular level. The activation of oncogenes by aberrant chromosomal translocations as well as the inactivation of tumour suppressor genes by chromosomal deletion or mutation are both important mechanisms of lymphomagenesis (Kuppers et al., 1999). Oncogenic viruses such as EBV and HTLV1 can also introduce foreign genetic sequences into the lymphocyte genome causing disruption of normal function (Neri et al., 1991).

There are a number of genetic, environmental, infectious and iatrogenic factors amongst patients with inflammatory bowel disease which can predispose to increased susceptibility to these mechanisms for the development of lymphoma:

- **Chronic inflammation** – The pathogenesis of IBD is not completely understood but aberrations in the innate and adaptive immune response to luminal antigens has been the focus of much research. It can be postulated that the dysregulation of these immune systems seen in the chronic inflammation associated with IBD may lead to antigen-driven lymphocyte proliferation and a relatively unhindered risk of genetic and chromosomal deviations (Sokol and Beaugerie, 2009). Another possibility is that the combination of metabolites, cytokines and chemokines seen in the mucosa of IBD patients promotes mutagenesis in bystander cells. These theories may help to explain the increased risk of lymphoma seen in a variety of different auto-immune conditions and their concordance to sites of inflammation (Smedby et al., 2006). EBV related lymphoma has been reported in longstanding pyothorax of over 20 years duration (Aozasa et al., 2005). This is a condition which is regarded to be due to chronic suppuration with no autoimmunity and it is suggested that any chronic inflammatory state may predispose to lymphoma development.
- **Genetic susceptibility** – Linkage studies and genome wide association studies have identified a large array of susceptibility genes for IBD (Barrett et al., 2008). These genetic changes may also be involved in the pathogenesis of lymphoma in certain individuals. For example, the first susceptibility gene identified, IBD1, encodes for the protein

NOD1 which in its wild-type activates nuclear factor kappa B (NF-κB) (Ogura et al., 2001). NF-κB is a tightly regulated mediator of T- and B-lymphocytes and alterations in its signalling pathway have been implicated in a number of malignancies including lymphoma (Jost and Ruland, 2007). Although some plausibility exists, this link remains to be established.

- **Therapeutic immune modulation** – Immunomodulatory drugs such as the thiopurines, (azathioprine and mercaptopurine), methotrexate, and the anti-TNF drugs (infliximab, adalimumab and certolizumab) have become standard treatment for complicated IBD. These drugs exert their effects through a number of mechanisms which are incompletely understood. It is recognised that AZA and its metabolites suppress intracellular inosinic acid synthesis which interferes with intracellular purine synthesis resulting in a down regulation of B- and T-cell proliferation (Bacon and Salmon, 1987). Thiopurine nucleotides also incorporate into lymphocyte DNA disrupting structure, repair mechanisms and promoting mutagenesis (Ling et al., 1992). There is also evidence that azathioprine renders DNA highly sensitive to damage to ultraviolet (UVA) radiation and this may account for the increased risk of non-melanomatous skin cancer in patients treated with thiopurines (O'Donovan et al., 2005). A recent study showed that IBD patients on thiopurine therapy had significantly more somatic mutations in circulating T-lymphocytes than in a thiopurine-naïve control group (Nguyen et al., 2009).

  The impact of anti-TNF drugs on the risk of mutagenesis has not been adequately studied. It is conceivable that interruption of TNF signalling disrupts immune surveillance mechanisms and alters the normal detection and elimination of cells with chromosomal abnormalities.

  At higher doses, methotrexate is cytotoxic, whereas the lower doses used in IBD patients are known to alter T-cell derived cytokines in inflammatory states. It inhibits pro-inflammatory cytokines such as interleukin-12, interferon-γ and tumour necrosis factor-α whilst promoting anti-inflammatory cytokines such as interleukin-10 (van Dieren et al., 2006). These cytokines have fundamental effects on lymphocyte proliferation and function but the specific mechanisms which may contribute to potential lymphoma development are not known.

- **Immunosuppression** – The increased risk of lymphoma in patients with immunodeficiency states such as HIV infection (Serraino et al., 1992) and post-transplant immunosuppression (Grulich et al., 2007a) is well recognised and many of these cases are EBV positive. The increased risk of opportunistic infections amongst IBD patients on immunomodulators therapy is also well documented. Toruner et al identified 100 cases of opportunistic infections over an 8 year period on their database of IBD patients from the Mayo Clinic and found that treatment with thiopurines conferred an Odds Ratio of 3.1 (Toruner et al., 2008). The majority of these opportunistic infections were caused by viruses including cytomegalovirus, Herpes simplex virus and Epstein-Barr virus.

  EBV is a widely disseminated human Herpes virus which has been associated with a number of different types of B-cell lymphoma, particularly mixed cellularity and lymphocyte depleted classical Hodgkin's lymphoma, Burkitt's lymphoma and post-transplant lymphoproliferative disorder (PTLD). EBV viral load can predict risk of PTLD (Stevens et al., 2001) and cases of infectious mononucleosis with early transformation to lymphoma have been described (Owen et al., 2010). Interestingly,

Wong et al describe a case of synchronous colonic adenocarcinoma and lymphoma and demonstrated that EBV was present in the lymphomatous tissue but not in the invasive adenomatous tissue (Wong et al., 2003). A series of IBD patients from the Mayo clinic identified 12 patients diagnosed with lymphoma between 1993 and 2000, half of whom were on azathioprine therapy. The lymphomas of five out of these six patients on azathioprine were EBV positive whereas only one out of the six azathioprine-naïve patients was EBV positive (Dayharsh et al., 2002). This study suggests a link between azathioprine therapy and EBV driven lymphoma in IBD though the numbers were too small to reach statistical significance. In the CESAME prospective study of over 21,000 French IBD patients, 9 of the 13 cases of lymphoma in patients on azathioprine were EBV positive with up to 16 years exposure to the drug (Beaugerie et al., 2009a). Reijasse et al measured EBV viral loads in patients with Crohn's disease and EBV sero-positive controls. There was no difference in viral loads between the two groups irrespective of immunomodulator or biological therapy but a minority of patients did have transient, very high EBV viral loads (Reijasse et al., 2004). It is not clear, whether these peaks in EBV viral load are associated with lymphoma risk but this does appear to be the case in post-transplant patients where EBV viral load can predict this outcome (Stevens et al., 2001).

The pathobiology of EBV and its role in lymphomagenesis is complex. The host-incorporated EBV genome encodes a number of proteins with similarities to a variety of cytokines, anti-apoptotic molecules and signal transducers that can immortalise and mutate infected cells (Sokol and Beaugerie, 2009).

The risk of other oncogenic viruses such as HLTV1 is not well described in the IBD literature. A recent meta-analysis suggested a lower prevalence of *Helicobacter Pylori* infection in IBD patients compared to control groups but its association with gastric MALT-oma is well documented (Luther et al., 2010).

5. Lymphoma risk in the literature

In order to evaluate any causality between IBD and the risk of lymphoma, it is extremely important to appreciate the quality of safety data available. Frequently, this information is flawed and difficult to interpret.

5.1 Quality of data

Randomised controlled drug trials collate information regarding adverse events but they are powered to elucidate differences in efficacy and not safety. They also tend to have relatively small numbers and a short follow up period which may not reflect the true incidence of late or delayed adverse events. Some useful safety information is available from observational studies of large populations. These have large numbers and long follow up but are susceptible to indication bias and often have other confounding factors. Case controlled series have an efficient methodology but may be hampered by the shortcomings of control selection. The most common form of safety data comes from case reports and case series which are able to identify rare risks. However, the inherent positive bias with this form of evidence, does not allow it to be utilised for risk quantification or for providing proof of causality. Post marketing surveillance, a form of *pharmaco-vigilence*, is another important source of safety data. This information may be made available through institutional reporting schemes, such as the FDA's Adverse Events Recording System (AERS) in the United States (FDA, 2011) or the MHRA's Yellow Card System in the United Kingdom (MHRA, 2011). Important information may come from drug specific data such as the TREAT registry (Lichtenstein et al., 2006), which is an on-going large-scale observational registry that was designed to examine the safety of Crohn's Disease therapies including infliximab. This type of data provides a *real world* experience with a heterogeneous group of patients suffering a variety of co-morbidities and taking concomitant medication. However, such schemes are generally voluntary systems which are prone to under-reporting and hence an under estimation of true incidence.

The low incidence of lymphoma, even in higher risk populations, poses a challenge to evaluating this risk. The incidence of all types of lymphoma diagnosed in the United Kingdom in 2007 was about 17 cases per 100,000 population (Cancer-Research-UK, 2011). A study of almost 3 million individuals would be necessary to detect an adverse event of this frequency with a confidence interval of 95%. No studies of this magnitude are available nor are likely to be available in the future.

5.2 Available data

The literature pertaining to the risk of lymphoma amongst IBD patients is dominated by case reports and case series. However, a number of large population studies have also been published over the last three decades which have been extremely valuable because they allow approximation of the risk of lymphoma (Loftus et al., 2000, Lewis et al., 2001, Beaugerie et al., 2009a, Greenstein et al., 1985). This information must be considered within the limitations of this type of study. A small number of meta-analyses have attempted to combine information from these population-based studies (Kandiel et al., 2005, Siegel et al., 2009). Post-marketing surveillance for drugs such as azathioprine, mercaptopurine and methotrexate are not available but some data regarding the newer anti-TNF therapies in IBD now exists (Lichtenstein et al., 2006).

Interest in the risk of developing lymphoma in the context of IBD and its treatment has grown exponentially (see Figure 3). This coincides with increasing use of immunomodulators in the management of IBD and concerns over their safety. Prior to the 1990s, only sporadic case reports and case series were available. More recently, a number of population based studies, review articles and meta-analyses have been published which are discussed in this report.

Additionally, changes in the classification of lymphoid neoplasia makes evaluation of the literature difficult in certain circumstances where there are overlapping features between diagnoses (Swerdlow et al., 2008).

6. Presentation of lymphoma in IBD

The presentation of lymphoma amongst IBD patients is very heterogenous and occurs in both Crohn's disease and ulcerative colitis.

There are abundant reports of lymphoma of the gastro-intestinal tract mimicking presentations of Crohn's disease (Kashi et al., 2010, Kang et al., 2007, Hurlstone, 2002, Jouini et al., 2001, Vincenzi et al., 2001, Camera et al., 1997, Maaravi et al., 1993, Scully et al., 1993,

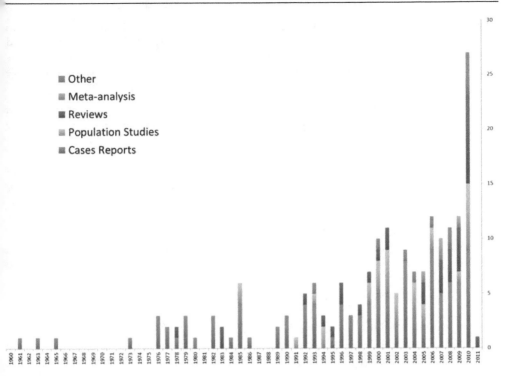

Fig. 3. Medline cited publications regarding lymphoma risk in IBD patients since 1950.

McCullough et al., 1992, Pohl et al., 1991, Bartram and Chrispin, 1973) and ulcerative colitis (Isomoto et al., 2003, Luo et al., 1997, Wagonfeld et al., 1976, Myerson et al., 1974, Parnes et al., 1974, Friedman et al., 1968, Federman et al., 1963). Clearly, lymphoma of the GI tract frequently occurs in the absence of inflammatory bowel disease. In a series from the Mayo Clinic spanning 40 years in the pre-biologic era, of the 2,332 cases of primary intestinal lymphoma identified, only 15 patients had concomitant inflammatory bowel disease (Holubar et al., 2010). These cases are not discussed further here.

6.1 Intestinal and extra-intestinal lymphoma

Lymphoma may present at a variety of sites amongst IBD patient but these can broadly be classified as intestinal and extra-intestinal.

Up to 15% of extra-nodal lymphoma involves the GI tract (Newton et al., 1997). In a series of 15 cases of intestinal lymphoma, 60% were colorectal, 27% involved the small bowel and there were individual cases in the stomach, duodenum and ileal pouch, each constituting 6.25% of this series (Holubar et al., 2010). In 80% of these cases, the location of the lymphoma was congruous to the site of IBD. In another series of 14 colorectal lymphomas, the commonest sites were the caecum and rectosigmoid but these were not IBD patients (Wong and Eu, 2006). Gastric mantle cell lymphoma has also been reported by Raderer et al in a patient with a 14 year history of Crohn's disease (Raderer et al., 2004). Ileal pouch lymphoma has also been reported in a number of other publications (Sengul et al., 2008,

Frizzi et al., 2000, Nyam et al., 1997) and one publication suggests EBV may be involved in the aetiology (Schwartz et al., 2006). Lymphoma at an ileostomy site has also been reported (Pranesh, 2002). Metachronous colonic lymphoma (Hill et al., 1993) as well as synchronous colonic adenocarcinoma and lymphoma (Hope-Ross et al., 1985, Nishigami et al., 2010) have been described in IBD patients.

In addition, a number of extra-intestinal sites of lymphoma amongst IBD patients have been reported. Hepatosplenic T-cell lymphoma (HSTCL) has become a concern amongst IBD physicians and this will be discussed in further detail. Owen et al reports a patient with UC treated with azathioprine who develops a B-cell lymphoproliferative disorder on her eyelid following a recent illness diagnosed as infectious mononucleosis (Owen et al., 2010). Deneau et al recently described the case of a child with an EBV-driven NK-cell lymphoma involving the skin and GI tract causing hepatosplenomegaly (Deneau et al., 2010). Other cutaneous lymphomas are described in the literature (Adams et al., 2004, Martinez Tirado et al., 2001). Vulval and peri-anal lymphoma has also been identified (Winnicki et al., 2009, Sivarajasingham et al., 2003). Kastner et al present a young lady with ulcerative colitis, previously treated with azathioprine, who presents with seizures and is found to have cerebral lesions of high grade B cell lymphoma (Kastner et al., 2007). Plamacytoma (a mature B-cell lymphoma) can present as a paravertebral mass (Redmond et al., 2007).

6.2 Clinical presentation

Many of the symptoms of intestinal lymphoma are very similar to those caused by inflammatory bowel disease. The most commonly presenting symptom is bloody diarrhoea occurring in almost three quarters of cases (Holubar et al., 2010, Wong and Eu, 2006). Other common symptoms include abdominal pain, weight loss and sweats. Presentation with bowel obstruction and perforation occurs less frequently (Holubar et al., 2010, Bourikas et al., 2008). Diagnosis of lymphoma is frequently made following laparotomy. Endoscopic appearances can be diverse, manifesting as ulceration, polyps or masses.

Duration of IBD before development of lymphoma appears to be very variable between individual cases. Shepherd et al reported 10 cases of colorectal lymphoma complicating inflammatory bowel disease (6 patients with UC and 4 with CD) (Shepherd et al., 1989). The duration of inflammatory bowel disease varied from 30 months to 20 years in these cases. In the CESAME study, there was between 1 to 16 years of exposure to thiopurines before lymphoma diagnosis (Beaugerie et al., 2009a).

More unusual presentations of lymphoma include jaundice due to a nodal mass at the porta hepatis in a patient with Crohn's disease (Parasher et al., 1999), spontaneous tumour lysis syndrome in a Crohn's patient with a plasmacytoma (Froilan Torres et al., 2009), nephrotic syndrome in a patient with Hodgkin's lymphoma and UC (Basic-Jukic et al., 2002), and jaundice due to vanishing bile duct syndrome in a patient with Hodgkin's lymphoma and IBD (DeBenedet et al., 2008).

7. Population and cohort studies

A number of population and cohort studies have been published and are described below. The standardised incidence ratio (SIR) is defined as the ratio between observed and expected events in a study population. This is a useful comparator to analyse the risk of lymphoma in IBD patients and has been used in much of the literature.

Incidence and Risk Factors for Lymphoma in a Single-Center Inflammatory Bowel Disease Population (Chiorean et al 2010)

A cohort study identified 3,585 patients attending a single IBD centre in Indianapolis, USA. Data was collected retrospectively between 1990 and 2005. Since 2005, the registry was updated prospectively. An electronic database was interrogated for diagnoses of Hodgkin's and non-Hodgkin's lymphoma and compared to expected age-standardised incident rates from the SEER registry. This study also used a case matched control group with a ratio of 1:10 to determine risk factors for lymphoma development. The population consisted of 2,277 Crohn's patients and 1,308 UC patients with no significant demographic differences between groups. 8 patients were identified with a diagnosis of lymphoma (6 NHL and 2 HL). Only 3 patients had thiopurine exposure but 2 of these patients had also received TNF antagonists and were EBV positive. The study did not find any statistically significant relationship between diagnosis of lymphoma with demographics, drug therapy, duration of treatment and length of diagnosis. Based on SEER statistics, the overall SIR for lymphoma was 1.6 (95% CI 0.6 to 3.0) but this was not significant. (Chiorean et al., 2010)

Risk of Cancer in Inflammatory Bowel Disease Treated with Azathioprine: A UK Population-Based Case-Control Study (Armstrong et al 2010)

This was a nested case-control study using the General Practice Research Database (GPRD) in the UK which was interrogated for patients with a diagnosis of IBD, any previous prescriptions for azathioprine or mercaptopurine and a subsequent diagnosis of any cancer. The GPRD is the largest longitudinal primary care database in the world containing approximately 50 million patient years of data. The control group consisted of all IBD patients who had not been diagnosed with a cancer. The total number of patients included in the study was 15,471 and 15 patients had diagnoses of lymphoma (2 HL, 6 NHL and 7 unspecified). The group found the risk of lymphoma for patients who had ever received thiopurines versus those that had never received such drugs was increased by an OR of 3.22 (95% CI 1.01 to 10.18). An SIR was not calculated for the risk of lymphoma compared to the background population in this study. (Armstrong et al., 2010)

Lymphoproliferative Disorders in an Inflammatory Bowel Disease Unit (Van Domselaar et al 2010)

This was a retrospective study of 911 patients attending a tertiary IBD clinic in Madrid followed up for a mean of 32.3 months. There were 7 cases of lymphoma identified in the cohort (6 NHL and 1 HL). The mean age at diagnosis was 53 years and the mean time from IBD to lymphoma diagnosis was 4.82 years (range 0 to 20 years). Three cases were associated with EBV. An SIR of 3.72 can be calculated from the figures presented though this was not calculated by the authors. (Van Domselaar et al., 2010)

Risk of Malignant Lymphoma in Patients with Inflammatory Bowel Diseases: A Dutch Nationwide Study (Vos et al)

The authors identified all IBD patients diagnosed with lymphoma between 1997 and 2004 from a Dutch nationwide histo- and cyto-pathology database known as PALGA. Age adjusted incidence of lymphoma was obtained from the Netherlands Central Bureau for

Statistics between these years. After excluding incomplete data, 44 cases of lymphoma were identified in 17,834 IBD patients. The calculated SIR was 1.27 (95% CI 0.92 to 1.68) and the authors concluded that there was no increased risk of lymphoma in IBD patients. However, the SIRs in the age groups 35-39 years and 45-49 years were 9.32 and 3.99 respectively and these did reach significance. Only 43% of patients were exposed to thiopurines. Of the patients in whom EBV status could be obtained, 92% (11/12) with EBV positive lymphoma were taking a thiopurine compared to 19% (4/21) who were EBV negative (p<0.001). (Vos et al., 2010)

Lymphoproliferative Disorders in Patients Receiving Thiopurines for Inflammatory Bowel Disease: A Prospective Observational Cohort Study (Beaugerie et al 2009)

This is a frequently quoted study which set out to objectively clarify the risk of cancer in IBD patients. 19,486 patients were enrolled into a prospective French nationwide database called CESAME (Cancers et Surrisque Associé aux Maladies inflammatoires intestinales En France) between May 2004 and June 2005 and followed up until 31st December 2007. This equated to almost 50,000 patient-years of follow up. Details regarding patient demographics, type of IBD, date of diagnosis, disease location, history of malignancy and exposure to immunosuppressive therapy including thiopurines, methotrexate and anti-TNF agents were collected. A total of 23 patients were identified who developed lymphoma (22 NHL, 1 HL). The SIR is not presented in this study but later discussed in a review article by the same author at 1.86 (95% CI 1.1 to 3.0) (Sokol and Beaugerie, 2009). The HR for patients taking AZA versus those who were not was 5.28 (95% CI 2.01 to 13.9). There was a trend towards increased risk of lymphoma with anti-TNF therapy but this did not reach statistical significance. No patients taking methotrexate developed lymphoma in this study. (Beaugerie et al., 2009a)

Risk of Haematopoietic Cancer in Patients with Inflammatory Bowel Disease (Askling et al 2005)

This was a huge population based cohort study using prospectively recorded data from a number of large Swedish IBD databases (Uppsala cohort, Stockholm County cohort, Stockholm pan-colitis register and Swedish in-patient register). 47, 679 patients were recruited in total and 180 lymphomas were detected. Compared to national Swedish cancer statistics, the calculated SIR was 1.09 in this study. (Askling et al., 2005)

Intestinal and Extra-Intestinal Cancer in Crohn's Disease: Follow-up of a Population-based Cohort in Copenhagen, Denmark (Jess et al 2004)

374 patients with a diagnosis of Crohn's disease were followed up for a median of 17 years in Copenhagen County. No lymphomas were observed in this population. (Jess et al., 2004)

Long-term Risk of Cancer in Ulcerative Colitis : A Population-based Cohort Study from Copenhagen County (Winther et al 2004)

This study is from the same cohort of patients investigated in the above study by Jess et al. In the sample of 1160 UC patients, the median follow up was 19 years. A total of 124 malignancies were observed including only 1 lymphoma. The SIR for lymphoma risk works out at 0.5 (95% CI 0.1 to 0.8) in this study. This suggests a protective role of UC in lymphomagenesis which is not demonstrated in any other studies. This result is likely to be artefactual due to the finding of only 1 case of lymphoma in the study. (Winther et al., 2004)

Inflammatory Bowel Disease is not Associated with an Increased Risk of Lymphoma (Lewis et al 2001)

This is an important large retrospective cohort study utilising the General Practice Research Database that was also used by Armstrong et al above. All patients coded with a diagnosis of UC or CD were eligible for inclusion and cross-matched for a diagnosis of HL and NHL. Prescriptions for AZA and 6MP were also analysed and an average dose per day was calculated. A control cohort was randomly selected but matched for age, sex and primary care practice. The study identified 6,605 patients with CD, 10,391 patients with UC and there were 60,506 patients in the control group. 18 patients were identified with lymphoma in this cohort compared with an expected 13.6 cases and an SIR of 1.32 (95% CI 0.78 to 2.10). The relative risk compared to the control group was 1.20 (96% CI 0.67 to 2.06). The authors concluded that IBD was not associated with an increased risk of lymphoma. Even on sub-analysis of patients prescribed thiopurines, there was no significant increased risk of lymphoma. (Lewis et al., 2001)

Cancer Risk in Patients with Inflammatory Bowel Disease – A Population-based Study (Bernstein et al 2001)

Population-based data was obtained from the University of Manitoba IBD database which was extracted from the Manitoba Health administrative databases in Winnipeg, Canada. An age and gender matched non-IBD control group was randomly selected with a ratio of 1:10. 5,529 patients were included in the study and the overall incidence of cancer was 690.2 per 100,000 population. 16 cases of NHL were identified but no cases of HL. This study found an incident rate ratio of 1.59 (95% CI 0.6 to 3.3) for the risk of lymphoma. The risk of developing lymphoma was highest in male patients with Crohn's disease where the IRR was calculated at 3.63 (95% CI 1.53 to 8.62). (Bernstein et al., 2001)

The Incidence of Lymphoid and Myeloid Malignancies Among Hospitalized Crohn's Disease Patients (Arseneau et al 2001)

This was a retrospective cohort study. Discharge data for all in-patients in the Commonwealth of Virginia and the State of California was analysed to identify patients who were admitted to hospital with a diagnosis code for Crohn's disease. These patients were then followed up for 2 years examining for new diagnostic codes for lymphoma. The patients were matched with a control group who had admissions to hospital over the same period with no history of CD. 5,426 patients were discharged from hospital in the study period with a diagnosis of CD. 10 cases of NHL were identified and an OR of 2.04 (95% CI 1.33 to 3.14) was calculated. (Arseneau et al., 2001)

Hodgkin's Disease Risk is Increased in Patients with Ulcerative Colitis (Palli et al 2000)

This is a population based study of all patients with IBD residing in Florence, Italy between 1978 and 1992. A total of 920 patients were followed up for a median of 11 years. An increased risk of Hodgkin's disease was observed in patients with UC with 6 cases identified and an SIR calculated at 9.3 (95% CI 2.5 to 23.8). The broad confidence interval makes it difficult to assess the validity of these findings in this study. (Palli et al., 2000)

Risk of Lymphoma in Inflammatory Bowel Disease (Loftus et al 2000)

This was a retrospective study of all incidence cases of IBD in Olmsted County, Minnesota between 1950 and 1993 examined for the diagnosis of lymphoma. The authors comment that the use of immunomodulators during this time frame was rare and hoped to be able to demonstrate the baseline risk of lymphoma in IBD patients. Expected cases of lymphoma were derived from published Olmsted County age-standardised incidence rates. 454 patients were diagnosed with IBD in the study period. Only 1 case of NHL was identified in the entire cohort and an SIR of 1.0 (95% CI 0.03 to 5.6) was calculated. The observed number of patients with lymphoma is so small in this study that the results are very difficult to interpret. (Loftus et al., 2000)

Increased Incidence of non-Hodgkin's Lymphoma in Inflammatory Bowel Disease Patients on Immunosuppressive Therapy but Overall Risk is Low (Farrell et al 2000)

This study interrogated an IBD database of 782 IBD patients in Dublin. 30% of patients were taking immunomodulators therapy with the majority on azathioprine. A total of 30 cancers were identified with 4 cases of NHL compared with the expected 0.53 cases. These figures produced an SIR of 31.2 (95% CI 2.0 to 85.0). All these patients were on immunosuppressive therapy (2 on MTX and 2 on AZA). Calculating an SIR for patients on immunosuppressive therapy, the authors found a 58.8 –fold increased risk. These rather alarming results have not been duplicated. The confidence intervals are very broad and difficult to interpret. A possible explanation for these outlying results is that this retrospective study was initiated shortly after two new cases of lymphoma had been identified in this cohort. This clustering of cases may have had a significant impact on risk calculations. (Farrell et al., 2000)

Increased Risk of Cancer in Ulcerative Colitis: A Population-based Cohort Study (Karlén et al 1999)

A cohort of 1547 patients with UC in Stockholm County diagnosed between 1955 and 1984 were followed on the National Cancer Register and the National Cause of Death Register until 1989. Comparisons were made with regional cancer statistics. 3 lymphomas were identified in the cohort with an SIR of 1.2 (95% CI 0.3 to 2.5). (Karlen et al., 1999)

Long-term Neoplasia Risk after Azathioprine Treatment in Inflammatory Bowel Disease (Connell et al 1994)

This study from St Mark's Hospital in London followed up 755 IBD patients taking azathioprine for a median of 12.5 months. The overall risk of cancer was similar to that of the background population with an SIR of 1.27 but there was an increased risk of colorectal malignancy with an SIR of 6.7. No cases of lymphoma were identified in this cohort. (Connell et al., 1994)

Crohn's Disease and Cancer: A Population-based Cohort Study (Persson et al 1994)

This study was performed by the same group and used similar methodology to the Karlén study from Stockholm described above. 1251 patients with Crohn's disease were followed up. There was an increased incidence of small bowel and upper GI tract malignancies. 4 cases of lymphoma were identified with an SIR of 1.4 (95% CI 0.4 to 3.5). (Persson et al., 1994)

Extracolonic Malignancies in Inflammatory Bowel Disease (Ekbom et al 1991)

This was a population based cohort with IBD consisting of 4776 patients from the Uppsala Health Care Region in central Sweden. All patients were followed up in the Swedish Cancer Registry and the Registry of Causes of Death for a diagnosis of malignancy. 9 cases of lymphoma were found in this cohort with an expected 8.9 cases. The SIR was 1.0 (95% CI 0.5 to 1.6). (Ekbom et al., 1991)

Extraintestinal Cancers in Inflammatory Bowel Disease (Greenstein et al 1985)

This was a retrospective case note review of patients with a diagnosis of IBD at the Mount Sinai Hospital, New York. 1961 patients were studied with a total of 8 lymphomas (6 NHL and 2 HL). The expected frequency of lymphoma expected was 1.67 giving an SIR of 4.79. (Greenstein et al., 1985)

8. Baseline risk of lymphoma in IBD

An estimate of the baseline lymphoma risk has been made for this chapter using a meta-analysis technique. Populations and cohort studies were identified using the MEDLINE database provided by the US National Library of Medicine (NLM). Statistical analysis was carried out using the Review Manager (RevMan) Version 5 software which is provided by The Cochrane Collaboration, Copenhagen, for preparing and maintaining Cochrane reviews and meta-analyses. Dichotomous data was entered and analysed using the Mantel-Haentszel statistical technique and a 95% confidence interval assuming a Poisson distribution of lymphoma incidence. Studies were only weighted by their size. Graphical representation of results is performed with a Forest plot indicating 95% confidence intervals.

A total of 145,208 patients from 16 trials were included in the meta-analysis (see Figure 4). This produced a cumulative Risk Ratio of 1.29 (95% CI of 1.10 to 1.51, p=0.002). However, this included hospital-based and specialist clinic cohorts which can introduce selection bias. The meta-analysis was repeated only including the 12 population-based studies (see Figure 5). 133,463 patients were included. This did not have a very large effect on the results and the Risk Ratio falls slightly to 1.23 (95% CI 1.05 to 1.45, p=0.01). In both analyses, the test for heterogeneity was not significant and the test for overall effect was 3.15 and 2.52 respectively.

Study or Subgroup	Observed Events	Total	Expected Events	Total	Weight	Risk Ratio M-H, Fixed, 95% CI	Year	Risk Ratio M-H, Fixed, 95% CI
Greenstein et al 1985	8	1961	2	1961	0.7%	4.00 [0.85, 18.81]	1985	
Ekbom et al 1991	9	4776	9	4776	3.3%	1.00 [0.40, 2.52]	1991	
Persson et al 1994	4	1251	3	1251	1.1%	1.33 [0.30, 5.95]	1994	
Karlen et al 1999	3	1547	3	1547	1.1%	1.00 [0.20, 4.95]	1999	
Farrell et al 2000	4	782	0	782	0.2%	9.00 [0.49, 166.88]	2000	
Loftus et al 2000	1	454	1	454	0.4%	1.00 [0.06, 15.94]	2000	
Arseneau et al 2001	10	5426	5	5426	1.8%	2.00 [0.68, 5.85]	2001	
Bernstein et al 2001	16	5529	10	5529	3.7%	1.60 [0.73, 3.52]	2001	
Lewis et al 2001	18	16996	14	16996	5.1%	1.29 [0.64, 2.58]	2001	
Winther et al 2004	1	1160	2	1160	0.7%	0.50 [0.05, 5.51]	2004	
Askling et al 2005	180	47679	166	47679	60.9%	1.08 [0.88, 1.34]	2005	
Beaugerie et al 2009	23	19846	12	19486	4.4%	1.88 [0.94, 3.78]	2009	
Armstrong et al 2010	15	15471	3	15471	1.1%	5.00 [1.45, 17.27]	2010	
Chiorean et al 2010	8	3585	5	3585	1.8%	1.60 [0.52, 4.89]	2010	
Vos et al 2010	44	17834	35	17834	12.8%	1.26 [0.81, 1.96]	2010	
Von Domselaar et al 2010	7	911	2	911	0.7%	3.50 [0.73, 16.80]	2010	
Total (95% CI)		145208		144848	100.0%	1.29 [1.10, 1.51]		
Total events	351		272					
Heterogeneity: Chi² = 15.74, df = 15 (P = 0.40); I² = 5%								
Test for overall effect: Z = 3.15 (P = 0.002)								

Fig. 4. Meta-analysis of population and cohort studies to evaluate the baseline risk of lymphoma.

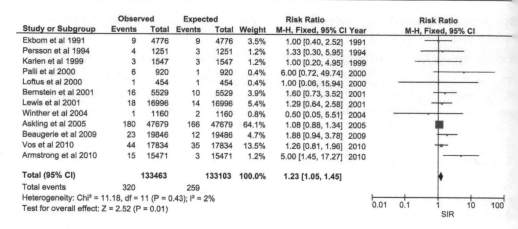

Fig. 5. Meta-analysis of population studies only to evaluate risk of lymphoma.

These findings would suggest that there is only a small (if any) increased risk of lymphoma in IBD patients compared to the general population.

9. Risk of lymphoma with thiopurines

The risk of lymphoma in patients treated with thiopurines has been analysed by including all cohort and population-based studies (see Figure 6). There were 35805 patients included from 7 studies. The test for heterogeneity was not significant and the test for overall effect was 4.03. Overall Risk Ratio is calculated at 3.54 (95% CI 1.91 to 6.54, p<0.0001) confirming the suspected increased risk of lymphoma in patients treated with azathioprine or mercaptopurine.

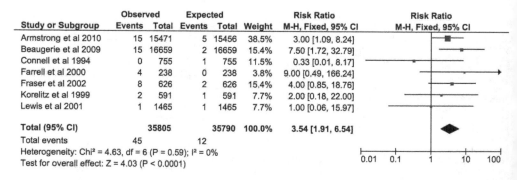

Fig. 6. Meta-analysis to evaluate the risk of lymphoma in patients treated with thiopurines.

10. Comparison to other published meta-analyses

Only three meta-analyses have investigated the background risk and the thiopurine-associated risk of lymphoma in IBD patients. Results from Von Roon et al and Kandiel et al support the findings of the meta-analyses produced here but the work by Masunaga et al shows some disparity.

The Risk of Cancer in Patients with Crohn's Disease (Von Roon et al 2007)

Meta-analytical techniques were used to quantify the risk of intestinal, extra-intestinal and haemopoietic malignancies in Crohn's patients. 34 studies were included with a total of 61,122 patients. Overall pooled estimates were obtained using a random-effects model. The relative risk of lymphoma was 1.42 (95% CI 1.16 to 1.73). This publication, similar to the meta-analysis presented in this dissertation, suggests only a slight increased baseline risk of lymphoma compared to the general population. (von Roon et al., 2007)

Increased Risk of Lymphoma among Inflammatory Bowel Disease Patients Treated with Azathioprine and 6-Mercaptopurine (Kandiel et al 2005)

This meta-analysis sought to provide an estimate of the relative risk of lymphoma among IBD patients treated with thiopurine therapy. Inclusion criteria were strict with only cohort studies in the English language, where the exposed group had received AZA or 6MP and the study had been specifically designed to evaluate the risk of cancer. 6 studies were included with a total of 3891 IBD patients. Similar methodology was used to the presented meta-analysis in this dissertation. Results were also pooled using a Mantzel-Haenszel method but weighting was proportioned to the inverse variance rather than the population size.

The pooled data identified 11 cases of lymphoma whilst the expected number of cases was 2.63, resulting in an SIR of 4.18 (95% CI 2.07 to 7.51). This is similar in magnitude to the SIR in the meta-analysis presented here at 3.54. However, Kandiel et al found a significant test of heterogeneity explained by the substantially higher rates of lymphoma in two of the included studies (Farrell et al 2000 and Connell et al 1994). Exclusion of these studies did not produce a large impact on the pooled SIR. (Kandiel et al., 2005)

Meta-Analysis of Risk of Malignancy with Immunosuppressive Drugs in Inflammatory Bowel Disease (Masunaga et al 2007)

This group aimed to compare the risks of developing malignancy in IBD patients receiving immunosuppressants with those who were not. 9 cohort studies met the inclusion criteria. Where a control group for comparison was not available in these studies, Masunaga et al compared incidence of lymphoma with that of the University of Manitoba IBD Database used by Bernstein et al in their population study. The meta-analysis technique calculated a Weighted Mean Difference (WMD) rather than SIR at 0.0 (95% CI -0.8 to 0.7). These results were not significant and the authors concluded that there was no increased risk of lymphoma in IBD patients treated with immunosuppressives. This result seems to deviate from the findings of the larger recent population studies (such as the CESAME study), that of the meta-analysis performed by Kandiel et al and the meta-analysis presented in this dissertation. This may be due to bias introduced by the arbitrary control method used to calculate expected lymphoma rates in control groups in this meta-analysis. (Masunaga et al., 2007)

11. Risk of lymphoma in patients treated with methotrexate

There is virtually no data for the risk of lymphoma in IBD patients taking methotrexate. Only 2 cases of lymphoma associated with MTX treatment for inflammatory bowel disease have been reported in the literature (Farrell et al., 2000). In this study, 31 patients were receiving methotrexate and two of them were subsequently diagnosed with lymphoma. One of these patients had also received cyclosporin A. As discussed earlier, the authors of this study found risk of lymphoma in their IBD cohort to be much higher than is reported elsewhere and this deviation may have resulted from a clustering of lymphoma diagnosis at the time of investigation. No reliable determination of risk can be obtained from this study.

In the large CESAME study, almost 700 patients (4%) had on-going or previous MTX use but no cases of lymphoma were identified in these patients (Beaugerie et al., 2009a).

Some information can be extrapolated from studies of other inflammatory conditions though this data must be applied with caution in IBD because the risk of the drug cannot be easily separated from the risk of the disease itself. Lymphoma associated with methotrexate has been reported in the rheumatology literature.

A large observational study of rheumatoid arthritis patients treated with methotrexate and/or anti-TNF drugs followed up 18,572 patients biannually found an SIR of 1.7 (95% CI 0.9 to 3.2). The authors concluded that there was no significant increased risk of lymphoma with methotrexate therapy over baseline (Wolfe and Michaud, 2004). A French 3 year prospective population study of RA patients treated with methotrexate identified 18 cases of NHL and 7 cases of HL. Compared to national population statistics, the authors found no increased risk of NHL but a Standardised Mortality Ratio of 7.4 (95% CI 3.0 to 15.3) for HL in their cohort (Mariette et al., 2002).

There are no similar studies in IBD and it is not possible to evaluate a relative or absolute risk of lymphoma with methotrexate therapy. However, it would appear that the risk of lymphoma in this patient group is low.

12. Risk of lymphoma in patients treated with anti-TNF drugs

It is difficult to assess the specific risk of anti-TNF drugs in IBD patients because most patients will have had thiopurine or methotrexate exposure prior to using this modality of treatment. The bulk of the literature regarding anti-TNF drugs is for the use of infliximab in Crohn's disease and little is known regarding differences in safety when used in UC.

A meta-analysis has recently been carried out by Siegel et al with very comprehensive methodology (Siegel et al., 2009). In this meta-analysis, 26 studies with a total of 8905 patients with 21,178 patient-years of exposure to anti-TNF drugs were included (see Table 2). 22 studies were regarding infliximab, 3 regarding adalimumab and only one regarding certolizumab. All the included studies were for the treatment of Crohn's disease through randomised controlled trials, cohort studies and case series. There were 13 cases of NHL with a mean age at presentation of 52 years and 62% male. 10 out of the 13 patients with NHL had received dual therapy with immunomodulators and anti-TNFs. The SIR for the risk of lymphoma in patients treated with anti-TNF drugs was 3.23 (95% CI 1.5 to 6.9) compared to SEER statistics (see Table 3). However, the majority of the lymphoma patients had previously had exposure to immunomodulators and the SIR calculated for anti-TNF therapy should actually be referred to as the risk of combination therapy. This numerical result is in the same order of magnitude as the risk for immunomodulator therapy alone (as calculated by the meta-analysis in this dissertation and other studies). This may suggest that immunomodulator therapy may play the dominant role in lymphoma risk even in settings where combination therapy is used.

Study	Year	Setting	Drug	N	Median f/u (weeks)	NHL cases
Colombel et al	2007	PRECISE RCT	CTZ	905	53	0
Colombel et al	2007	OLE of GAIN and CHARM	ADA	1169	58	0
Sandborn et al	2007	CLASSIC II RCT	ADA	276	56	1
Lemann et al	2006	RCT IXB + AZA	IXB	57	52	0
Schroder et al	2006	Controlled pilot study of IXB + MTX	IXB	19	48	0
Mantzaris et al	2004	RCT IXB + AZA	IXB	45	60	0
Sands et al	2004	IXB for fistulising CD	IXB	282	54	0
Hanauer et al	2002	ACCENT I	IXB	573	54	1
Rutgeerts et al	1999	RCT	IXB	73	48	6
Lichtenstein et al	2007	TREAT registry	IXB	3396	201	0
Biancome et al	2006	Matched pair study	IXB	404	109	1
Doumit et al	2004	Cohort study	IXB	322	104	0
Carbone et al	2007	Case series	IXB	34	52	0
Peyrin-Biroulet et al	2007	Case series for switch to ADA	ADA	52	52	0
Hyder et al	2006	Case series for fistulising CD	IXB	22	91	0
Pacault et al	2006	Case series	IXB	137	150	0
Talbot et al	2005	Case series for perianal CD	IXB	21	87	0
Choi et al	2005	Case series from Korea	IXB	13	57	0
Ardizzone et al	2004	Case series for perianal CD	IXB	20	67	0
Colombel et al	2004	Case series from Mayo Clinic	IXB	500	74	1
Rodrigo et al	2004	Case series for fistulising CD	IXB	44	72	0
Schroder et al	2004	Case series IXBMTX in fistulising CD	IXB	12	57.6	0
Sciderer et al	2004	Cohort study	IXB	92	113	0
Ljung et al	2003	Population-based cohort	IXB	191	52	3
Kinney et al	2003	Case series	IXB	117	52	0
Cohen et al	2000	Case series	IXB	129	52	0

Table 2. Studies included in meta-analysis By Siegel et al 2009. (ADA adalimumab; CTZ certolizumab, MTX methotrexate, AZA azathioprine, CD Crohn's disease, RCT randomised controlled trial, f/u follow up, OLE open label extension).

	NHL rate per 10,000 patient-years	SIR	95% CI
SEER (all ages)	1.9		
IM alone	3.6		
Anti-TNF vs SEER	6.1	3.23	1.5 to 6.9
Anti-TNF vs IM alone	6.1	1.7	0.5 to 7.1

Table 3. Results of meta-analysis by Siegel et al 2009.

The majority of these studies have relatively small numbers of patients, short follow up and were not designed to evaluate efficacy. However, the TREAT registry data includes the largest number of patients and has the longest follow up. The TREAT (Crohn's Therapy, Resource, Evaluation and Assessment Tool) registry is a large prospective, observational, multi-centre, long-term registry of Crohn's disease patients designed to evaluate the safety of infliximab and is a form of post-marketing surveillance. The TREAT registry is hoped to represent *real world* patients without the biases inherent to patients included in trials. No cases of lymphoma were reported in the registry.

The CESAME study data was not included in the meta-analysis by Siegel et al. Beaugerie et al calculated SIRs depending on anti-TNF and thiopurine combination or mono-therapy as well as whether drugs were continued or discontinued (Beaugerie et al., 2009a). These results are presented in Table 4. The results cannot confirm an increased risk of lymphoma in those continuing anti-TNF therapy because the confidence interval crosses 1.0. However, there does appear to be an increased risk when anti-TNF drugs have been used with thiopurines, particularly when combination therapy is continued.

	NHL cases	SIR	95% CI
Continuing anti-TNF therapy	2	4.53	0.55 to 16.4
Discontinued anti-TNF therapy	3	6.92	1.43 to 20.2
Continuing thiopurines and anti-TNF therapy	2	10.2	1.24 to 36.9
Continuing thiopurines but discontinued or never anti-TNFs	13	6.53	3.48 to 11.2

Table 4. SIRs in patients treated with thiopurines and anti-TNF drugs (Beaugerie et al 2009)

13. Hepatosplenic T-cell lymphoma

Hepatosplenic T-cell lymphoma (HSTCL) is a rare form of peripheral non-Hodgkin's lymphoma. In the majority of incidences, it results from a clonal expansion of γ/δ T-cells but α/β T-cell receptors can also be expressed in some cases (Gaulard et al., 1990). Only 100 to 200 cases of HSTCL in the entire medical literature have been reported (Belhadj et al., 2003) but there has been recent concern regarding the safety of thiopurines and anti-TNF therapy, particularly when used in combination, for the management of IBD. To date, 36 cases of HSTCL have been reported in IBD patients (Kotlyar et al., 2011), mostly affecting young men and the prognosis has been invariably fatal. Despite treatment with chemotherapy and stem cell transplantation, median survival is only 11 months (Falchook et al., 2009) but novel treatment strategies have shown some promise in isolated cases (Jaeger et al., 2008, Tey et al., 2008). Diagnosis is made by liver, splenic or bone marrow biopsy exhibiting atypical medium-sized lymphoid cells with round nuclei, small distinct nucleoli, loosely condensed chromatin, moderate pale cytoplasm and particular immunophenotypic expression which will be discussed further (Swerdlow et al., 2008).

13.1 Clinical presentation

The aberrant cells infiltrate into the sinusoids of the spleen, liver and bone marrow resulting in the classical presentation of hepatosplenomegaly with thrombocytopenia but no lymphadenopathy. Systemic B symptoms of fever, night sweats and weight loss may affect up to 80% of patients. Other findings may include anaemia, abnormal liver function tests and less frequently atypical lymphocytes on peripheral blood film (Falchook et al., 2009).

13.2 Immunophenotypic and genetic features

The tumour cells express CD2, surface CD3, CD7 and CD16 but there is absence of CD4, CD5, CD8 and the B-cell surface marker CD20 (Swerdlow et al., 2008). Most cases express the γ/δ T-cell receptor (TCR-γ positive) but rarer cases express the α/β T-cell receptor (TCR-β positive) and studies demonstrate clonal rearrangements of the TCR gene.

A recent systematic review investigating chromosomal abnormalities in IBD patients diagnosed with HSTCL identified the development of isochrome 7q in 57.1%, aberrations of chromosome 8 in 35.7%, trisomy 8 in 21.4% and loss of the Y chromosome in 14.3 % of cases (Kotlyar et al., 2010). The group were intrigued by the cases with loss of the Y chromosome as almost all cases of HSTCL have presented in men. These chromosomal abnormalities are not specific to IBD patients.

13.3 HSTCL in IBD

HSTCL is not linked to EBV infection. However, the risk of HSTCL does seem to be related to thiopurine and anti-TNF therapy. DNA damage specific to chromosome 7 has been seen in a dose dependent manner with thiopurine agents (Piccin et al., 2010) and inhibition of TNF may result in decreased effectiveness of immune surveillance eliminating cells with aberrant abnormal chromosomal pattern (Shale et al., 2008).

Early concern was regarding a risk of HSTCL in IBD patients who had previous exposure to both thiopurines and anti-TNF drugs but more and more cases have been identified with only thiopurine exposure. Anti-TNF drugs are frequently used in non-IBD conditions, such as rheumatoid arthritis, ankylosing spondylitis and psoriasis, but they are rarely used in combination with other immunomodulators. It is interesting that, HSTCL has only been reported in a single non-IBD patient who received adalimumab for rheumatoid arthritis (Shale et al., 2008). Conversely, there are a number of case reports of patients developing HSTCL whilst on immunosuppression in the post-transplant setting (Roelandt et al., 2009, Tey et al., 2008, Steurer et al., 2002) where anti-TNF drugs are not used.

Kotlyar et al recently presented a systematic review investigating medications, duration of therapy and ages of IBD patients diagnosed with HSTCL (Kotlyar et al., 2011). 36 cases of HSTCL have occurred in IBD patients since 1996, all of whom had a history of thiopurine exposure. 20 of these patients also had also received anti-TNF therapy. Four patients had previously received both infliximab and adalimumab and an additional patient had received a third biologic, natalizumab. There were no patients who had received an anti-TNF drug alone. Most patients had received at least 2 years therapy with a thiopurine and of those patients who had received infliximab, the number of previous infusions ranged from 1 to 20 up to 5 years prior to the diagnosis of HSTCL. The age range of patients was 12 to 58 years with a median of 23 years. The majority of patients were under 35 years old and the older patient appears to be an isolated case. Of the 31 patients in whom gender was known, only two were female.

13.4 Clinical application

From the limited information available, HSTCL seems to be linked to previous prolonged thiopurine exposure and the risk may be higher in those who have also received an anti-TNF drug. This seems to compete with conclusions drawn from recent efficacy trials. The SONIC trial found that combination therapy with azathioprine and infliximab reached significantly higher rates of steroid-free clinical remission than either of these drugs as monotherapy for a cohort of naïve patients with moderate to severe Crohn's disease (24.1% vs 34.9% vs 46.2% AZA vs IXB vs AZA+IXB at 50 weeks) (Colombel et al., 2010).

Whilst it is not possible to estimate the relative risk of HSTCL in IBD patients, Kotlyar et al attempted to derive the absolute risk of HSTCL in men using epidemiology data from the US and Europe as well as an estimate of thiopurine use in IBD patients from the French CESAME trial (Beaugerie et al., 2009a, Kotlyar et al., 2010). The group concluded that more than 99.99% of patients in immunomodulatory treatment will not develop HSTCL. Further reassurance comes from the CESAME study in that no cases of HSTCL were found despite analysis of over 50,000 patient-years follow up.

A vigilant approach must be taken when using thiopurines for the treatment of male patients under 35 years. Kotlyar et al recommended careful monitoring in patients who have been on thiopurine treatment for more than 2 years but this may be difficult to put in to practice as no pre-malignant markers have been identified. Decisions between the use of combination or monotherapy must be made in the context of clinical severity of disease and poor prognostic markers for complicated IBD. The risk of HSTCL is extremely low and patients should be made aware of this when making choices regarding their treatment. Highly efficacious therapeutic strategies should not be rejected based entirely on the low risk of HSTCL. Somewhat reassuringly, despite the rapidly increasing number of patients on anti-TNF drugs, exceeding 5 million patient-years exposure, the rate at which new cases of HSTCL have been diagnosed has not changed over the last 15 years.

14. Confounding factors and limitations

There are a number of limitations to the data which has been pooled for the meta-analyses presented in this chapter. There are also confounding factors which are not taken in to account by the source studies.

14.1 Age

Data from the US and UK clearly demonstrates that the incidence of non-Hodgkin's lymphoma, the predominant form of lymphoid neoplasm seen in IBD patients, increases with advancing age (see Figure 2). Most of the studies reviewed in this chapter use age standardised statistics to estimate risk of lymphoma in IBD patients. An earlier meta-analysis carried out by Kandiel et al, found a relative risk for the development of lymphoma in IBD patients treated with thiopurines of 4.18 (95% CI 2.07 to 7.51) which is comparable to the findings of the meta-analysis presented here. The authors went on to calculate the number of patients that would need to be treated for each new diagnosis of lymphoma i.e. the number needed to harm (NNH). Approximating to a relative risk of 4, the NNH varied from 4357 in 20-29 year olds to just 355 in 70-79 year olds (Kandiel et al., 2005). The risk of lymphoma is not uniform across all age groups and this needs to be taken in to account when this information is applied to a clinical setting.

14.2 Gender

Gender also appears to be a further factor when analysing the risk of both Hodgkin's and non-Hodgkin's lymphoma. Although other autoimmune conditions tend to affect more women, the gender difference for IBD is small. Men have an increased risk of lymphoma (see Figure 2 and Figure 3) but the magnitude of the gender difference varies with age and type of lymphoma. In NHL there is only a slight preponderance for males but in HL, the incidence is three times greater in males in certain age groups. As discussed, HSTCL occurs almost exclusively in young men. Many of the studies in this analysis did not separate results for male and female patients but this may have made analysis difficult because of the generally small number of cases of lymphoma detected in these cohorts. Vos et al, in their nationwide Dutch study, calculated SIRs for male and female patients separately but did not find a substantial difference when they took both groups as a whole. However, in the 35-39 years age range, males had an SIR of 10.25 (95% CI 2.56 to 23.05) and females, 6.74 (95% CI 1.20 to 16.77) and this difference was significant (Vos et al., 2010).

14.3 Type of lymphoma

Non-Hodgkin's lymphoma appears to be the predominant lymphoid malignancy detected in IBD patients, particularly diffuse large B-cell lymphoma (DLBCL). The CESAME study group found 22 cases of NHL and only 1 HL in their large cohort of patients from France (Beaugerie et al., 2009a). Few studies have attempted to separate findings for HL and NHL. Palli et al did find an increased risk of HL in patients with UC but the confidence interval was large and the validity of these results has been put in to question (Palli et al., 2000).

14.4 Type of IBD

Whether Crohn's disease or ulcerative colitis confers a higher risk of lymphoma has not been established. Two publications from the same population-based cohort in Copenhagen, Denmark distinguished their analysis between CD and UC patients. In the CD group no lymphomas were identified and only 1 lymphoma was found in the UC group (SIR 0.5) (Winther et al., 2004, Jess et al., 2004). A further population-based cohort from Stockholm, Sweden also analysed UC and CD separately in two different publications. Again no cases of lymphoma were seen in the CD group but there were 3 in the UC group (SIR 1.2) (Persson et al., 1994, Karlen et al., 1999). Interpreting these findings with such small numbers is fraught with difficulty. In the CESAME study, 16 of the 23 lymphomas were in patients with Crohn's disease (Beaugerie et al., 2009a).

14.5 Exposure to immunomodulators

Not all studies have attempted to evaluate the risk of lymphoma associated with immunomodulator therapy. The studies which have attempted to make this estimation are heterogenous and frequently there is a lack of distinction between lifetime exposure to these drugs, the cumulative doses received and whether cessation of a drug returns any lymphoma risk back to baseline. The CESAME study group attempted to answer some of these questions (Beaugerie et al., 2009a) by analysing patients who have *continuing*, *discontinued* or *never received* thiopurines. The SIRs for these three groups were 6.86 (95% CI 3.94 to 11.31), 1.44 (95% CI 0.17 to 5.20) and 1.43 (CI 95% 0.53 to 3.12) respectively. This may suggest that discontinuation of thiopurines returns risk to baseline but the results were not statistically significant.

14.6 Disease severity

It is not clear whether it is the disease itself, its treatment or a combination of the two which might put IBD patients at increased risk of lymphoma. It is possible that the use of drugs such as thiopurines and biologics are a marker of more aggressive disease and it is disease severity which disposes to lymphoma development. However, modern management of IBD has led to earlier use of these drugs, often in patients who do not have severe disease but possess risk factors for complicated disease, in an attempt to alter the natural history of the condition.

Severity of disease as a risk factor for lymphoma has not been analysed in any depth in IBD patients but there is some evidence available from other autoimmune diseases. A study of 378 RA patients diagnosed with lymphoma found no significant association with individual drugs but a marked increased risk with high disease activity which conferred a 70-fold increased risk (Baecklund et al., 2006). The authors concluded that it was the disease activity, not its treatment that was important in lymphomagenesis. In the CESAME study, some data regarding disease activity was collated but was not linked to lymphoma risk (Beaugerie et al., 2009a).

15. Other risk factors for lymphoma development

It is important to recognise a number of other risk factors for lymphoma development which are relevant to the IBD population but have not been well studied yet.

15.1 Pharmacogenomics of thiopurine therapy

Azathioprine is a pro-drug which is metabolised to 6-mercaptopurine and then to a number of further metabolites including 6-thioguanine (6TG) and 6-methylmercaptopurine (6MMP) which are associated with myelo- and hepato-toxicity when they accumulate at high levels. Important enzymes in this pathway include thiopurine methyl transferase (TPMT) and hypoxanthine phosphoribosyltransferase (HPRT). It is recognised that polymorphisms of TPMT can influence TPMT activity and hence levels of 6TG and 6MMP. About 1 in 300 individuals have homozygote TPMT mutations and AZA or 6MP therapy results in very high levels of 6TG causing myelo-toxicity. Those with heterozygote mutations have intermediate TPMT activity and dose adjustment of AZA and 6MP may be required.

Thiopurines are also commonly used drugs for the management of acute lymphoblastic leukaemia (ALL) in paediatric patients. Following treatment, these patients have an increased risk of subsequently developing secondary myelodysplasia or acute myeloid leukaemia but it had been thought that this risk is associated with alkylating agents, epipodophyllotoxins or radiation therapy rather than due to AZA. However, Bo et al showed that paediatric patients with allelic variations of the TPMT gene (and lower TPMT levels) had a higher rate of secondary leukaemias in this setting (Bo et al., 1999). Thiopurines result in the incorporation of 6TG, a purine analogue, into lymphocyte DNA which can activate DNA repair mechanisms. This introduces the risk of point mutations and chromosomal abnormalities during repair processes. It follows that higher levels of 6TG may increase this risk further, possibly explaining the link with lymphomagenesis in IBD patients treated with thiopurines.

Disanti et al made an interesting observation in a cohort of IBD patients treated with 6MP over a 37 year period. The investigators divided the group of over 600 patients in to those who developed a sustained leukopenia of $<4.0 \times 10^9/l$ for 20 or more days and those who did not. They found that there was an increased risk of haematological malignancies in the group with sustained leukopenia (p=0.014) (Disanti et al., 2006).

Although, the TPMT levels were not known in these patients, further investigation in to the association between TPMT and lymphoma risk may be intriguing.

15.2 Radiation exposure

The use of imaging modalities such as computed tomography and fluoroscopy have been an important component for the diagnosis and assessment of IBD but there has been increasing concern regarding the cancer risk associated with diagnostic ionising radiation (Brenner and Hall, 2007). Much of the risk of medical radiation exposure is extrapolated from studies of populations near nuclear explosions and occupational exposure but there is some evidence in certain medical settings (Brenner et al., 2003). For example, young patients with scoliosis who have had repeated chest x-rays were at increased risk of breast malignancy (Doody et al., 2000).

Recent evidence suggests that CT imaging is being used more frequently in IBD patients, particularly those with Crohn's disease (Newnham et al., 2007, Kroeker et al., 2011). Leukaemia is well recognised as a long term consequence of radiation exposure and this risk is higher in children (Darby et al., 1992, Shimizu et al., 1990). However, there is little evidence to confirm an increased risk of lymphoma in patients exposed to diagnostic ionising radiation though the mechanisms of oncogenesis may be similar. There was no increased risk of lymphoma seen in patients receiving radiotherapy for uterine cancer nor amongst tuberculosis patients with repeated pneumothorax who had an average of 77 chest x-rays on follow up (Boice, 1992). A study including 318 NHL patients found no increased exposure to diagnostic radiation compared to controls if imaging from the 12 months immediately prior to lymphoma diagnosis was excluded. The authors felt that radiological procedures within this period were performed to investigate the lymphoma rather than a causative factor (Boice et al., 1991).

15.3 Vitamin D and sunlight exposure

Vitamin D deficiency is common amongst IBD patients. Recent studies have shown suboptimal levels of Vitamin D in 57 to 78% of recently diagnosed patients with IBD (Leslie et al., 2008, Bours et al., 2010). The protective role of Vitamin D has been investigated in a number of malignancies including prostate, colon, lung, pancreatic, endometrial, breast and even skin cancer (Schwartz and Skinner, 2007). The paracrine and autocrine effects of extra-renal 25-hydroxy-Vitamin-D$_3$ via the nuclear Vitamin D Receptor (VDR) include regulation of cell cycle proliferation, induction of apoptosis and increased cell differentiation signalling.

Recent epidemiologic studies demonstrate a reduction in NHL risk with increased sunlight exposure (Armstrong and Kricker, 2007). As sunlight is a major vitamin D source, it has been suggested that vitamin D status may mediate this observed association. A recent review of the literature could not conclude or dismiss a link between vitamin D insufficiency and lymphoma due to confounding findings in a number of studies and the limitations on the accuracy of dietary history taking which was the most frequent methodology in these studies (Kelly et al., 2009).

The role of Vitamin D in lymphomagenesis in the IBD population has not been investigated and warrants further study.

16. Summary of findings and application to clinical practice

This systematic review and the meta-analyses carried out in this chapter have made some key findings:

- There is only a small (if any) increased overall risk of lymphoma in IBD patients.
- Thiopurine therapy results in a 3 to 4-fold increased risk of lymphoma in IBD patients.
- The risk of lymphoma with methotrexate therapy cannot be evaluated adequately but appears to be low.
- Treatment with anti-TNF drugs appears to confer an increased risk of lymphoma in IBD patients. However, this may reflect previous or concurrent immunomodulator exposure rather than the risk of anti-TNFs alone.
- HSTCL is associated with long term thiopurine therapy. Additionally, anti-TNF therapy may increase this risk.

It is the role of the IBD physician to help patients balance up the risks and benefits of these drugs and make the right choice for themselves. Due to the significant morbidity associated with IBD, simply avoiding these drugs is frequently not an option. It is mandatory to provide clear communication of risks and benefits and to individualise this to the patient because lymphoma risk in IBD patients is not uniform nor is the risk of complicated disease. A recent study found that patients were more likely to tolerate the risk of adverse events due to IBD drug therapy for moderately symptomatic Crohn's disease than gastroenterologists would choose for their patients (Johnson et al., 2010).

Patient selection is paramount. The risk of most forms of lymphoma appears to be higher in males and in older age groups. HSTCL is particularly relevant to men under the age of 35 years. Special consideration of the risks must be made in these groups. A number of predictors for severe or complicated disease are now being identified which should allow selection of patients who are most likely to gain from aggressive treatment (Beaugerie et al., 2006).

There is ample evidence that immunomodulators and anti-TNF drugs are very effective for the treatment of IBD. In a 30 year review, Fraser et al found that there were 64% and 87% remission rates at 6 months for patients treated with AZA for Crohn's disease and ulcerative colitis respectively (Fraser et al., 2002). Feagan et al found 65% remission at 40 weeks with MTX for Crohn's disease (Feagan et al., 2000). In the SONIC study, there was 57% remission at 1 year for combined AZA and IXB therapy (Colombel et al., 2010). The CHARM study and its open label extension, ADHERE, for adalimumab in Crohn's disease found improved fistula healing rates, 57% decreased hospitalisation and improved Work Productivity Scores (Panaccione et al., 2010). A Markov model found that the benefits of azathioprine for the treatment of Crohn's disease outweighed the risk of lymphoma but such calculations are inherently based on estimations and assumptions (Lewis et al., 2000).

Additionally, there is evidence that stopping these drugs may be harmful to patients. Azathioprine withdrawal leads to relapse within 18 months at 21% vs 8% (p=0.02, NNH=8) (Lemann et al., 2005). Methotrexate withdrawal leads to relapse within 40 weeks in 61% vs 35% (p=0.04, NNH=4) (Feagan et al., 2000). Infliximab withdrawal leads to hospitalisation within 1 year in 38% vs 23% (p=0.05, NNH=7) (Rutgeerts et al., 2004). However, the CESAME study did suggest that stopping immunomodulator therapy did return the risk of lymphoma back to baseline.

No form of screening is able to predict lymphoma development. Although, the role of vitamin D status and TPMT expression on lymphoma risk is intriguing, there is insufficient evidence to recommend the routine testing of these parameters to guide patient management. Prophylactic use of antivirals in renal transplant recipients has been shown to reduce the risk of post-transplant lymphoproliferative disorders by as much as 83% and the use of this strategy in IBD patients on immunosuppression is warranted (Funch et al., 2005).

The morbidity associated with IBD, the efficacy of these drugs and the risks of stopping them are important factors in making management decisions with patients. In many patients, the benefits will outweigh the risks.

17. References

Adams, A. E., Zwicker, J., Curiel, C., Kadin, M. E., Falchuk, K. R., Drews, R. & Kupper, T. S. 2004. Aggressive cutaneous T-cell lymphomas after TNFalpha blockade. *J Am Acad Dermatol*, 51, 660-2.

Altekruse, S., Kosary, C., Krapcho, M., Neyman, N., Aminou, R., Waldron, W., Ruhl, J., Howlander, N., Tatalovich, Z., Cho, H., Mariotto, A., Eisner, M., Lewis, D., Cronin, K., Chen, H., Feuer, E., Stinchcomb, D. & Edwards, B. 2010. SEER Cancer Statistics Review, 1975-2007. National Cancer Institute.

Altieri, A., Bermejo, J. L. & Hemminki, K. 2005. Familial risk for non-Hodgkin lymphoma and other lymphoproliferative malignancies by histopathologic subtype: the Swedish Family-Cancer Database. *Blood*, 106, 668-72.

Aozasa, K., Takakuwa, T. & Nakatsuka, S. 2005. Pyothorax-associated lymphoma: a lymphoma developing in chronic inflammation. *Adv Anat Pathol*, 12, 324-31.

Ardizzone, S., Maconi, G., Colombo, E., Manzionna, G., Bollani, S. & Bianchi Porro, G. 2004. Perianal fistulae following infliximab treatment: clinical and endosonographic outcome. *Inflamm Bowel Dis*, 10, 91-6.

Armstrong, B. K. & Kricker, A. 2007. Sun exposure and non-Hodgkin lymphoma. *Cancer Epidemiol Biomarkers Prev*, 16, 396-400.

Armstrong, R. G., West, J. & Card, T. R. 2010. Risk of cancer in inflammatory bowel disease treated with azathioprine: a UK population-based case-control study. *Am J Gastroenterol*, 105, 1604-9.

Arseneau, K. O., Stukenborg, G. J., Connors, A. F., Jr. & Cominelli, F. 2001. The incidence of lymphoid and myeloid malignancies among hospitalized Crohn's disease patients. *Inflamm Bowel Dis*, 7, 106-12.

Askling, J., Brandt, L., Lapidus, A., Karlen, P., Bjorkholm, M., Lofberg, R. & Ekbom, A. 2005. Risk of haematopoietic cancer in patients with inflammatory bowel disease. *Gut*, 54, 617-22.

Aydogan, A., Corapcioglu, F., Elemen, E. L., Oncel, S., Gurbuz, Y. & Tugay, M. 2010. Childhood non-Hodgkin's lymphoma arising as a complication early in the course of Crohn's disease. *Turk J Pediatr*, 52, 411-5.

Bacon, P. A. & Salmon, M. 1987. Modes of action of second-line agents. *Scand J Rheumatol Suppl*, 64, 17-24.

Baecklund, E., Iliadou, A., Askling, J., Ekbom, A., Backlin, C., Granath, F., Catrina, A. I., Rosenquist, R., Feltelius, N., Sundstrom, C. & Klareskog, L. 2006. Association of chronic inflammation, not its treatment, with increased lymphoma risk in rheumatoid arthritis. *Arthritis Rheum*, 54, 692-701.

Bargen, J. 1928. Chronic ulcerative colitis associated with malignant disease. *Arch Surg*, 17, 561-576.

Barrett, J. C., Hansoul, S., Nicolae, D. L., Cho, J. H., Duerr, R. H., Rioux, J. D., Brant, S. R., Silverberg, M. S., Taylor, K. D., Barmada, M. M., Bitton, A., Dassopoulos, T., Datta, L. W., Green, T., Griffiths, A. M., Kistner, E. O., Murtha, M. T., Regueiro, M. D., Rotter, J. I., Schumm, L. P., Steinhart, A. H., Targan, S. R., Xavier, R. J., Libioulle, C., Sandor, C., Lathrop, M., Belaiche, J., Dewit, O., Gut, I., Heath, S., Laukens, D., Mni, M., Rutgeerts, P., Van Gossum, A., Zelenika, D., Franchimont, D., Hugot, J. P., De Vos, M., Vermeire, S., Louis, E., Cardon, L. R., Anderson, C. A., Drummond, H., Nimmo, E., Ahmad, T., Prescott, N. J., Onnie, C. M., Fisher, S. A., Marchini, J., Ghori, J., Bumpstead, S., Gwilliam, R., Tremelling, M., Deloukas, P., Mansfield, J., Jewell, D., Satsangi, J., Mathew, C. G., Parkes, M., Georges, M. & Daly, M. J. 2008. Genome-wide association defines more than 30 distinct susceptibility loci for Crohn's disease. *Nat Genet*, 40, 955-62.

Bartram, C. & Chrispin, A. R. 1973. Primary lymphosarcoma of the ileum and caecum. *Pediatr Radiol*, 1, 28-33.

Basic-Jukic, N., Radman, I., Roncevic, T. & Jakic-Razumovic, J. 2002. Hodgkin s disease with nephrotic syndrome as a complication of ulcerative colitis: case report. *Croat Med J*, 43, 573-5.

Beaugerie, L., Brousse, N., Bouvier, A. M., Colombel, J. F., Lemann, M., Cosnes, J., Hebuterne, X., Cortot, A., Bouhnik, Y., Gendre, J. P., Simon, T., Maynadie, M.,

Hermine, O., Faivre, J. & Carrat, F. 2009a. Lymphoproliferative disorders in patients receiving thiopurines for inflammatory bowel disease: a prospective observational cohort study. *Lancet,* 374, 1617-25.

Beaugerie, L., Seksik, P. & Carrat, F. 2009b. Thiopurine therapy is associated with a three-fold decrease in the incidence of advanced neoplaisa in IBD patients with longstanding extensive colitis: the CESAME prospective data. *Journal of Crohn's and Colitis,* 3.

Beaugerie, L., Seksik, P., Nion-Larmurier, I., Gendre, J. P. & Cosnes, J. 2006. Predictors of Crohn's disease. *Gastroenterology,* 130, 650-6.

Beaugerie, L., Sokol, H. & Seksik, P. 2009c. Noncolorectal malignancies in inflammatory bowel disease: more than meets the eye. *Dig Dis,* 27, 375-81.

Belhadj, K., Reyes, F., Farcet, J. P., Tilly, H., Bastard, C., Angonin, R., Deconinck, E., Charlotte, F., Leblond, V., Labouyrie, E., Lederlin, P., Emile, J. F., Delmas-Marsalet, B., Arnulf, B., Zafrani, E. S. & Gaulard, P. 2003. Hepatosplenic gammadelta T-cell lymphoma is a rare clinicopathologic entity with poor outcome: report on a series of 21 patients. *Blood,* 102, 4261-9.

Bernstein, C. N. 2010. Epidemiologic clues to inflammatory bowel disease. *Curr Gastroenterol Rep,* 12, 495-501.

Bernstein, C. N., Blanchard, J. F., Kliewer, E. & Wajda, A. 2001. Cancer risk in patients with inflammatory bowel disease: a population-based study. *Cancer,* 91, 854-62.

Biancone, L., Orlando, A., Kohn, A., Colombo, E., Sostegni, R., Angelucci, E., Rizzello, F., Castiglione, F., Benazzato, L., Papi, C., Meucci, G., Riegler, G., Petruzziello, C., Mocciaro, F., Geremia, A., Calabrese, E., Cottone, M. & Pallone, F. 2006. Infliximab and newly diagnosed neoplasia in Crohn's disease: a multicentre matched pair study. *Gut,* 55, 228-33.

Bo, J., Schroder, H., Kristinsson, J., Madsen, B., Szumlanski, C., Weinshilboum, R., Andersen, J. B. & Schmiegelow, K. 1999. Possible carcinogenic effect of 6-mercaptopurine on bone marrow stem cells: relation to thiopurine metabolism. *Cancer,* 86, 1080-6.

Boice, J. D., Jr. 1992. Radiation and non-Hodgkin's lymphoma. *Cancer Res,* 52, 5489s-5491s.

Boice, J. D., Jr., Morin, M. M., Glass, A. G., Friedman, G. D., Stovall, M., Hoover, R. N. & Fraumeni, J. F., JR. 1991. Diagnostic x-ray procedures and risk of leukemia, lymphoma, and multiple myeloma. *JAMA,* 265, 1290-4.

Bourikas, L. A., Tzardi, M., Hatzidakis, A. & Koutroubakis, I. E. 2008. Small bowel perforation due to non-Hodgkin-lymphoma in a patient with ulcerative colitis and systemic lupus erythematosus. *Dig Liver Dis,* 40, 144.

Bours, P. H., Wielders, J. P., Vermeijden, J. R. & Van De Wiel, A. 2010. Seasonal variation of serum 25-hydroxyvitamin D levels in adult patients with inflammatory bowel disease. *Osteoporos Int.*

Brenner, D. J. & Hall, E. J. 2007. Computed tomography--an increasing source of radiation exposure. *N Engl J Med,* 357, 2277-84.

Brenner, D. J., Doll, R., Goodhead, D. T., Hall, E. J., Land, C. E., Little, J. B., Lubin, J. H., Preston, D. L., Preston, R. J., Puskin, J. S., Ron, E., Sachs, R. K., Samet, J. M., Setlow, R. B. & Zaider, M. 2003. Cancer risks attributable to low doses of ionizing radiation: assessing what we really know. *Proc Natl Acad Sci U S A,* 100, 13761-6.

Camera, L., Della Noce, M. & Cirillo, L. C. 1997. [Primary ileo-cecal lymphoma mimicking Crohn's disease. Report of a case]. *Radiol Med,* 94, 122-4.

Cancer-Research-UK. 2011. *Cancer Research UK* [Online]. Available: http://www.cancerresearchuk.org/.

Carbone, J., Gonzalez-Lara, V., Sarmiento, E., Chean, C., Perez, J. L., Marin, I., Rodriguez-Molina, J. J., Gil, J. & Fernandez-Cruz, E. 2007. Humoral and cellular monitoring to predict the development of infection in Crohn's disease patients beginning treatment with infliximab. *Ann N Y Acad Sci,* 1107, 346-55.

Chandesris, M. O., Malamut, G., Verkarre, V., Meresse, B., Macintyre, E., Delarue, R., Rubio, M. T., Suarez, F., Deau-Fischer, B., Cerf-Bensussan, N., Brousse, N., Cellier, C. & Hermine, O. 2010. Enteropathy-associated T-cell lymphoma: a review on clinical presentation, diagnosis, therapeutic strategies and perspectives. *Gastroenterol Clin Biol,* 34, 590-605.

Chang, E. T., Smedby, K. E., Hjalgrim, H., Porwit-Macdonald, A., Roos, G., Glimelius, B. & Adami, H. O. 2005. Family history of hematopoietic malignancy and risk of lymphoma. *J Natl Cancer Inst,* 97, 1466-74.

Chiorean, M. V., Pokhrel, B., Adabala, J., Helper, D. J., Johnson, C. S. & Juliar, B. 2010. Incidence and Risk Factors for Lymphoma in a Single-Center Inflammatory Bowel Disease Population. *Dig Dis Sci.*

Cho, J. H. 2008. The genetics and immunopathogenesis of inflammatory bowel disease. *Nat Rev Immunol,* 8, 458-66.

Cohen, R. D. 2001. Efficacy and safety of repeated infliximab infusions for Crohn's disease: 1-year clinical experience. *Inflamm Bowel Dis,* 7 Suppl 1, S17-22.

Coleman, J. R. 1999. Cancer Survival Trends in England & Wales, 1971-1995 by deprivation and NHS region. *The Stationary Office.*

Colombel, J. F., Loftus, E. V., Jr., Tremaine, W. J., Egan, L. J., Harmsen, W. S., Schleck, C. D., Zinsmeister, A. R. & Sandborn, W. J. 2004. The safety profile of infliximab in patients with Crohn's disease: the Mayo clinic experience in 500 patients. *Gastroenterology,* 126, 19-31.

Colombel, J. F., Sandborn, W. J., Reinisch, W., Mantzaris, G. J., Kornbluth, A., Rachmilewitz, D., Lichtiger, S., D'haens, G., Diamond, R. H., Broussard, D. L., Tang, K. L., Van Der Woude, C. J. & Rutgeerts, P. 2010. Infliximab, azathioprine, or combination therapy for Crohn's disease. *N Engl J Med,* 362, 1383-95.

Connell, W. R., Kamm, M. A., Dickson, M., Balkwill, A. M., Ritchie, J. K. & Lennard-Jones, J. E. 1994. Long-term neoplasia risk after azathioprine treatment in inflammatory bowel disease. *Lancet,* 343, 1249-52.

Cosnes, J., Nion-Larmurier, I., Beaugerie, L., Afchain, P., Tiret, E. & Gendre, J. P. 2005. Impact of the increasing use of immunosuppressants in Crohn's disease on the need for intestinal surgery. *Gut,* 54, 237-41.

Dal Maso, L. & Franceschi, S. 2006. Hepatitis C virus and risk of lymphoma and other lymphoid neoplasms: a meta-analysis of epidemiologic studies. *Cancer Epidemiol Biomarkers Prev,* 15, 2078-85.

Darby, S. C., Olsen, J. H., Doll, R., Thakrar, B., Brown, P. D., Storm, H. H., Barlow, L., Langmark, F., Teppo, L. & Tulinius, H. 1992. Trends in childhood leukaemia in the

Nordic countries in relation to fallout from atmospheric nuclear weapons testing. *BMJ*, 304, 1005-9.

Dayharsh, G. A., Loftus, E. V., Jr., Sandborn, W. J., Tremaine, W. J., Zinsmeister, A. R., Witzig, T. E., Macon, W. R. & Burgart, L. J. 2002. Epstein-Barr virus-positive lymphoma in patients with inflammatory bowel disease treated with azathioprine or 6-mercaptopurine. *Gastroenterology*, 122, 72-7.

Debenedet, A. T., Berg, C. L., Enfield, K. B., Woodford, R. L., Bennett, A. K. & Northup, P. G. 2008. A case of vanishing bile duct syndrome and IBD secondary to Hodgkin's lymphoma. *Nat Clin Pract Gastroenterol Hepatol*, 5, 49-53.

Deneau, M., Wallentine, J., Guthery, S., O'gorman, M., Bohnsack, J., Fluchel, M., Bezzant, J. & Pohl, J. F. 2010. Natural killer cell lymphoma in a pediatric patient with inflammatory bowel disease. *Pediatrics*, 126, e977-81.

D'haens, G. R. 2009. Top-down therapy for Crohn's disease: rationale and evidence. *Acta Clin Belg*, 64, 540-6.

Diebold, D. 2001. World Health Organisation Classification of Malignant Lymphomas. *Experimental Oncology*, 23, 101-103.

Disanti, W., Rajapakse, R. O., Korelitz, B. I., Panagopoulos, G. & Bratcher, J. 2006. Incidence of neoplasms in patients who develop sustained leukopenia during or after treatment with 6-mercaptopurine for inflammatory bowel disease. *Clin Gastroenterol Hepatol*, 4, 1025-9.

Doody, M. M., Lonstein, J. E., Stovall, M., Hacker, D. G., Luckyanov, N. & Land, C. E. 2000. Breast cancer mortality after diagnostic radiography: findings from the U.S. Scoliosis Cohort Study. *Spine (Phila Pa 1976)*, 25, 2052-63.

Ekbom, A., Helmick, C., Zack, M. & Adami, H. O. 1991. Extracolonic malignancies in inflammatory bowel disease. *Cancer*, 67, 2015-9.

Ekstrom Smedby, K., Vajdic, C. M., Falster, M., Engels, E. A., Martinez-Maza, O., Turner, J., Hjalgrim, H., Vineis, P., Seniori Costantini, A., Bracci, P. M., Holly, E. A., Willett, E., Spinelli, J. J., La Vecchia, C., Zheng, T., Becker, N., De Sanjose, S., Chiu, B. C., Dal Maso, L., Cocco, P., Maynadie, M., Foretova, L., Staines, A., Brennan, P., Davis, S., Severson, R., Cerhan, J. R., Breen, E. C., Birmann, B., Grulich, A. E. & Cozen, W. 2008. Autoimmune disorders and risk of non-Hodgkin lymphoma subtypes: a pooled analysis within the InterLymph Consortium. *Blood*, 111, 4029-38.

Epstein, M. A., Achong, B. G. & Barr, Y. M. 1964. Virus Particles in Cultured Lymphoblasts from Burkitt's Lymphoma. *Lancet*, 1, 702-3.

Falchook, G. S., Vega, F., Dang, N. H., Samaniego, F., Rodriguez, M. A., Champlin, R. E., Hosing, C., Verstovsek, S. & Pro, B. 2009. Hepatosplenic gamma-delta T-cell lymphoma: clinicopathological features and treatment. *Ann Oncol*, 20, 1080-5.

Farrell, R. J., Ang, Y., Kileen, P., O'briain, D. S., Kelleher, D., Keeling, P. W. & Weir, D. G. 2000. Increased incidence of non-Hodgkin's lymphoma in inflammatory bowel disease patients on immunosuppressive therapy but overall risk is low. *Gut*, 47, 514-9.

FDA. 2011. *FDA* [Online]. Available: http://www.fda.gov/.

Feagan, B. G., Fedorak, R. N., Irvine, E. J., Wild, G., Sutherland, L., Steinhart, A. H., Greenberg, G. R., Koval, J., Wong, C. J., Hopkins, M., Hanauer, S. B. & Mcdonald, J.

W. 2000. A comparison of methotrexate with placebo for the maintenance of remission in Crohn's disease. North American Crohn's Study Group Investigators. *N Engl J Med*, 342, 1627-32.

Federman, J., Goldstein, M. E. & Weingarten, B. 1963. Malignant lymphoma of over fifteen years' duration masquerading as ulcerative colitis. *Am J Roentgenol Radium Ther Nucl Med*, 89, 771-8.

Fraser, A. G., Orchard, T. R. & Jewell, D. P. 2002. The efficacy of azathioprine for the treatment of inflammatory bowel disease: a 30 year review. *Gut*, 50, 485-9.

Friedman, H. B., Silver, G. M. & Brown, C. H. 1968. Lymphoma of the colon simulating ulcerative colitis. Report of four cases. *Am J Dig Dis*, 13, 910-7.

Frizzi, J. D., Rivera, D. E., Harris, J. A. & Hamill, R. L. 2000. Lymphoma arising in an S-pouch after total proctocolectomy for ulcerative colitis: report of a case. *Dis Colon Rectum*, 43, 540-3.

Froilan Torres, C., Castro Carbajo, P., Pajares Villarroya, R., Plaza Santos, R., Gomez Senent, S., Martin Arranz, M. D., Adan Merino, L., Martin Arranz, E., Mancenido Marcos, N., Peces, R. & Benito Lopez, D. 2009. Acute spontaneous tumor lysis syndrome in a patient with Crohn's disease taking immunosuppressants. *Rev Esp Enferm Dig*, 101, 288-94.

Funch, D. P., Walker, A. M., Schneider, G., Ziyadeh, N. J. & Pescovitz, M. D. 2005. Ganciclovir and acyclovir reduce the risk of post-transplant lymphoproliferative disorder in renal transplant recipients. *American journal of transplantation : official journal of the American Society of Transplantation and the American Society of Transplant Surgeons*, 5, 2894-900.

Gaulard, P., Bourquelot, P., Kanavaros, P., Haioun, C., Le Couedic, J. P., Divine, M., Goossens, M., Zafrani, E. S., Farcet, J. P. & Reyes, F. 1990. Expression of the alpha/beta and gamma/delta T-cell receptors in 57 cases of peripheral T-cell lymphomas. Identification of a subset of gamma/delta T-cell lymphomas. *Am J Pathol*, 137, 617-28.

Ghosh, S. & Mitchell, R. 2007. Impact of inflammatory bowel disease on quality of life: Results of the European Federation of Crohn's and Ulcerative Colitis Associations (EFCCA) patient survey. *J Crohns Colitis*, 1, 10-20.

Glaser, S. L. 1991. Black-white differences in Hodgkin's disease incidence in the United States by age, sex, histology subtype and time. *Int J Epidemiol*, 20, 68-75.

Goldin, L. R., Pfeiffer, R. M., Gridley, G., Gail, M. H., Li, X., Mellemkjaer, L., Olsen, J. H., Hemminki, K. & Linet, M. S. 2004. Familial aggregation of Hodgkin lymphoma and related tumors. *Cancer*, 100, 1902-8.

Greenstein, A. J., Gennuso, R., Sachar, D. B., Heimann, T., Smith, H., Janowitz, H. D. & Aufses, A. H., JR. 1985. Extraintestinal cancers in inflammatory bowel disease. *Cancer*, 56, 2914-21.

Grulich, A. E., Vajdic, C. M. & Cozen, W. 2007a. Altered immunity as a risk factor for non-Hodgkin lymphoma. *Cancer Epidemiol Biomarkers Prev*, 16, 405-8.

Grulich, A. E., Van Leeuwen, M. T., Falster, M. O. & Vajdic, C. M. 2007b. Incidence of cancers in people with HIV/AIDS compared with immunosuppressed transplant recipients: a meta-analysis. *Lancet*, 370, 59-67.

Hanauer, S. B., Feagan, B. G., Lichtenstein, G. R., Mayer, L. F., Schreiber, S., Colombel, J. F., Rachmilewitz, D., Wolf, D. C., Olson, A., Bao, W. & Rutgeerts, P. 2002. Maintenance infliximab for Crohn's disease: the ACCENT I randomised trial. *Lancet*, 359, 1541-9.

Hanauer, S. B., Sandborn, W. J., Rutgeerts, P., Fedorak, R. N., Lukas, M., Macintosh, D., Panaccione, R., Wolf, D. & Pollack, P. 2006. Human anti-tumor necrosis factor monoclonal antibody (adalimumab) in Crohn's disease: the CLASSIC-I trial. *Gastroenterology*, 130, 323-33; quiz 591.

Hemminki, K., Li, X., Sundquist, J. & Sundquist, K. 2008. Cancer risks in ulcerative colitis patients. *Int J Cancer*, 123, 1417-21.

Hill, D. H., Mills, J. O. & Maxwell, R. J. 1993. Metachronous colonic lymphomas complicating chronic ulcerative colitis. *Abdom Imaging*, 18, 369-70.

Hjalgrim, H., Askling, J., Sorensen, P., Madsen, M., Rosdahl, N., Storm, H. H., Hamilton-Dutoit, S., Eriksen, L. S., Frisch, M., Ekbom, A. & Melbye, M. 2000. Risk of Hodgkin's disease and other cancers after infectious mononucleosis. *J Natl Cancer Inst*, 92, 1522-8.

Holubar, S. D., Dozois, E. J., Loftus, E. V., Jr., Teh, S. H., Benavente, L. A., Harmsen, W. S., Wolff, B. G., Cima, R. R. & Larson, D. W. 2010. Primary intestinal lymphoma in patients with inflammatory bowel disease: A descriptive series from the prebiologic therapy era. *Inflamm Bowel Dis*.

Hope-Ross, M., Magee, D. J., O'donoghue, D. P. & Murphy, J. J. 1985. Ulcerative colitis complicated by lymphoma and adenocarcinoma. *Br J Surg*, 72, 22.

Hurlstone, D. P. 2002. Early phase mantle cell lymphoma: macroscopic similarities to terminal ileal Crohn's disease. *Am J Gastroenterol*, 97, 1577-8.

Isomoto, H., Furusu, H., Onizuka, Y., Kawaguchi, Y., Mizuta, Y., Maeda, T. & Kohno, S. 2003. Colonic involvement by adult T-cell leukemia/lymphoma mimicking ulcerative colitis. *Gastrointest Endosc*, 58, 805-8.

Jaeger, G., Bauer, F., Brezinschek, R., Beham-Schmid, C., Mannhalter, C. & Neumeister, P. 2008. Hepatosplenic gammadelta T-cell lymphoma successfully treated with a combination of alemtuzumab and cladribine. *Ann Oncol*, 19, 1025-6.

Jaffe, E., Harris, N., Stein, H. & Vardiman, J. (eds.) 2001. *World Health Organisation Classification of Tumours. Pathology and Genetics of Tumours of Haemopoietic and Lymphoid Tissues*: IARC Press, Lyon.

Jarnerot, G., Hertervig, E., Friis-Liby, I., Blomquist, L., Karlen, P., Granno, C., Vilien, M., Strom, M., Danielsson, A., Verbaan, H., Hellstrom, P. M., Magnuson, A. & Curman, B. 2005. Infliximab as rescue therapy in severe to moderately severe ulcerative colitis: a randomized, placebo-controlled study. *Gastroenterology*, 128, 1805-11.

Jarrett, A. F., Armstrong, A. A. & Alexander, E. 1996. Epidemiology of EBV and Hodgkin's lymphoma. *Ann Oncol*, 7 Suppl 4, 5-10.

Jess, T., Loftus, E. V., Jr., Velayos, F. S., Harmsen, W. S., Zinsmeister, A. R., Smyrk, T. C., Schleck, C. D., Tremaine, W. J., Melton, L. J., 3rd, Munkholm, P. & Sandborn, W. J. 2006. Risk of intestinal cancer in inflammatory bowel disease: a population-based study from olmsted county, Minnesota. *Gastroenterology*, 130, 1039-46.

Jess, T., Winther, K. V., Munkholm, P., Langholz, E. & Binder, V. 2004. Intestinal and extra-intestinal cancer in Crohn's disease: follow-up of a population-based cohort in Copenhagen County, Denmark. *Aliment Pharmacol Ther*, 19, 287-93.

Johnson, F. R., Hauber, B., Ozdemir, S., Siegel, C. A., Hass, S. & Sands, B. E. 2010. Are gastroenterologists less tolerant of treatment risks than patients? Benefit-risk preferences in Crohn's disease management. *J Manag Care Pharm*, 16, 616-28.

Jost, P. J. & Ruland, J. 2007. Aberrant NF-kappaB signaling in lymphoma: mechanisms, consequences, and therapeutic implications. *Blood*, 109, 2700-7.

Jouini, S., Ayadi, K., Mokrani, A., Wachuku, E., Hmouda, H. & Gourdie, R. 2001. [Mediterranean lymphoma mimicking Crohn's disease]. *J Radiol*, 82, 855-8.

Kandiel, A., Fraser, A. G., Korelitz, B. I., Brensinger, C. & Lewis, J. D. 2005. Increased risk of lymphoma among inflammatory bowel disease patients treated with azathioprine and 6-mercaptopurine. *Gut*, 54, 1121-5.

Kang, H. Y., Hwang, J. H., Park, Y. S., Bang, S. M., Lee, J. S., Chung, J. H. & Kim, H. 2007. Angioimmunoblastic T-cell lymphoma mimicking Crohn's disease. *Dig Dis Sci*, 52, 2743-7.

Karlen, P., Lofberg, R., Brostrom, O., Leijonmarck, C. E., Hellers, G. & Persson, P. G. 1999. Increased risk of cancer in ulcerative colitis: a population-based cohort study. *Am J Gastroenterol*, 94, 1047-52.

Kashi, M. R., Belayev, L. & Parker, A. 2010. Primary extranodal Hodgkin lymphoma of the colon masquerading as new diagnosis of Crohn's disease. *Clin Gastroenterol Hepatol*, 8, A20.

Kastner, F., Paulus, W., Deckert, M., Schlegel, P., Evers, S. & Husstedt, I. W. 2007. [Primary CNS lymphoma in azathioprine therapy for autoimmune diseases: review of the literature and case report]. *Nervenarzt*, 78, 451-6.

Kawashima, K., Hayashi, K., Ohnoshi, T., Teramoto, N. & Kimura, I. 1994. Epstein-Barr virus-associated post-transplant non-Hodgkin's lymphoma: establishment and characterization of a new cell line. *Jpn J Cancer Res*, 85, 1080-6.

Kelly, J. L., Friedberg, J. W., Calvi, L. M., Van Wijngaarden, E. & Fisher, S. G. 2009. Vitamin D and non-Hodgkin lymphoma risk in adults: a review. *Cancer Invest*, 27, 942-51.

Kinney, T., Rawlins, M., Kozarek, R., France, R. & Patterson, D. 2003. Immunomodulators and "on demand" therapy with infliximab in Crohn's disease: clinical experience with 400 infusions. *Am J Gastroenterol*, 98, 608-12.

Kotlyar, D. S., Blonski, W., Diamond, R. H., Wasik, M. & Lichtenstein, G. R. 2010. Hepatosplenic T-cell lymphoma in inflammatory bowel disease: a possible thiopurine-induced chromosomal abnormality. *Am J Gastroenterol*, 105, 2299-301.

Kotlyar, D. S., Osterman, M. T., Diamond, R. H., Porter, D., Blonski, W. C., Wasik, M., Sampat, S., Mendizabal, M., Lin, M. V. & Lichtenstein, G. R. 2011. A systematic review of factors that contribute to hepatosplenic T-cell lymphoma in patients with inflammatory bowel disease. *Clin Gastroenterol Hepatol*, 9, 36-41 e1.

Kroeker, K. I., Lam, S., Birchall, I. & Fedorak, R. N. 2011. Patients with IBD are exposed to high levels of ionizing radiation through CT scan diagnostic imaging: a five-year study. *J Clin Gastroenterol*, 45, 34-9.

Kuppers, R., Klein, U., Hansmann, M. L. & Rajewsky, K. 1999. Cellular origin of human B-cell lymphomas. *N Engl J Med,* 341, 1520-9.

Lal, S. & Steinhart, A. H. 2006. Antibiotic therapy for Crohn's disease: a review. *Can J Gastroenterol,* 20, 651-5.

Langmead, L. & Rampton, D. S. 2006. Review article: complementary and alternative therapies for inflammatory bowel disease. *Aliment Pharmacol Ther,* 23, 341-9.

Larsson, S. C. & Wolk, A. 2007. Obesity and risk of non-Hodgkin's lymphoma: a meta-analysis. *Int J Cancer,* 121, 1564-70.

Lemann, M., Mary, J. Y., Colombel, J. F., Duclos, B., Soule, J. C., Lerebours, E., Modigliani, R. & Bouhnik, Y. 2005. A randomized, double-blind, controlled withdrawal trial in Crohn's disease patients in long-term remission on azathioprine. *Gastroenterology,* 128, 1812-8.

Lemann, M., Mary, J. Y., Duclos, B., Veyrac, M., Dupas, J. L., Delchier, J. C., Laharie, D., Moreau, J., Cadiot, G., Picon, L., Bourreille, A., Sobahni, I. & Colombel, J. F. 2006. Infliximab plus azathioprine for steroid-dependent Crohn's disease patients: a randomized placebo-controlled trial. *Gastroenterology,* 130, 1054-61.

Leslie, W. D., Miller, N., Rogala, L. & Bernstein, C. N. 2008. Vitamin D status and bone density in recently diagnosed inflammatory bowel disease: the Manitoba IBD Cohort Study. *Am J Gastroenterol,* 103, 1451-9.

Lewis, J. D., Bilker, W. B., Brensinger, C., Deren, J. J., Vaughn, D. J. & Strom, B. L. 2001. Inflammatory bowel disease is not associated with an increased risk of lymphoma. *Gastroenterology,* 121, 1080-7.

Lewis, J. D., Schwartz, J. S. & Lichtenstein, G. R. 2000. Azathioprine for maintenance of remission in Crohn's disease: benefits outweigh the risk of lymphoma. *Gastroenterology,* 118, 1018-24.

Lichtenstein, G. R., Feagan, B. G., Cohen, R. D., Salzberg, B. A., Diamond, R. H., Chen, D. M., Pritchard, M. L. & Sandborn, W. J. 2006. Serious infections and mortality in association with therapies for Crohn's disease: TREAT registry. *Clin Gastroenterol Hepatol,* 4, 621-30.

Ling, Y. H., Chan, J. Y., Beattie, K. L. & Nelson, J. A. 1992. Consequences of 6-thioguanine incorporation into DNA on polymerase, ligase, and endonuclease reactions. *Mol Pharmacol,* 42, 802-7.

Ljung, T., Karlen, P., Schmidt, D., Hellstrom, P. M., Lapidus, A., Janczewska, I., Sjoqvist, U. & Lofberg, R. 2004. Infliximab in inflammatory bowel disease: clinical outcome in a population based cohort from Stockholm County. *Gut,* 53, 849-53.

Lofstrom, B., Backlin, C., Sundstrom, C., Ekbom, A. & Lundberg, I. E. 2007. A closer look at non-Hodgkin's lymphoma cases in a national Swedish systemic lupus erythematosus cohort: a nested case-control study. *Ann Rheum Dis,* 66, 1627-32.

Loftus, E. V., Jr., Tremaine, W. J., Habermann, T. M., Harmsen, W. S., Zinsmeister, A. R. & Sandborn, W. J. 2000. Risk of lymphoma in inflammatory bowel disease. *Am J Gastroenterol,* 95, 2308-12.

Long, M. D., Herfarth, H. H., Pipkin, C. A., Porter, C. Q., Sandler, R. S. & Kappelman, M. D. 2010. Increased risk for non-melanoma skin cancer in patients with inflammatory bowel disease. *Clin Gastroenterol Hepatol,* 8, 268-74.

Luo, J. C., Hwang, S. J., Li, C. P., Liu, J. H., Chen, P. M., Liu, S. M., Chiang, J. H., Chang, F. Y. & Lee, S. D. 1997. Primary low grade B-cell lymphoma of colon mimicking inflammatory bowel disease: a case report. *Zhonghua Yi Xue Za Zhi (Taipei)*, 59, 367-71.

Luther, J., Dave, M., Higgins, P. D. & Kao, J. Y. 2010. Association between Helicobacter pylori infection and inflammatory bowel disease: a meta-analysis and systematic review of the literature. *Inflamm Bowel Dis*, 16, 1077-84.

Maaravi, Y., Wengrower, D. & Leibowitz, G. 1993. A unique presentation of lymphoma of the colon. *J Clin Gastroenterol*, 17, 49-51.

Mack, T. M., Cozen, W., Shibata, D. K., Weiss, L. M., Nathwani, B. N., Hernandez, A. M., Taylor, C. R., Hamilton, A. S., Deapen, D. M. & Rappaport, E. B. 1995. Concordance for Hodgkin's disease in identical twins suggesting genetic susceptibility to the young-adult form of the disease. *N Engl J Med*, 332, 413-8.

Mariette, X., Cazals-Hatem, D., Warszawki, J., Liote, F., Balandraud, N. & Sibilia, J. 2002. Lymphomas in rheumatoid arthritis patients treated with methotrexate: a 3-year prospective study in France. *Blood*, 99, 3909-15.

Martinez Tirado, P., Redondo Cerezo, E., Gonzalez Aranda, Y., M, J. C. T., Nogueras Lopez, F. & Gomez Garcia, M. 2001. [Ki-1 lymphoma of the skin in a patient with Crohn's disease undergoing treatment with azathioprine]. *Gastroenterol Hepatol*, 24, 271-2.

Masunaga, Y., Ohno, K., Ogawa, R., Hashiguchi, M., Echizen, H. & Ogata, H. 2007. Meta-analysis of risk of malignancy with immunosuppressive drugs in inflammatory bowel disease. *Ann Pharmacother*, 41, 21-8.

Mccullough, J. E., Kim, C. H. & Banks, P. M. 1992. Mantle zone lymphoma of the colon simulating diffuse inflammatory bowel disease. Role of immunohistochemistry in establishing the diagnosis. *Dig Dis Sci*, 37, 934-8.

Merhi, M., Raynal, H., Cahuzac, E., Vinson, F., Cravedi, J. P. & Gamet-Payrastre, L. 2007. Occupational exposure to pesticides and risk of hematopoietic cancers: meta-analysis of case-control studies. *Cancer Causes Control*, 18, 1209-26.

MHRA. 2011. *MHRA* [Online]. Available: http://www.mhra.gov.uk/index.htm.

Miligi, L., Costantini, A. S., Benvenuti, A., Kriebel, D., Bolejack, V., Tumino, R., Ramazzotti, V., Rodella, S., Stagnaro, E., Crosignani, P., Amadori, D., Mirabelli, D., Sommani, L., Belletti, I., Troschel, L., Romeo, L., Miceli, G., Tozzi, G. A., Mendico, I. & Vineis, P. 2006. Occupational exposure to solvents and the risk of lymphomas. *Epidemiology*, 17, 552-61.

Myerson, P., Myerson, D., Miller, D., Deluca, V. A., Jr. & Lawson, J. P. 1974. Lymphosarcoma of the bowel masquerading as ulcerative colitis: report of a case. *Dis Colon Rectum*, 17, 710-5.

Neri, A., Barriga, F., Inghirami, G., Knowles, D. M., Neequaye, J., Magrath, I. T. & Dalla-Favera, R. 1991. Epstein-Barr virus infection precedes clonal expansion in Burkitt's and acquired immunodeficiency syndrome-associated lymphoma. *Blood*, 77, 1092-5.

Newnham, E., Hawkes, E., Surender, A., James, S. L., Gearry, R. & Gibson, P. R. 2007. Quantifying exposure to diagnostic medical radiation in patients with inflammatory bowel disease: are we contributing to malignancy? *Aliment Pharmacol Ther*, 26, 1019-24.

Newton, R., Ferlay, J., Beral, V. & Devesa, S. S. 1997. The epidemiology of non-Hodgkin's lymphoma: comparison of nodal and extra-nodal sites. *Int J Cancer*, 72, 923-30.

Nguyen, T., Vacek, P. M., O'neill, P., Colletti, R. B. & Finette, B. A. 2009. Mutagenicity and potential carcinogenicity of thiopurine treatment in patients with inflammatory bowel disease. *Cancer Res*, 69, 7004-12.

Nishigami, T., Kataoka, T. R., Torii, I., Sato, A., Tamura, K., Hirano, H., Hida, N., Ikeuchi, H. & Tsujimura, T. 2010. Concomitant adenocarcinoma and colonic non-Hodgkin's lymphoma in a patient with ulcerative colitis: a case report and molecular analysis. *Pathol Res Pract*, 206, 846-50.

Nyam, D. C., Pemberton, J. H., Sandborn, W. J. & Savcenko, M. 1997. Lymphoma of the pouch after ileal pouch-anal anastomosis: report of a case. *Dis Colon Rectum*, 40, 971-2.

O'donovan, P., Perrett, C. M., Zhang, X., Montaner, B., Xu, Y. Z., Harwood, C. A., Mcgregor, J. M., Walker, S. L., Hanaoka, F. & Karran, P. 2005. Azathioprine and UVA light generate mutagenic oxidative DNA damage. *Science*, 309, 1871-4.

Ogura, Y., Bonen, D. K., Inohara, N., Nicolae, D. L., Chen, F. F., Ramos, R., Britton, H., Moran, T., Karaliuskas, R., Duerr, R. H., Achkar, J. P., Brant, S. R., Bayless, T. M., Kirschner, B. S., Hanauer, S. B., Nunez, G. & Cho, J. H. 2001. A frameshift mutation in NOD2 associated with susceptibility to Crohn's disease. *Nature*, 411, 603-6.

Oruc, N., Ozutemiz, O., Tekin, F., Sezak, M., Tuncyurek, M., Krasinskas, A. M. & Tombuloglu, M. 2010. Celiac disease associated with B-cell lymphoma. *Turk J Gastroenterol*, 21, 168-71.

Owen, C. E., Callen, J. P. & Bahrami, S. 2010. Cutaneous Lymphoproliferative Disorder Complicating Infectious Mononucleosis in an Immunosuppressed Patient. *Pediatr Dermatol*.

Packey, C. D. & Sartor, R. B. 2008. Interplay of commensal and pathogenic bacteria, genetic mutations, and immunoregulatory defects in the pathogenesis of inflammatory bowel diseases. *J Intern Med*, 263, 597-606.

Palli, D., Trallori, G., Bagnoli, S., Saieva, C., Tarantino, O., Ceroti, M., D'albasio, G., Pacini, F., Amorosi, A. & Masala, G. 2000. Hodgkin's disease risk is increased in patients with ulcerative colitis. *Gastroenterology*, 119, 647-53.

Panaccione, R., Colombel, J. F., Sandborn, W. J., Rutgeerts, P., D'haens, G. R., Robinson, A. M., Chao, J., Mulani, P. M. & Pollack, P. F. 2010. Adalimumab sustains clinical remission and overall clinical benefit after 2 years of therapy for Crohn's disease. *Aliment Pharmacol Ther*, 31, 1296-309.

Parasher, G., Jaswal, S., Golbey, S., Grinberg, M. & Iswara, K. 1999. Extraintestinal non-Hodgkin's lymphoma presenting as obstructive jaundice in a patient with Crohn's disease. *Am J Gastroenterol*, 94, 226-8.

Parkin, D. M. 2006. The global health burden of infection-associated cancers in the year 2002. *Int J Cancer*, 118, 3030-44.

Parnes, I. H., Warner, R. R., Berman, R. & Sanders, M. 1974. Diffuse lymphosarcoma of the colon simulating ulcerative colitis. *Mt Sinai J Med*, 41, 802-6.

Persson, P. G., Karlen, P., Bernell, O., Leijonmarck, C. E., Brostrom, O., Ahlbom, A. & Hellers, G. 1994. Crohn's disease and cancer: a population-based cohort study. *Gastroenterology*, 107, 1675-9.

Peyrin-Biroulet, L., Laclotte, C. & Bigard, M. A. 2007. Adalimumab maintenance therapy for Crohn's disease with intolerance or lost response to infliximab: an open-label study. *Aliment Pharmacol Ther*, 25, 675-80.

Piccin, A., Cortelazzo, S., Rovigatti, U., Bourke, B. & Smith, O. P. 2010. Immunosuppressive treatments in Crohn's disease induce myelodysplasia and leukaemia. *Am J Hematol*, 85, 634.

Pohl, C., Eidt, S., Ziegenhagen, D. & Kruis, W. 1991. [Immunoproliferative disease of the small intestine. A rare differential diagnosis of Crohn's disease]. *Dtsch Med Wochenschr*, 116, 1265-9.

Pranesh, N. 2002. Lymphoma in an ileostomy. *Postgrad Med J*, 78, 368-9.

Raderer, M., Puspok, A., Birkner, T., Streubel, B. & Chott, A. 2004. Primary gastric mantle cell lymphoma in a patient with long standing history of Crohn's disease. *Leuk Lymphoma*, 45, 1459-62.

Redmond, M., Quinn, J., Murphy, P., Patchett, S. & Leader, M. 2007. Plasmablastic lymphoma presenting as a paravertebral mass in a patient with Crohn's disease after immunosuppressive therapy. *J Clin Pathol*, 60, 80-1.

Reijasse, D., Le Pendeven, C., Cosnes, J., Dehee, A., Gendre, J. P., Nicolas, J. C. & Beaugerie, L. 2004. Epstein-Barr virus viral load in Crohn's disease: effect of immunosuppressive therapy. *Inflamm Bowel Dis*, 10, 85-90.

Rodrigo, L., Perez-Pariente, J. M., Fuentes, D., Cadahia, V., Garcia-Carbonero, A., Nino, P., De Francisco, R., Tojo, R., Moreno, M. & Gonzalez-Ballina, E. 2004. Retreatment and maintenance therapy with infliximab in fistulizing Crohn's disease. *Rev Esp Enferm Dig*, 96, 548-54; 554-8.

Roelandt, P. R., Maertens, J., Vandenberghe, P., Verslype, C., Roskams, T., Aerts, R., Nevens, F. & Dierickx, D. 2009. Hepatosplenic gammadelta T-cell lymphoma after liver transplantation: report of the first 2 cases and review of the literature. *Liver Transpl*, 15, 686-92.

Rubin, G. P., Hungin, A. P., Chinn, D. J. & Dwarakanath, D. 2004. Quality of life in patients with established inflammatory bowel disease: a UK general practice survey. *Aliment Pharmacol Ther*, 19, 529-35.

Rubin, G. P., Hungin, A. P., Kelly, P. J. & Ling, J. 2000. Inflammatory bowel disease: epidemiology and management in an English general practice population. *Aliment Pharmacol Ther*, 14, 1553-9.

Rutgeerts, P., D'haens, G., Targan, S., Vasiliauskas, E., Hanauer, S. B., Present, D. H., Mayer, L., Van Hogezand, R. A., Braakman, T., Dewoody, K. L., Schaible, T. F. & Van Deventer, S. J. 1999. Efficacy and safety of retreatment with anti-tumor necrosis factor antibody (infliximab) to maintain remission in Crohn's disease. *Gastroenterology*, 117, 761-9.

Rutgeerts, P., Van Assche, G. & Vermeire, S. 2004. Optimizing anti-TNF treatment in inflammatory bowel disease. *Gastroenterology*, 126, 1593-610.

Rutter, M. D., Saunders, B. P., Wilkinson, K. H., Rumbles, S., Schofield, G., Kamm, M. A., Williams, C. B., Price, A. B., Talbot, I. C. & Forbes, A. 2006. Thirty-year analysis of a colonoscopic surveillance program for neoplasia in ulcerative colitis. *Gastroenterology*, 130, 1030-8.

Sandborn, W. J., Feagan, B. G., Stoinov, S., Honiball, P. J., Rutgeerts, P., Mason, D., Bloomfield, R. & Schreiber, S. 2007a. Certolizumab pegol for the treatment of Crohn's disease. *N Engl J Med*, 357, 228-38.

Sandborn, W. J., Hanauer, S. B., Rutgeerts, P., Fedorak, R. N., Lukas, M., Macintosh, D. G., Panaccione, R., Wolf, D., Kent, J. D., Bittle, B., Li, J. & Pollack, P. F. 2007b. Adalimumab for maintenance treatment of Crohn's disease: results of the CLASSIC II trial. *Gut*, 56, 1232-9.

Sands, B. E., Anderson, F. H., Bernstein, C. N., Chey, W. Y., Feagan, B. G., Fedorak, R. N., Kamm, M. A., Korzenik, J. R., Lashner, B. A., Onken, J. E., Rachmilewitz, D., Rutgeerts, P., Wild, G., Wolf, D. C., Marsters, P. A., Travers, S. B., Blank, M. A. & Van Deventer, S. J. 2004. Infliximab maintenance therapy for fistulizing Crohn's disease. *N Engl J Med*, 350, 876-85.

Sartor, R. B. 2008. Microbial influences in inflammatory bowel diseases. *Gastroenterology*, 134, 577-94.

Satsangi, J., Silverberg, M. S., Vermeire, S. & Colombel, J. F. 2006. The Montreal classification of inflammatory bowel disease: controversies, consensus, and implications. *Gut*, 55, 749-53.

Schroder, O., Blumenstein, I. & Stein, J. 2006. Combining infliximab with methotrexate for the induction and maintenance of remission in refractory Crohn's disease: a controlled pilot study. *Eur J Gastroenterol Hepatol*, 18, 11-6.

Schroder, O., Blumenstein, I., Schulte-Bockholt, A. & Stein, J. 2004. Combining infliximab and methotrexate in fistulizing Crohn's disease resistant or intolerant to azathioprine. *Aliment Pharmacol Ther*, 19, 295-301.

Schwartz, G. G. & Skinner, H. G. 2007. Vitamin D status and cancer: new insights. *Curr Opin Clin Nutr Metab Care*, 10, 6-11.

Schwartz, L. K., Kim, M. K., Coleman, M., Lichtiger, S., Chadburn, A. & Scherl, E. 2006. Case report: lymphoma arising in an ileal pouch anal anastomosis after immunomodulatory therapy for inflammatory bowel disease. *Clin Gastroenterol Hepatol*, 4, 1030-4.

Scully, C., Eveson, J. W., Witherow, H., Young, A. H., Tan, R. S. & Gilby, E. D. 1993. Oral presentation of lymphoma: case report of T-cell lymphoma masquerading as oral Crohn's disease, and review of the literature. *Eur J Cancer B Oral Oncol*, 29B, 225-9.

Seiderer, J., Goke, B. & Ochsenkuhn, T. 2004. Safety aspects of infliximab in inflammatory bowel disease patients. A retrospective cohort study in 100 patients of a German University Hospital. *Digestion*, 70, 3-9.

Sengul, N., Berho, M., Baig, M. K. & Weiss, E. 2008. Ileal pouch lymphoma following restorative proctocolectomy for ulcerative colitis. *Inflamm Bowel Dis*, 14, 584.

Serraino, D., Salamina, G., Franceschi, S., Dubois, D., La Vecchia, C., Brunet, J. B. & Ancelle-Park, R. A. 1992. The epidemiology of AIDS-associated non-Hodgkin's lymphoma in the World Health Organization European Region. *Br J Cancer*, 66, 912-6.

Shale, M., Kanfer, E., Panaccione, R. & Ghosh, S. 2008. Hepatosplenic T cell lymphoma in inflammatory bowel disease. *Gut,* 57, 1639-41.

Shepherd, N. A., Hall, P. A., Williams, G. T., Codling, B. W., Jones, E. L., Levison, D. A. & Morson, B. C. 1989. Primary malignant lymphoma of the large intestine complicating chronic inflammatory bowel disease. *Histopathology,* 15, 325-37.

Shimizu, Y., Kato, H. & Schull, W. J. 1990. Studies of the mortality of A-bomb survivors. 9. Mortality, 1950-1985: Part 2. Cancer mortality based on the recently revised doses (DS86). *Radiat Res,* 121, 120-41.

Siegel, C. A., Marden, S. M., Persing, S. M., Larson, R. J. & Sands, B. E. 2009. Risk of lymphoma associated with combination anti-tumor necrosis factor and immunomodulator therapy for the treatment of Crohn's disease: a meta-analysis. *Clin Gastroenterol Hepatol,* 7, 874-81.

Silano, M., Volta, U., Vincenzi, A. D., Dessi, M. & Vincenzi, M. D. 2008. Effect of a gluten-free diet on the risk of enteropathy-associated T-cell lymphoma in celiac disease. *Dig Dis Sci,* 53, 972-6.

Sivarajasingham, N., Adams, S. A., Smith, M. E. & Hosie, K. B. 2003. Perianal Hodgkin's lymphoma complicating Crohn's disease. *Int J Colorectal Dis,* 18, 174-6.

Smedby, K. E., Hjalgrim, H., Askling, J., Chang, E. T., Gregersen, H., Porwit-Macdonald, A., Sundstrom, C., Akerman, M., Melbye, M., Glimelius, B. & Adami, H. O. 2006. Autoimmune and chronic inflammatory disorders and risk of non-Hodgkin lymphoma by subtype. *J Natl Cancer Inst,* 98, 51-60.

Smith, M. A., Irving, P. M., Marinaki, A. M. & Sanderson, J. D. 2010. Review article: malignancy on thiopurine treatment with special reference to inflammatory bowel disease. *Aliment Pharmacol Ther,* 32, 119-30.

Sokol, H. & Beaugerie, L. 2009. Inflammatory bowel disease and lymphoproliferative disorders: the dust is starting to settle. *Gut,* 58, 1427-36.

Steinmaus, C., Smith, A. H., Jones, R. M. & Smith, M. T. 2008. Meta-analysis of benzene exposure and non-Hodgkin lymphoma: biases could mask an important association. *Occup Environ Med,* 65, 371-8.

Steurer, M., Stauder, R., Grunewald, K., Gunsilius, E., Duba, H. C., Gastl, G. & Dirnhofer, S. 2002. Hepatosplenic gammadelta-T-cell lymphoma with leukemic course after renal transplantation. *Hum Pathol,* 33, 253-8.

Stevens, S. J., Verschuuren, E. A., Pronk, I., Van Der Bij, W., Harmsen, M. C., The, T. H., Meijer, C. J., Van Den Brule, A. J. & Middeldorp, J. M. 2001. Frequent monitoring of Epstein-Barr virus DNA load in unfractionated whole blood is essential for early detection of posttransplant lymphoproliferative disease in high-risk patients. *Blood,* 97, 1165-71.

Swerdlow, S., Campo, E., Harris, N., Jaffe, E., Pileri, S., Stein, H., Thiele, J. & Vardiman, J. (eds.) 2008. *World Health Organisation Classification of Tumours of the Haemopoietic and Lymphoid Tissues,* Lyon: IARC Press.

Talbot, C., Sagar, P. M., Johnston, M. J., Finan, P. J. & Burke, D. 2005. Infliximab in the surgical management of complex fistulating anal Crohn's disease. *Colorectal Dis,* 7, 164-8.

Tey, S. K., Marlton, P. V., Hawley, C. M., Norris, D. & Gill, D. S. 2008. Post-transplant hepatosplenic T-cell lymphoma successfully treated with HyperCVAD regimen. *Am J Hematol*, 83, 330-3.

Theander, E., Henriksson, G., Ljungberg, O., Mandl, T., Manthorpe, R. & Jacobsson, L. T. 2006. Lymphoma and other malignancies in primary Sjogren's syndrome: a cohort study on cancer incidence and lymphoma predictors. *Ann Rheum Dis*, 65, 796-803.

Thompson, C. A., Habermann, T. M., Wang, A. H., Vierkant, R. A., Folsom, A. R., Ross, J. A. & Cerhan, J. R. 2010. Antioxidant intake from fruits, vegetables and other sources and risk of non-Hodgkin's lymphoma: the Iowa Women's Health Study. *Int J Cancer*, 126, 992-1003.

Toruner, M., Loftus, E. V., Jr., Harmsen, W. S., Zinsmeister, A. R., Orenstein, R., Sandborn, W. J., Colombel, J. F. & Egan, L. J. 2008. Risk factors for opportunistic infections in patients with inflammatory bowel disease. *Gastroenterology*, 134, 929-36.

Travis, L. B., Curtis, R. E., Boice, J. D., Jr., Hankey, B. F. & Fraumeni, J. F., JR. 1991. Second cancers following non-Hodgkin's lymphoma. *Cancer*, 67, 2002-9.

Travis, L. B., Curtis, R. E., Glimelius, B., Holowaty, E., Van Leeuwen, F. E., Lynch, C. F., Adami, J., Gospodarowicz, M., Wacholder, S., Inskip, P. & Et Al. 1993. Second cancers among long-term survivors of non-Hodgkin's lymphoma. *J Natl Cancer Inst*, 85, 1932-7.

Van Dieren, J. M., Kuipers, E. J., Samsom, J. N., Nieuwenhuis, E. E. & Van Der Woude, C. J. 2006. Revisiting the immunomodulators tacrolimus, methotrexate, and mycophenolate mofetil: their mechanisms of action and role in the treatment of IBD. *Inflamm Bowel Dis*, 12, 311-27.

Van Domselaar, M., Lopez San Roman, A., Bastos Oreiro, M. & Garrido Gomez, E. 2010. [Lymphoproliferative disorders in an inflammatory bowel disease unit]. *Gastroenterol Hepatol*, 33, 12-6.

Vincenzi, B., Finolezzi, E., Fossati, C., Verzi, A., Santini, D., Tonini, G., Arullani, A. & Avvisati, G. 2001. Unusual presentation of Hodgkin's disease mimicking inflammatory bowel disease. *Leuk Lymphoma*, 42, 521-6.

Von Roon, A. C., Reese, G., Teare, J., Constantinides, V., Darzi, A. W. & Tekkis, P. P. 2007. The risk of cancer in patients with Crohn's disease. *Dis Colon Rectum*, 50, 839-55.

Vos, A. C., Bakkal, N., Minnee, R. C., Casparie, M. K., De Jong, D. J., Dijkstra, G., Stokkers, P., Van Bodegraven, A. A., Pierik, M., Van Der Woude, C. J., Oldenburg, B. & Hommes, D. W. 2010. Risk of malignant lymphoma in patients with inflammatory bowel diseases: A Dutch nationwide study. *Inflamm Bowel Dis*.

Wagonfeld, J. B., Baker, A. L., Reed, J. S., Platz, C. E. & Kirsner, J. B. 1976. Acute dilation of the colon in malignant lymphoma. *Gastroenterology*, 70, 264-7.

Winnicki, M., Gariepy, G., Sauthier, P. G. & Funaro, D. 2009. Hodgkin lymphoma presenting as a vulvar mass in a patient with crohn disease: a case report and literature review. *J Low Genit Tract Dis*, 13, 110-4.

Winther, K. V., Jess, T., Langholz, E., Munkholm, P. & Binder, V. 2004. Long-term risk of cancer in ulcerative colitis: a population-based cohort study from Copenhagen County. *Clin Gastroenterol Hepatol*, 2, 1088-95.

Wolfe, F. & Michaud, K. 2004. Lymphoma in rheumatoid arthritis: the effect of methotrexate and anti-tumor necrosis factor therapy in 18,572 patients. *Arthritis Rheum,* 50, 1740-51.

Wong, M. T. & Eu, K. W. 2006. Primary colorectal lymphomas. *Colorectal Dis,* 8, 586-91.

Wong, N. A., Herbst, H., Herrmann, K., Kirchner, T., Krajewski, A. S., Moorghen, M., Niedobitek, F., Rooney, N., Shepherd, N. A. & Niedobitek, G. 2003. Epstein-Barr virus infection in colorectal neoplasms associated with inflammatory bowel disease: detection of the virus in lymphomas but not in adenocarcinomas. *J Pathol,* 201, 312-8.

Xue, F. B., Xu, Y. Y., Wan, Y., Pan, B. R., Ren, J. & Fan, D. M. 2001. Association of H. pylori infection with gastric carcinoma: a Meta analysis. *World J Gastroenterol,* 7, 801-4.

Zachos, M., Tondeur, M. & Griffiths, A. M. 2007. Enteral nutritional therapy for induction of remission in Crohn's disease. *Cochrane Database Syst Rev,* CD000542.

Zhang, S. M., Hunter, D. J., Rosner, B. A., Giovannucci, E. L., Colditz, G. A., Speizer, F. E. & Willett, W. C. 2000. Intakes of fruits, vegetables, and related nutrients and the risk of non-Hodgkin's lymphoma among women. *Cancer Epidemiol Biomarkers Prev,* 9, 477-85.

4

Development, Optimization and Absorption Mechanism of DHP107, Oral Paclitaxel Formulation for Single-Agent Anticancer Therapy

In-Hyun Lee, Jung Wan Hong, Yura Jang,
Yeong Taek Park and Hesson Chung
*Korea Institute of Science and Technology
and Daehwa Pharmaceutical
Korea*

1. Introduction

Paclitaxel, administered as intravenous infusion currently, is an effective anticancer drug belonging to the taxane family (Figure 1) and used in the treatment of a wide variety of cancers including breast and ovarian cancers (Rowinsky et al., 1995). Researchers have been looking for more effective and convenient ways to administer paclitaxel with less formulation-related toxicities than the commercially available formulations like Taxol® by Bristol-Meyers Squibb. It is well known that some of the limitations of the current formulation come from Cremophor EL, a polyoxyethylated castor oil. This particular component is known to cause hypersensitivity (Weiss et al., 1990), to be responsible for nonlinear pharmacokinetic behavior (Kearns et al., 1995; Gianni, 1995) and to cause paclitaxel precipitation oftentimes when diluted during the infusion process (Pfeifer, 1993). Formulations for paclitaxel and its analogs have been prepared in many different ways for various administration procedures (Kim et al., 2006; Xie et al., 2007; Sugahara et al., 2007; Singla et al., 2002; Hennenfent & Govindan, 2006). Several years ago, Abraxane®, a suspension of albumin nanoparticles containing paclitaxel, obtained approval to treat metastatic breast cancer patients (Ibrahim et al., 2002; Garber, 2004). Abraxane®, a solvent-

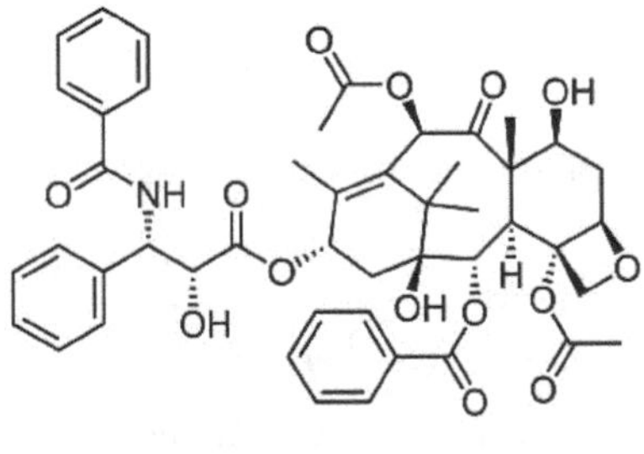

Fig. 1. Structure of paclitaxel

Formulation	AUC (µg·h/ml)	Cmax (µg/ml)	Dose (mg/kg)	Rodent species	Ref
Without inhibitors					
Taxol	0.50 (0-8*)	0.14	10	mice	Sparreboom et al., 1997
Taxol	0.37 (0-4)	0.13***	10	mice	Bardelmeijer et al., 2004
Taxol	1.89 (0-∞)	0.11	50	rat	Choi & Li, 2005
Taxol	0.41 (0-6)	0.12	10	mice	Bardelmeijer et al., 2000
Cremophor/ethanol	0.51 (0-24)	0.10	5	mice	Asperen et al., 1998
Supersaturable-SEDDS	0.44 (0-∞)	0.28	10	rat	Gao et al., 2003
SMEDDS	0.81 (0-24)	0.05	2	rat	Yang et al., 2004
SMEDDS	0.97 (0-24)	0.05	10	rat	Yang et al., 2004
microemulsion	0.45 (0-24)	0.05	25	rat	Woo et al., 2003
Suspension in Tween 80	1.65 (0-24)	0.11	40	rat	Choi et al., 2004a, 2004b
Lipid nanocapsule	1.05 (0-∞)	0.37	10	rat	Peltier et al., 2006
With inhibitors					
Cremophor/Ethanol +Cyclosporine A (50**)	6.68 (0-24)	0.73	10	mice	Asperen et al., 1998
Supersaturable-SEDDS +cyclosporine A (30)	1.05 (0-∞)	0.31	10	rat	Gao et al., 2003
SMEDDS+cyclosporine A (40)	1.14 (0-24)	0.16	2	rat	Yang et al., 2004
Taxol+verapamil (15)	4.27 (0-∞)	0.19	50	rat	Choi & Li, 2005
Microemulsion+KR-30031 (20)	3.37 (0-24)	0.22	25	rat	Woo et al., 2003
Surfactant mix + KR30031 (5)	0.39 (0-12)	0.06	5	rat	Kim et al., 2004
Suspension in Tween 80 + quercetin (20)	5.00 (0-24)	0.28	40	rat	Choi et al., 2004b
Taxol+cyclosporine A (50)	3.61 (0-4)	0.82***	10	mice	Bardelmeijer et al., 2004
Taxol+PSC 833 (50)	2.71 (0-4)	1.47***	10	mice	Bardelmeijer et al., 2004
Taxol+GF120918 (25)	1.39 (0-4)	0.55***	10	mice	Bardelmeijer et al., 2004
Taxol+LY335979 (80)	1.41 (0-4)	0.42***	10	mice	Bardelmeijer et al., 2004
Taxol+R101933 (80)	0.93 (0-4)	0.32***	10	mice	Bardelmeijer et al., 2004
Taxol+GF120918 (25)	2.65 (0-10)	0.77	10	mice	Bardelmeijer et al., 2000
Taxol+PSC 833 (50)				mice	Asperen et al., 1997

* Time-interval used for the calibration of AUC,
** Dose of the inhibitor in mg/kg, and
*** Estimated concentration

Table 1. Mini-review: Selective pharmacokinetic data of paclitaxel after oral administration to rodents.

free formulation has a number of improved features such as shorter infusion time and no hypersensitivity without premedication (Garber, 2004).

Since an oral route would clearly be an attractive alternative to injection for patients as well as for medical personnel, there have been many attempts to prepare effective oral paclitaxel

Development, Optimization and Absorption Mechanism of DHP107, Oral Paclitaxel Formulation
or Single-Agent Anticancer Therapy

93

formulations. Paclitaxel, however, is known to be absorbed poorly in the gastrointestinal tract when administered orally (Sparreboom et al., 1997; Bardelmeijer et al., 2004; Choi & Li, 2005; Bardelmeijer et al., 2000). The reasons for poor absorption were identified to be drug metabolism by cytochrome P450 (CYP) and the existence of the efflux system, such as P-glycoproteins in intestinal epithelial cells and liver (Schellens et al., 2000). Tellingen and co-workers identified that the epithelial efflux system composed of P-glycoproteins lowered the drug absorption by demonstrating that orally administered paclitaxel can be absorbed well in mice with a homozygously disrupted mdr1a gene (mdr1a(-/-) mice) (Sparreboom et al., 1997). Proof-of-concept experiments in mice and man have also shown that oral absorption of paclitaxel could be increased dramatically by concomitant administration of a P-glycoprotein inhibitor, cyclosporine A (Schellens et al., 2000; Asperen et al., 1998; Meerum Terwogt et al., 1999). Other P-glycoprotein blockers that could also serve as CYP 450 inhibitors also boosted the oral absorption of paclitaxel (Sparreboom et al., 1997; Bardelmeijer et al., 2004; Choi & Li, 2005; Kim et al., 2004; Asperen et al., 1997). Formulations that do not contain Cremophor EL, that could lower the *in vivo* toxicity and increase solubilization of paclitaxel, were shown to deliver paclitaxel efficiently via oral administration especially when P-glycoprotein inhibitors were given simultaneously (Kim et al., 2004; Gao et al., 2003; Yang et al., 2004; Woo et al., 2003; Choi et al., 2004a, 2004b; Peltier et al., 2006).

In Table 1, we reviewed the literature on oral paclitaxel formulations and summarized the pharmacokinetic data of paclitaxel obtained from the small-animal experiments (FVB mice and Sprague-Dawley rats). In the Table, we have listed Area under the plasma concentration vs. time curve (AUC) value, maximum drug concentration in the blood (C_{max}) and oral dose. One has to keep in mind that the data from different papers may not be compared directly since the AUC values in the literature were estimated for different time intervals and drug doses while the pharmacokinetics of paclitaxel is known to be non-linear (Kearns et al., 1995; Gianni, 1995). Different time intervals could not be normalized due to lack of information in the pharmacokinetics data to make such estimations and thus must be viewed with caution. Another important point to note is that Cremophor EL in Taxol®, used for intravenous administration in some cases (Sparreboom et al., 1997; Bardelmeijer et al., 2004; Asperen et al., 1998; Gao et al., 2003; Yang et al., 2004; Peltier et al., 2006), causes nonlinear pharmacokinetic behavior (Sparreboom et al., 1996). Also, paclitaxel dissolved in Tween 80, also used for intravenous controls in others (Choi & Li, 2005; Bardelmeijer et al., 2000; Woo et al., 2003; Choi et al., 2004a, 2004b), does show linear pharmacokinetic behavior, but has *ca.* 5~10 times lower AUC values when compared to diluted Taxol® (Sparreboom et al., 1996). For these reasons, it was impossible to list the bioavailability values in Table 1.

In the past several years, we have been developing paclitaxel formulations with biocompatible oils, lipids and emulsifiers (Lee et al. Hong et al., 2004; I. H. Lee et al., 2005; S. J. Lee et al., 2005). Paclitaxel dissolved in a stable Lipiodol formulation was shown to retard the growth of hepatocellular carcinoma efficiently when transcatheter arterial chemoembolization was performed in rabbits (Yoon et al., 2003). Also, a paclitaxel formulation prepared with monoolein, tricaprylin and Tween 80 was mucoadhesive when given intravesically (S. J. Lee et al., 2005). Paclitaxel in this formulation penetrated to lamina propria and close to the muscle layer of the bladder while the paclitaxel concentration was low throughout the depth of the bladder tissue when Taxol® was used. We also have shown that this mucoadhesive formulation can deliver paclitaxel effectively when given by oral route without additional active pharmaceutical ingredient as an absorption enhancer (Lee et al., 2004; Hong et al., 2004; I. H. Lee et al., 2005, Shin et al., 2009). As an endeavor to formulate more efficient oral paclitaxel formulations, we have prepared oil-based paclitaxel formulations with monoolein, saturated triglycerides and emulsifiers. Monoolein was included in the formulation as a main ingredient due to its high bioadhesiveness (Nielsen et al., 1998) and its ability to release the encapsulated drug in a controlled fashion (Clogston et al., 2005a, 2005b). Triglycerides were added since they can solubilize paclitaxel efficiently (Kan et al., 1999). To access the effectiveness of the formulations, pharmacokinetic and anti-tumor efficacy studies were performed in mice models.

2. Materials and methods

2.1 Materials

Distilled monoolein (RYLO™ MG 19, > 90 % pure) was purchased from Danisco Ingredients, Denmark. Paclitaxel was obtained from Samyang Genex (Korea) and Indena S.P.A. (Italy). Cremophor EL, Tween 80 and triglycerides (triacetin, tributyrin, tricaproin, tricaprylin, tricaprin and trilaurin) were purchased from Sigma Chemical Co. (St. Louis, MO).

2.2 Preparation of oral paclitaxel formulations

The compositions of the oral paclitaxel formulations used in the experiments are summarized in Tables 2 and 3. Paclitaxel formulations with various triglycerides (Table 2) were prepared as follows: Paclitaxel in amorphous form was dissolved completely at 10 mg/ml in mixtures of oils consisting of monoolein, triglycerides and Tween 80 by sonication for 30 s. Some of the oral paclitaxel formulations were semi-solid or solid wax at ambient temperatures with the melting points of 30 ~ 50 °C, and therefore had to be warmed before oral feeding.

In Table 3, Paclitaxel, amorphous or crystalline, was dissolved completely in excess amount of methylene chloride and mixed subsequently with tricaprylin. Methylene chloride was evaporated completely to prepare paclitaxel/tricaprylin solution by vacuum evaporation (BUCHI rotavapor R-200, Germany) at 40 °C for 1 h. The content of methylene chloride was determined by gas chromatography and was less than 100 ppm in the paclitaxel/tricaprylin solution. Monoolein and Tween 80 were added to the paclitaxel/tricaprylin solution and mixed completely by sonication for 30 s. A formulation that does not contain paclitaxel, eG2, was also prepared for control. The oral paclitaxel formulations were semi-solid wax with the melting temperature of 33 ~ 35 °C, and were warmed to body temperature before feeding.

Dispersions of the oral paclitaxel formulations (G8, G9, and G10) were prepared by adding 2.3 times (by volume) of distilled water or syrup to the formulation G2 (also will be referred to as DHP107) and by vortexing or sonicating for 1 min.

2.3 Animals

Male ICR and Balb/c athymic mice, 7 weeks old, were purchased from Orient Bio Co. (Seoul, Korea) and Japan SLC (Japan), respectively, and maintained 1 week. Animal care

Development, Optimization and Absorption Mechanism of DHP107, Oral Paclitaxel Formulation
for Single-Agent Anticancer Therapy

95

and handling followed institutional guidelines (Korea Institute of Science and Technology). Mice were maintained with free access to food and water under a 12-h light/dark cycle.

2.4 Differential scanning calorimetry

Differential scanning calorimetry (DSC) was performed to obtain the heating thermograms of paclitaxel and the formulations in Table 2 (DSC 821e, Mettler Toledo, Columbus, OH, equipped with Intracooler, Haake EK90/MT, Haake, Denmark) at a heating scan rate of 5 °C/min. Scans were made with samples contained in hermetically sealed aluminum crucibles (ME-27331, Mettler Toledo). Initial heating scans were reported for paclitaxel and the formulations in Table 2. In case of the formulations, thermal history did not alter the heating thermograms if the samples were cooled to – 20 °C before reheating.

2.5 Determination of the particle size in the dispersion

The average particle size in the dispersions G8, G9 and G10 in Table 3 was determined by quasielastic laser light scattering with a Malvern Zetasizer® (Malvern Instruments Limited, England). The dispersions were diluted by 300 times in water before the measurement. The size determination was repeated 3 times/sample. The average size and the size distribution were estimated from the log-normal size distribution function as shown previously (Chung et al., 2001)

2.6 Oral administration of paclitaxel formulations

Paclitaxel formulations in Tables 2 and 3 were liquefied at 37 ~ 50 °C and administered orally at doses of 25, 50, 75, and 100 mg/kg with a blunt needle via the esophagus into the stomach. The male ICR mice were fasted for 8 h prior to oral administration except for the group G3. Taxol® prepared by dissolving paclitaxel in an equivolume mixture of Cremophor EL and ethanol at 6 mg/ml (Taxol®) was diluted by 6 times with the saline solution, and was administered via bolus tail-vein injection at a dose of 10 mg/kg as a positive control. Blood samples were collected at various time points (n=6) after drug administration, and were stored at -70 °C until analysis.

2.7 Analysis of paclitaxel concentrations in blood

Whole blood (200 µl) was spiked with irbesartan (0.5 µg/ml; internal standard), mixed and added to acetonitrile (400 µl) to precipitate proteins. After centrifugation at 14,000 RCF for 20 min, the supernatant was collected and mixed with the mobile phase to adjust the volume to 0.6 ml. Ten microliters of the blood was injected into the LC/MS/MS system. Analyses were performed with a Thermo-Finnigan Discovery Max LC/MS/MS (San Jose, CA, USA). The LC system was performed at 35 °C on a Capcellpak C18 column (150 X 2.0 mm i.d., 5 µm particle size, Shisheido, Japan) equipped with a Zorbax SB-Aq (12.5 X 2.1 mm i.d.) guard column. The mobile phase consisted of 55 % acetonitrile, 0.08 % formic acid and 44.92 % water, and the flow rate was 0.4 ml/min. The instrument was operated in SRM mode (positive ion), monitoring the ion transitions from m/z 854 $\rightarrow$ 285 (paclitaxel) and m/z 429 $\rightarrow$ 195 (internal standard). The paclitaxel LC/MS/MS assay was linear over the range of 2 ~ 1000 ng/ml with a lower quantitation limit of 2 ng/ml in blood. Paclitaxel concentrations in blood were calculated based on a standard curve of paclitaxel in blank pooled animal blood with the internal standard.

2.8 Tumor experiment

Suspension of NCI-H358 human non-small cell lung cancer cells (1.2×10^7 cells/mouse), purchased from American Type Culture Collection (ATCC, Manassas, VA), was injected subcutaneously to the dorsal flank of male Balb/c athymic mice (8 weeks). When the tumor volume (length × width × height × 0.5236) reached *ca.* 100 mm³ in 10 days after the injection (day 0), the experimental groups were divided at random into three groups (n=8). On days 1, 2, 3, 4 and 5, G2 formulation (DHP107) was administered orally at a dose of 50 mg/kg (G2). For controls, mice injected intravenously with diluted Taxol® (Taxol, 10 mg/kg) and fed orally with the vehicle only (eG2) on days 1, 2, 3, 4 and 5 were also observed.

2.9 Characterization of crystalline forms of paclitaxel

X-Ray diffraction (XRD) measurements were made by using an x-ray diffractometer (D8 Discover, Bruker, Karlsruhe, Germany) with the general area detector diffraction system (GADDS, Bruker, Karlsruhe, Germany). The Cu K$_\alpha$ radiation of wavelength 1.542 Å was provided by the x-ray generator (FL CU 4 KE, Bruker, Karlsruhe, Germany) operating at 40 kV and 45 mA. Sample-to-detector distance was 300 mm. Exposure time was 1 ~ 5 h. To avoid air scattering, the beam path was filled with helium. The surface morphology of paclitaxel was observed by scanning electron microscopy (SEM; Hitachi S-2460N, Japan) at an accelerating voltage of 15 kV after Pt/Au sputter coating (Hitachi E1010 Ion sputter, Japan).

3. Results

3.1 Characterization of crystalline forms of paclitaxel

Crystalline forms of paclitaxel obtained from different sources were determined by DSC, x-ray diffraction and scanning electron microscopy. Paclitaxel can exist as different polymorphs having distinct physical properties, which could influence the manufacturing process of the formulations (Liggins et al., 1997; Lee et al., 2001). Paclitaxel obtained from Samyang Genex (Genexol, Korea) had the glass transition temperature at 150 °C and an exothermic transition at 220 °C whereas paclitaxel obtained from Indena had the melting transition at 210 °C as shown in Figure 2, corresponding to amorphous and anhydrous crystalline forms, respectively, as shown in the literature (Liggins et al., 1997). X-ray diffraction data revealed the differences in the crystallinity of paclitaxel. Diffraction pattern of Genexol showed two broad scattering peaks centered at *ca.* 10° and 20° characteristic of the amorphous form. Paclitaxel from Indena, on the other hand, revealed a pattern with strong and sharp diffraction peaks at 5.7° and 12.6° indicating a highly ordered structure. Surface morphology was also visualized by SEM. Genexol was observed to be in the powder form with highly contoured surfaces. We note that the grain size or the surface area of the powder varied depending on the lot numbers of Genexol (data not shown). For instance, Genexol 131 was composed of powders with wrinkled surfaces whereas Genexol 183 contained smooth and round particles as well when observed by SEM. Needle-like crystals were observed for paclitaxel from Indena. Based on DSC, XRD and SEM experiments,

Development, Optimization and Absorption Mechanism of DHP107, Oral Paclitaxel Formulation
for Single-Agent Anticancer Therapy

97

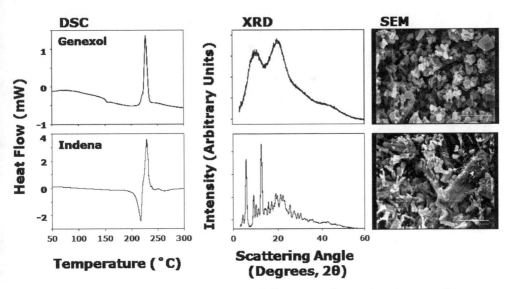

Fig. 2. Differential Scanning calorimetry, x-ray diffraction and scanning electron microscopy
of paclitaxel obtained from of Genexol (upper panels) and Indena (lower panels).

we confirmed that Paclitaxel from Samyang Genex and Indena were in amorphous and
anhydrous crystalline forms, respectively.

Due to the differences in the grain size and crystalline forms, we used two different
procedures in preparing the oral formulations. Genexol 131 was readily soluble in all of the
lipid mixtures in Table 2 when sonicated for *ca.* 30 s. Genexol 183, which had larger grains
than Genexol 131, and paclitaxel from Indena did not dissolve in the lipid mixture. In these
cases, paclitaxel was solubilized completely in the mixture of methylene chloride and
triglyceride. Methylene chloride was evaporated completely from the mixture before other
ingredients were added to prepare the formulations in Table 3.

3.2 Physical properties of oral paclitaxel formulations

Oral paclitaxel formulations existed as oil/wax mixtures at ambient temperatures, but
formed clear liquid at 37 °C except for the Formulation T12 (Table 2). The T12 formulation
existed as solid wax at ambient temperatures. Thermal behavior of the formulations
containing different triglycerides was investigated by performing DSC (Figure 3A).

The thermograms were identical with or without paclitaxel in the formulations, and those
with paclitaxel are shown in the Figure. Tween 80, liquid at room temperature, did not show
any phase transition in the temperature range from 0 to 60 °C. Lamellar crystalline-to-fluid
isotropic, or the chain melting, phase transition of monoolein was observed at 32 °C, which
is similar to the values reported for pure monoolein (Briggs et al., 1996; Qiu & Caffrey, 2000)
or Myverol 18-99K (Clogston, 2000) in the literature. The chain melting transition of
monoolein for the monoolein/Tween 80 (55.0:16.5 by weight) mixture was observed at 26 °C,
since Tween 80 lowered the transition temperature of monoolein. In the formulations T2, T4
and T6, only the chain melting transition of monoolein was observed because triacetin,

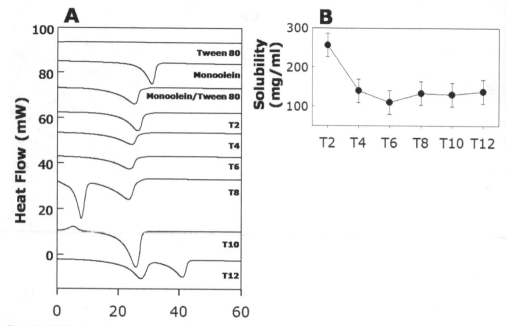

Fig. 3. A) Heating thermograms obtained from the formulations prepared with different triglycerides (T2 ~ T12, in Table 2), Tween 80, monoolein and monoolein/Tween 80 mixture (55.0:16.5 by weight). The concentration of paclitaxel was 1 %(w/w) in all formulations. B) Solubility of paclitaxel in the formulations containing monoolein, triglyceride and Tween 80 at 55.0:27.5:16.5 by weight at 37 °C.

tributyrin and tricaprin were immiscible with solid monoolein. We could identify visually the phase separation of these triglycerides below *ca.* 26 °C. In T8 formulation, chain melting transitions of tricaprylin and monoolein were observed at 8 and 23 °C, respectively. In case of T10 formulation, single transition peak from the melting transition of the eutectic mixture of monoolein and tricaprin (2:1 by weight) was observed at 26 °C (Roh et al., 2004). The chain melting transitions of monoolein and trilaurin were observed at 32 and 41 °C, respectively, for T12 formulation. Results show that all the formulations existed as solid/liquid or solid/solid mixtures at room temperature, but transforms into the single-phase liquid when heated to the body temperature for T2 ~ T10 formulations or above 45 °C for T12 formulation. Paclitaxel was solubilized well inside all of the formulations in the temperature range studied when observed by polarized light microscopy (data not shown).

3.3 Solubility of paclitaxel in oral formulations

The solubility of paclitaxel in the oral formulations with different triglycerides was determined at 37 °C. Mixtures of monoolein/triglyceride/Tween 80 were prepared at 55.0:27.5:16.5 by weight and warmed to melt. Paclitaxel in powder form (Genexol, Samyang Genex, lot G131) was added stepwise to these mixtures until undissolved aggregates were observed. The mixtures were vortexed for 10 s and sonicated for 3 min after each addition at 37 °C. The formulation containing trilaurin was heated to 60 °C and cooled to 37 °C to obtain

Development, Optimization and Absorption Mechanism of DHP107, Oral Paclitaxel Formulation
or Single-Agent Anticancer Therapy

99

the undercooled liquid for the measurement. Solubility of paclitaxel was *ca.* 250 ± 30 mg/ml for the formulation containing triacetin, but was *ca.* 120 ± 40 mg/ml for those with other triglycerides (Figure 3B).

3.4 Pharmacokinetics of oral paclitaxel administration and intravenous Taxol injection

Oral paclitaxel formulations were warmed to body temperature and administered to male ICR mice. We note that not the dispersions but the oily formulations were administered, and no other active pharmaceutical ingredients were given to the animals. Diluted Taxol® was given intravenously as a control. Paclitaxel concentration in blood after oral administration of formulation G2 (DHP107, paclitaxel dose of 50 mg/kg) and intravenous injection of Taxol® (10 mg/kg) was plotted as a function of time in Figure 4A (normal scale) and Figure 4B (logarithmic scale). Paclitaxel concentration in blood was 60.2 µg/ml in 1 min after intravenous injection, and dropped to *ca.* 6.2 and 0.8 µg/ml and in 0.5 and 3 h, respectively. Paclitaxel concentration in blood increased and became 1.2 and 2.1 µg/ml at 1 and 3 h, respectively, after oral administration of DHP107. Pharmacokinetic parameters are listed in Table 2. The bioavailability [(BA) (%) = (AUC_{oral} / AUC_{iv}) · ($Dose_{iv}$/ $Dose_{oral}$) ×100] of DHP107 in mice was *ca.* 14 %. Since the plasma concentration of paclitaxel above a threshold value of 85.3 ng/ml (dashed line in Figure 4B) was proven to be pharmacologically active, DHP107 could be effective for more than 8 h (Huizing et al., 1997).

Treatment group	Triglyceride type	T_{max} (h)	C_{max} (µg/ml)	AUC_{0-9} (µg·h /ml)
T2	Triacetin	3	0.4	1.6
T4	Tributyrin	3	1.5	5.4
T6	Tricaproin	3	3.1	12.0
T8	Tricaprylin	1	2.7	8.9
T10	Tricaprin	1	2.2	8.4
T12	Trilaurin	1	1.5	4.9

Table 2. Pharmacokinetic parameters of paclitaxel after oral administration (50 mg/kg dose) of the formulations containing different triglycerides to Balb/c mice. The composition of the formulations was paclitaxel:monoolein:triglyceride:Tween 80 = 1.0:55.0:27.5:16.5 by weight.

3.5 Oral administration of formulations with different triglycerides

Paclitaxel formulations prepared with various triglycerides (paclitaxel: monoolein: triglyceride:Tween 80 = 1.0:55.0:27.5:16.5 by weight) were administered orally at 50 mg/kg dose to male ICR mice (Table 2, Figure 4C). AUC values were 12.1 ± 2.6, 8.9 ± 1.8 and 8.4 ± 2.7 µg·h/ml for T6, T8 and T10 groups, respectively, with no statistical differences (p<0.15 by Student *t*-test). In case of T2, T4 and T12 groups, AUC of paclitaxel was 1.6 ± 0.5 (p<0.003 compared the AUC with T6 formulation), 5.4 ± 0.7 (p<0.01) and 4.9 ±1.6 µg·h/ml (p<0.01), respectively. Maximum concentration of paclitaxel in blood (C_{max}) was also the highest for the formulation with tricaproin (T6) and was 3.2 ± 0.7 µg·h/ml. Interestingly, the time to reach C_{max} (T_{max}) was 3 h for the formulations with shorter chain triglycerides (T2, T4 and T6) and 1 h for T8, T10 and T12 groups.

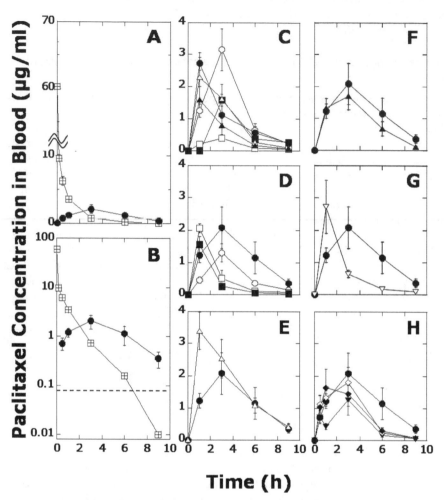

Fig. 4. Mean blood concentration of paclitaxel after intravenous administration of Taxol®
and administration of oral formulations. Comparison between intravenous Taxol (⊞, 10
mg/kg) and oral DHP107 (G2, ●, 50 mg/kg) is shown in normal (A) and logarithmic (B)
scales. The dashed line in B) indicates the pharmacologically effective concentration (85.3
ng/ml). Oral administration of paclitaxel formulations C) with different triglycerides (T2: □,
T4: ■, T6: ○, T8: ●, T10: △, T12: ▲), D) with different paclitaxel contents (G1: ○, 5 mg
paclitaxel/ml formulation, G2, DHP107: ●, 10 mg/ml, G3: □, 15 mg/kg, G4: ■, 20 mg/ml),
E) under the fasting (G2, DHP107: ●) and non-fasting (G5: △) conditions, F) prepared with
crystalline (G6: ▲) and amorphous (G2, DHP107: ●) paclitaxel, G) with (G2, DHP107: ●) or
without (G7: ▽) Tween 80, and H) dispersed in syrup (G8: ▼) or in water (G9: ◇) by
vortexing and in water by sonication (G10: ◆) or given per se (G2, DHP107: ●). The oral
dose of paclitaxel was 50 mg/kg except for G1 (25 mg/kg), G3 (75 mg/kg) and G4 (100
mg/kg).

Treatment group	Paclitaxel Dose (mg/kg)	Composition [%(w/w)]						T_{max} (h)	C_{max} (µg/ml)	AUC_{0-9} (µg h /ml)	Crystallinity of paclitaxel
		Paclitaxel	Monoolein	Tricaprylin	Tween 80	Cremophor EL	Ethanol				
G1	25 (p.o.)	0.5	55.5	27.5	16.5	-	-	3	1.3	5.2	Amorphous
G2 (DHP107)	50 (p.o.)	1.0	55.0	27.5	16.5	-	-	3	2.0	11.0	Amorphous
G3	75 (p.o.)	1.5	54.5	27.5	16.5	-	-	1	2.0	4.7	Amorphous
G4	100 (p.o.)	2.0	54.0	27.5	16.5	-	-	1	1.5	3.1	Amorphous
G5 (DHP107, Non-fasting)	50 (p.o.)	1.0	55.0	27.5	16.5	-	-	1	3.4	15.3	Amorphous
G6	50 (p.o.)	1.0	55.0	27.5	16.5	-	-	3	1.6	8.3	Crystalline
G7	50 (p.o.)	1.0	66.0	33.0	-	-	-	1	2.7	6.3	Amorphous
eG2	0 (p.o.)	0.0	56.0	27.5	16.5	-	-	-	-	-	-
Taxol	10 (i.v.)	0.6	-	-	-	57.0	42.4	0.016	60.2	15.7	Amorphous

Treatment group	Paclitaxel Dose (mg/kg)	Composition [%(w/w)]						T_{max} (h)	C_{max} (µg/ml)	AUC_{0-9} (µg h /ml)	Dispersing method
		Paclitaxel	Monoolein	Tricaprylin	Tween 80	Syrup	Water				
G8	50 (p.o.)	0.3	16.2	8.0	5.5	70	-	3	1.2	4.6	Vortex
G9	50 (p.o.)	0.3	16.2	8.0	5.5	-	70	3	1.8	7.5	Vortex
G10	50 (p.o.)	0.3	16.2	8.0	5.5	-	70	1	1.6	7.1	Sonication

Table 3. Compositions of paclitaxel formulations and pharmacokinetic parameters of paclitaxel after intravenous or oral administration in Balb/c mice.

3.6 Oral administration of formulations with different paclitaxel contents

We prepared the formulations with different Paclitaxel contents while fixing the weight ratio of monoolein:tricaprylin:Tween 80 to 55.0:27.5:16.5 by weight (G1, G2, G3 and G4 in Table 3, Figure 4D). Bioavailability was 13 % and 14 % when the concentration of paclitaxel was 0.5 and 1 %(w/w), respectively, in the formulation. When the concentration was 1.5 and 2.0 %(w/w), bioavailability decreased with increasing paclitaxel dose and was 4 % and 2 %, respectively.

3.7 Fasting vs. non-fasting conditions

When the formulation is given orally, the fullness of stomach can influence the pharmacokinetics of the administered drug. Throughout the experiments, we administered the oral formulations after 8 h of fasting. In G5, however, we fed DHP107 to mice with free access to food and water before and after the drug administration in order to observe the influence of stomach emptiness on the absorption of the drug. Under the non-fasting condition, C_{max} increased to 3.4 µg/ml when compared to the fasting condition (2.0 µg/ml) and T_{max} was reduced to 1 h (Figure 4E). The AUC values for non-fasting and fasting conditions were 15.3 (20 % BA) and 11.0 µg·h /ml (14 % BA), respectively. We could conclude that the food in the gastrointestinal tract did not interfere with, but rather helped the absorption of paclitaxel.

3.8 Crystalline vs. amorphous paclitaxel

The formulations made with crystalline and amorphous paclitaxel were administered orally to mice (Figure 4F). The pharmacokinetic profiles were virtually identical for these two formulations. We expected that the crystallinity of the drug would not affect the degree of oral absorption since paclitaxel was dissolved completely in tricaprylin/dichloromethane mixture before adding other ingredients, and therefore, the final products would be identical.

3.9 Formulation without Tween 80

Oral formulations with (G2, DHP107, Table 3) or without Tween 80 (G7) were prepared. Pharmacokinetic profiles were different for these two formulations (Figure 4G). When the formulation without Tween 80 was administered, T_{max} was 1 h instead of 3, and the AUC value was reduced to 6.3 µg·h / ml, which was *ca.* 56 % of that for DHP107.

3.10 Oral administration of the aqueous dispersions of DHP107

Even though our oral paclitaxel formulations including DHP107 can be taken *per se*, they can also be mixed with water or taste-masking syrups for administration. To examine how the absorption of paclitaxel changes upon feeding the dispersion, DHP107 was mixed with water or syrup at 3:7 by weight. DHP107 was dispersed spontaneously in water to produce emulsion droplets having average diameter of 6-8 µm. By vortexing the mixture of DHP107 and water or syrup for 1 min, the diameters of emulsion droplets were reduced to 6 (polydispersity = 1) or 3 (polydispersity = 1) µm, respectively. By sonicating DHP107/water mixture at 180 KW for 1 min, we also obtained the dispersion with the oil droplets having 1.4 µm (polydispersity = 1) in diameter.

When the dispersions were orally administered, pharmacokinetic profiles did not change significantly except for the fact that the AUC values were reduced to *ca.* 40 ~ 70 % of the original G2 formulation.

3.11 Antitumor efficacy of DHP107 in experimental animals

To evaluate the antitumor activity of DHP107 in mice, suspension of NCI-H358 cells was injected subcutaneously to Balb/c athymic mice. All of the mice inoculated with the human non-small cell lung cancer cells developed progressively growing tumors. The mice were administered orally with DHP107 (G2, 50 mg/kg) or intravenously with Taxol® (10 mg/kg) for 5 consecutive days 10 days after the inoculation. The entire tumor tissue was removed surgically after the experiment and photographed as shown in Figure 5A. In the group administered with oral DHP107 and intravenous Taxol®, the tumor size was reduced gradually from *ca.* 100 to 15 ± 3 and 19 ± 5 mm³, respectively, in *ca.* 25 days after the administration of the drug and remained unchanged for the duration of the experiment (Figure 5B). The tumor size data for these two groups were indifferent statistically. In the control group administered orally with the vehicle only, the tumor grew continuously to *ca.* 360 ± 20 mm³ in 45 days.

4. Discussion

In current study, we prepared oil formulations for oral administration of paclitaxel and examined their physical properties, pharmacokinetic profiles and antitumor activities.

Development, Optimization and Absorption Mechanism of DHP107, Oral Paclitaxel Formulation
for Single-Agent Anticancer Therapy

103

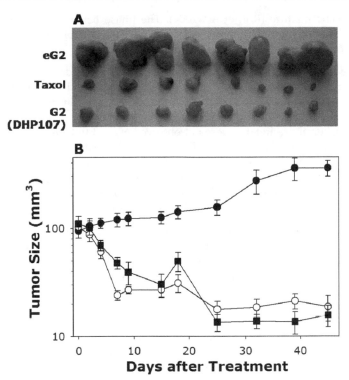

Fig. 5. Antitumor activity of DHP107 in male Balb/c athymic mice, subcutaneously injected
with suspension of NCI-H358 cells (1.2×10⁷ cells/mouse). A) The entire tumor tissue
removed surgically after the experiment. B) The volume of tumor for the oral vehicle control
(eG2, ●), intravenous Taxol® (○, 10mg/kg) and oral DHP107 (G2, ■, 50 mg/kg).

Paclitaxel was commercially available in at least two different polymorphs. Amorphous
paclitaxel was readily soluble in our oral formulations at 10 mg/ml when sonicated for 30 s.
Crystalline paclitaxel, on the other hand, did not dissolve in the oily formulations directly. We
had to dissolve crystalline paclitaxel in the tricaprylin/methylene chloride mixture completely,
and to remove the solvent in turn to obtain the oily solution of paclitaxel/tricaprylin before
adding monoolein and Tween 80. Even though paclitaxel could also be dissolved in methylene
chloride/tricaprylin/monoolein/Tween 80 as well as in methylene chloride/tricaprylin,
monoolein and Tween 80 were not added to the mixture until after evaporating the solvent to
minimize the oxidation of these materials containing unsaturated hydrocarbons.
Pharmacokinetic study showed that AUC values were identical statistically when paclitaxel
from different vendors or different preparation processes was used (Figure 4F).

DSC study was performed for the formulations with different triglycerides. In the heating
thermograms, two endothermic transitions were observed corresponding to the chain
melting transitions of monoolein and triglycerides for T8 and T12 formulations. Chain
melting transition of triacetin, tributyrin and tricaproin were not observed since the phase
transition temperatures of these triglycerides were below 0 °C. There was only a single
endothermic transition for the tricaprin/monoolein mixture at the weight ratio of 2:1 since

they formed a eutectic mixture (Roh et al., 2004). The phase behavior of monoolein and triglycerides could be explained by the classical binary eutectic phase diagram of two immiscible solid phases and a completely miscible melt.

We could conclude from the DSC data that monoolein and tricaprylin do not mix below *ca.* 30 °C where monoolein exists as lamellar crystalline phase. Monoolein and Tween 80 did not mix in this temperature range either. Above 30 °C, however, all three ingredients, tricaprylin, monoolein and Tween 80 existed as liquid and mixed homogeneously. Two important things to note were that paclitaxel precipitates were not observed even at 0 °C by microscopy in any of the oral formulations and that the formulations could be heated and cooled in cycles between -20 and 40 °C without compromising the effectiveness of the drug. These results are significant in that the oral formulation (possibly in a soft capsule) can be stored in the shelf and orally administered in the phase-separated form, but transforms into a homogenous liquid solution by the body heat while traveling inside the gastrointestinal tract.

In our oral formulations, monoolein was included due to its well-known mucoadhesive property (Nielsen et al., 1998). Monoolein and other monoglycerides have been used in oral drug delivery formulations since they can enhance absorption of small molecules and even proteins through the epithelial cells (Ganem-Quintanar et al., 2000; Chung et al., 2002). The absorption enhancing mechanism is not clearly known. Nanopore induction or the membrane perturbation (Anderson, 2005), and the intermediate phases formed in the intestine (Kossena et al., 2005) were considered important. *In vitro* study showed that monoglycerides can enhance the cellular absorption of drugs by inhibition of P-glycoproteins (Konishi et al., 2004). Further studies are required to explain the absorption enhancing mechanism of monoolein unequivocally.

In the previous study, we administered intravesically the dispersion of DHP107 in water to experimental rabbits and observed that the formulation adhered tightly to the bladder mucosa, and paclitaxel penetrated through the physical barrier imposed by the uroepithelium (S. J. Lee et al., 2005). Histological examination of the bladder and other tissues did not reveal any local or systemic toxicity to the rabbits.

Oral administration of formulations containing different triglycerides showed that those with tricaproin, tricaprylin and tricaprin had higher AUC values than others. The formulation with tricaproin had the highest AUC value. We must note that paclitaxel was mixed directly with the vehicles and sonicated for 30 s to obtain the formulations in Table 2. When the preparation process was changed to add and to remove methylene chloride in turn in order to solubilize crystalline as well as amorphous paclitaxel, the AUC value of tricaprylin/monoolein/Tween 80/paclitaxel formulation (G2, DHP107) increased from 8.9 to 11.0 μg·h/ml, which was similar to that of tricaproin/monoolein/Tween 80/paclitaxel formulation in Table 2 (T6) statistically. We proceeded with the tricaprylin/monoolein/Tween 80/paclitaxel formulation for further experiments because the toxicity of tricaprylin (LD50 = 3700 mg/kg; intravenous and 26600 mg/kg; oral) was much lower than that of tricaproin (LD50 = 122 mg/kg; intravenous) for mice according to the Material Safety Data Sheets for tricaprylin (T9126) and tricaproin (T4137) provided by Sigma (www.sigma-aldrich.com).

We also performed the pharmacokinetic study with the formulations having different contents of the drug, under fasting or non-fasting conditions, by changing the commercial source of paclitaxel, with or without the emulsifier, Tween 80 and in the form of dispersions

Development, Optimization and Absorption Mechanism of DHP107, Oral Paclitaxel Formulation
or Single-Agent Anticancer Therapy

105

in syrup or in water. From these experiments, we could conclude that the optimum concentration of paclitaxel in the formulation was 10 mg/ml, and the tricaprylin/monoolein/Tween 80/paclitaxel formulation was the most effective when given directly to the non-fasting animals. Under the fasting conditions, T_{max} was 3 h. T_{max}, however, was 1 h when the animal had free access to food and water. In a separate experiment, we observed that the bile salts helped the micronization and micellization of DHP107. It is possible that the micronization process of DHP107 was fastened by the secreted bile salts already existing under the non-fasting condition. When the formulation was fed to the empty stomach, on the other hand, bile salt secretion would start after the oily DHP107 reaches the upper intestine.

Our liquid type formulations were very effective in delivering paclitaxel orally, easy to prepare, biocompatible, and physically stable. Preclinical studies have demonstrated superior antitumor efficacy and high bioavailability. Most notably, the blood paclitaxel concentration was high after the oral administration even though the P-glycoprotein inhibitors were not co-administered when compared to the formulations reported in the literature (Table 1). The results show that the blood paclitaxel concentration reached as high as *ca.* 3 µg/ml and higher than 1 µg/ml for 4~6 hours in Balb/c mice after oral administration of 50 mg/kg of paclitaxel dose. Also the bioavailability of paclitaxel was *ca.* 14 % and 20 % when compared to Taxol® injection under fasting and non-fasting conditions, respectively.

Antitumor experiment also showed that the tumor regression rate of the oral DHP107 group (50 mg/kg) was similar to that of the intravenous Taxol® group (10 mg/kg). Also, the tumor size of an established non-small cell lung cancer was significantly reduced after the oral treatment. Considering that the bioavailability of DHP107 was *ca.* 14 ~ 20 % compared to Taxol® injection, similar regression rate was expected to a degree.

5. Conclusions

In conclusion, we prepared oral paclitaxel formulations that do not contain P-glycoprotein inhibitors as active pharmaceutical ingredients. The formulations are liquid at body temperature and can solubilize paclitaxel effectively. The oral bioavailability of paclitaxel was 14 ~ 20 % when compared to the intravenous Taxol® formulation without concomitant administration of P-glycoprotein inhibitors. Preclinical efficacy study on mice showed that the tumor size was reduced significantly for the human non-small cell lung carcinoma. In separate studies, we have determined the tissue distribution of paclitaxel after oral administration (manuscript in preparation) and performed pre-clinical antitumor efficacy studies in mice with several tumor types (manuscript in preparation). Regulatory preclinical experiments to initiate the clinical evaluations of DHP107 have also been carried out.

6. References

Anderson, D. (2005) Reversed liquid crystalline phases with non-paraffin hydrophobes. European Patent 1539099A2, 2005

Bardelmeijer, H. A., Beijnen, J. H., Brouwer, K. R., Rosing, H., Nooijen, W. J., Schellens, J. H. M., & van Tellingen, O. (2000) Increased oral bioavailability of paclitaxel by GF120918 in mice through selective modulation of P-glycoprotein. *Clin. Cancer Res.*, Vol. 6. pp. 4416-4421

Bardelmeijer, H. A., Ouwehand, M., Beijnen, J. H., Schellens, J. H. M,. & van Tellingen, O. (2004) Efficacy of novel P-glycoprotein inhibitors to increase the oral uptake of paclitaxel in mice. *Inves. New Drugs,* Vol. 22. pp. 219–229

Briggs, J., Chung, H., & Caffrey, M. (1996) The temperature-composition phase diagram and mesophase structure characterization of the monoolein/water system. *J. Phys. II France,* Vol. 6. pp. 723-751

Choi, J. S., & Li, X. (2005) The effect of verapamil on the pharmacokinetics of paclitaxel in rats. *Eur. J. Pharm. Sci.,* Vol. 24. pp. 95-100

Choi, J. -S., Choi, H. -K., & Shin, S. -C. (2004) Enhanced bioavailability of paclitaxel after oral coadministration with flavone in rats. *Int. J. Pharm.,* Vol. 275. pp. 165-170

Choi, J. -S., Jo, B. -W., & Kim, Y. -C. (2004) Enhanced paclitaxel bioavailability after oral administration paclitaxel or prodrug to rats pretreated with quercetin. *Eur. J. Pharm. Biopharm.,* Vol. 57. pp. 313-318

Chung, H., Kim, J.-s., Um, J. Y., Kwon, I. C., & Jeong, S. Y. (2002) Self-assembled "nanocubicle" as a carrier for peroral insulin delivery. *Diabetologia,* Vol. 45. pp. 448-451

Chung, H., Kim, T. W., Kwon, M., Kwon, I. C., & Jeong, S. Y. (2001) Oil components modulate physical characteristics and function of the natural oil emulsions as drug or gene delivery system. *J. Control. Rel.,* Vol. 71. pp. 339-350

Clogston, J., Craciun, G., Hart D.J., & Caffrey, M. (2005) Controlling release from the lipidic cubic phase by selective alkylation. *J. Cont. Rel.,* Vol. 102. pp. 441-461

Clogston, J., & Caffrey, M. (2005) Controlling release from the lipidic cubic phase. Amino acids, peptides, proteins and nucleic acids. *J. Cont. Rel.,* Vol. 107. pp. 97-111

Clogston, J., Rathman, J., Tomasko, D., Walker, H., & Caffrey, M. (2000) Phase behavior of a monoacylglycerol (Myverol 18-99K)/water system. *Chem. Phys. Lipids,* Vol. 107. pp. 191-220

Ganem-Quintanar, A., Quintanar-Guerrero, & D., Buri, P. (2000) Monoolein: A review of pharmaceutical applications. *Drug Dev. Indust. Pham.,* Vol. 26. pp. 809-820

Gao, P., Rush, B. D., Pfund, W. P., Huang, T., Bauer, J. M., Morozowich, W., Kuo, M. -S., & Hageman, M. J. (2003) Development of a supersaturable SEDDS (S-SEDDS) formulation of paclitaxel with improved oral bioavailability. *J. Pharm. Sci.,* Vol. 92. pp. 2386-2398

Garber, K. (2004) Improved paclitaxel formulation hints at new chemotherapy approach. *J. Natl. Cancer Inst.,* Vol. 96. pp. 90-91

Gianni, L., Kearns, C. M., Giani, A., Capri, G., Vigano, L., Lacatelli, A., Bonadonna, G., & Egorin, M. J. (1995). Nonlinear pharmacokinetics and metabolism of paclitaxel and its pharmacokinetic/pharmacodynamic relationships in humans. *J. Clin. Oncol.,* Vol. 13. pp. 180-190

Hennenfent, K. L., & Govindan, R. (2006) Novel formulations of taxanes: a review. Old wine in a new bottle? *Ann. Oncol.,* Vol. 17. pp. 735 - 749

Hong, J. W., Lee, I. H., Kwok, Y. H., Park, Y. T., Kwon, I. C., Jeong, S. Y., & Chung, H. (2004) The tissue distribution of paclitaxel after peroral administration of mucoadhesive formulation, *Proceedings of Controlled Release Society 31st Annual Meeting,* Honolulu, HA, 2004

Huizing, M. T., Giaccone, G., Van Warmerdam, L. J. C., Rosing, H., Bakker, P. J. M., Vermorken, J. B., Postmus, P. E., Zandwijk, N., van Koolen, M. G. J., ten Bokkel Huinink, W. W., van der Vijgh, W. J., Bierhorst, F. J., Lai, A., Dalesio, O., Pinedo, H. M., Veenhof, C. H., & Beijnen, J. H. (1997) Pharmacokinetics of paclitaxel and carboplatin in a dose escalating and dose sequencing study in patients with non small cell lung cancer. *J. Clin. Oncol.*, Vol. 15. pp. 317–329

Ibrahim, N. K., Desai, N., Legha, S., Soon-Shiong, P., Theriault, R. L., Rivera, E., Esmaeli, B., Ring, S. E., Bedikian, A., Hortobagyi, G. N., & Ellerhorst, J. A. (2002) Phase I and pharmacokinetic study of ABI-007, a Cremophor-free, protein-stabilized, nanoparticle formulation of paclitaxel. *Clin. Cancer Res.*, Vol. 8. pp. 1038-1044

Kan, P., Chen, Z. B., Lee, C. J., & Chu, I. M. (1999) Development of nonionic surfactant/ phospholipids o/w emulsion as a paclitaxel delivery system. *J. Control. Rel.*, Vol. 58. pp. 271– 278

Kearns, C. M., Gianni, L., & Egorin, M. J. (1995). Paclitaxel pharmacokinetics and pharmacodynamics. *Semin. Oncol.*, Vol. 3. pp. 16-23

Kim, D. W., Kwon, J. S., Kim, Y. G., Kim, M. S., Lee, G. S., Youn, T. J., & Cho, M. -C. (2004) Novel oral formulation of paclitaxel inhibits neointimal hyperplasia in a rat carotid artery injury model. *Circulation,* Vol. 109. pp. 1558-1563

Kim, J.-H., Kim, Y.-S., Kim, S., Park, J. H., Kim, K., Choi, K., Chung, H., Jeong, S. Y., Park, R.-W., Kim, I.-S., & Kwon, I. C. (2006) Hydrophobically modified glycol chitosan nanoparticles as carriers for paclitaxel. *J. Cont. Rel.*, Vol. 111. pp. 228-234

Konishi, T., Satsu, H., Hatsugai, Y., Aizawa, K., Inakuma, T., Nagata, S., Sakuda, S.-h., Nagasawa, H., & Shimizu, M. (2004) Inhibitory effect of a bitter melon extract on the P-glycoprotein activity in intestinal Caco-2 cells. *Brit. J. Pharm.*, Vol. 143. pp. 379-387

Kossena, G. A., Charman, W. N., Boyd, B. J., & Porter, C. J. H. (2005) Influence of the intermediate digestion phases of common formulation lipids on the absorption of a poorly water-soluble drug. *J. Pharm. Sci.*, Vol. 94. pp. 481-492

Lee, I. H., Hong, J. W., Y. H., Kwak, Y. H., Park, Y. T., Kwon, I. C., Jeong, S. Y., & Chung, H. (2004) Oral paclitaxel delivery systems, *Proceedings of Controlled Release Society 31st Annual Meeting*, Honolulu, HA, 2004

Lee, I.-H., Park, Y. T., Roh, K., Chung, H., Kwon, I. C., & Jeong, S. Y. (2005) Stable paclitaxel formulations in oily contrast medium. *J. Cont. Rel.*, Vol. 102. pp. 415-425

Lee, J. H., Gi, U.-S., Kim, J.-H., Kim, Y., Kim, S.-H., Oh, H., & Min, B. (2001) Preparation and characterization of solvent induced dihydrated, anhydrous, and amorphous paclitaxel. *Bull. Korean Chem. Soc.*, Vol. 22. pp. 925-928

Lee, S.-J., Kim, S. W., Chung, H., Park, Y. T., Choi, Y. W., Cho, Y.-H., & Yoon, M. S. (2005) Bioadhesive drug delivery system using glyceryl monooleate for the intravesical administration of paclitaxel. *Chemotherapy,* Vol. 51. pp. 311–318

Liggins, R.T., Hunter, W. L., & Burt, H. M. (1997) Solid-state characterization of paclitaxel. *J. Pharm. Sci.,* 86 pp. 1458-1463

Meerum Terwogt, J. M., Malingre, M. M., Beijnen, J. H., ten Bokkel Huinink, W. W., Rosing, H., Koopman, F. J., van Tellingen, O., Swart, M., & Schellens, J. H. M. (1999) Coadministration of oral cyclosporin A enables oral therapy with paclitaxel. *Clin. Cancer Res.*, Vol. 5. pp. 3379– 3384

Nielsen, L. S., Schubert, L., & Hansen, J. (1998) Bioadhesive drug delivery systems. I. Characterisation of mucoadhesive properties of systems based on glyceryl mono-oleate and glyceryl monolinoleate. *Eur. J. Pharm. Sci.*, Vol. 6. pp. 231-239

Peltier, S., Oger, J.-M., Lagarce, F., Couet, W., Benoît, J.-P. (2006) Enhanced oral paclitaxel bioavailability after administration of paclitaxel-loaded lipid nanocapsules. *Pharm. Res.*, Vol. 23. pp. 1243-1250

Pfeifer, R.W., Hale, K.N., Cronquist, & S. E., Daniels, M. (1993) Precipitation of paclitaxel during infusion by pump. *Am. J. Hosp. Pharm.*, Vol. 50. pp. 2518–2521

Qiu, H., & Caffrey, M. (2000) The phase diagram of the monoolein/water system: metastability and equilibrium aspects. *Biomaterials*, Vol. 21. pp. 223-234

Roh, K. H., Lee, S. Y., Kwon, I. C., Jeong, S. Y., & Chung, H. (2004) Hydrophilic polymers stabilize eutectic mixture of monoglyceride and triglyceride. *Proceedings of Biophysical Society 48th Annual Meeting*, Baltimore, MD, 2004

Rowinsky, E. K. & Donehower, R. C. (1995). Paclitaxel (Taxol), *N. Engl. J. Med.*, Vol. 332. pp. 1004-1014

Schellens, J. H. M., Malingre, M. M., Kruijtzer, C. M. F., Bardelmeijer, H. A., van Tellingen, O., Schinkel, A. H., & Beijnen, J. H. (2000) Modulation of oral bioavailability of anticancer drugs: from mouse to man. *Eur. J. Pharm. Sci.*, Vol. 12. pp. 103-110

Shin, B. S., Kim, H. J., Hong, S. H., Lee, J. B., Hwang, S. W., Lee, M. H., & Yoo, S. D. (2009) Enhanced absorption and tissue distribution of paclitaxel following oral administration of DHP 107, a novel mucoadhesive lipid dosage form. *Cancer Chemoth. Pharm.* Vol. 64. Pp. 87-94

Singla, A. K., Garg, A., & Aggarwal, D. (2002) Paclitaxel and its formulations. *Int. J. Pharm.*, Vol. 235. pp. 179-192

Sparreboom, A., Van Asperen, J., Mayer, U., Schinkel, A. H., Smit, J. W., Meijer, D. K. F., Borst, P., Nooijen, W. J., Beijnen, J. H., & Van Tellingen, O. (1997) Limited oral bioavailability and active epithelial excretion of paclitaxel (Taxol) caused by P-glycoprotein in the intestine. *Proc. Natl. Acad. Sci. USA*, Vol. 94. pp. 2031-2035

Sparreboom, A., van Tellingen, O., Nooijen, W. J., & Beijnen, J. H. (1996) Nonlinear pharmacokinetics of paclitaxel in mice results from the pharmaceutical vehicle Cremophor EL. *Cancer Res.*, Vol. 56. pp. 2112-2115

Sugahara, S.-i., Kajiki, M., Kuriyama, H., & obayashi, T.-r. (2007) Complete regression of xenografted human carcinomas by a paclitaxel–carboxymethyl dextran conjugate (AZ10992). *J. Cont. Rel.*, Vol. 117. pp. 40-50

van Asperen, J., van Tellingen, O., Sparreboom, A., Schinkel, A. H., Borst, P., Nooijen, W. J., Beijnen, J. H. (1997) Enhanced oral bioavailability of paclitaxel in mice treated with the P-glycoprotein blocker SDZ PSC 833. *Br. J. Cancer*, Vol. 76. pp. 1181-1183

Van Asperen, J., van Tellingen, O., van der Valk, M. A., Rozenhart, M., & Beijnen, J. H. (1998) Enhanced oral absorption and decreased elimination of paclitaxel in mice cotreated with cyclosporine A. *Clin. Cancer Res.*, Vol. 4. pp. 2293-2297

Weiss, R. B., Donehower, R. C., Wiernik, P. H. T., Ohnuma, R. J., Trump, D. L., Baker Jr, J. R., Van Echo, D. A., Von Hoff, D. D. & Leyland-Jones, B. (1990). Hypersensitivity reactions from taxol, *J. Clin. Oncol.*, Vol. 8. pp. 1263-1268

Woo. J. S., Lee, C. H., Shim, C. K., & Hwang, S. -J. (2003) Enhanced oral bioavailability of paclitaxel by coadministration of the P-glycoprotein inhibitor KR30031. *Pharm. Res.*, Vol. 20. pp. 24-30

Xie, Z., Guan, H., Chen, X., Lu, C., Chen, L., Hu, X., Shi, Q., & Jing, X. A (2007) novel polymer–paclitaxel conjugate based on amphiphilic triblock. *J. Cont. Rel.*, Vol. 117. pp. 210-216

Yang, S., Gursoy, R. N., Lambert, G., & Benita, S. (2004) Enhanced oral absorption of paclitaxel in a novel self-microemulsifying drug delivery system with or without concomitant use of P-glycoprotein inhibitors. *Pharm. Res.*, Vol. 21. pp. 261-270

Yoon, C. J., Chung, J. W., Park, J. H., Yoon, Y. H., Lee, J. W., Jeong, S. Y., & Chung, H. (2003) Transcatheter arterial chemoembolization with paclitaxel-lipiodol solution in rabbit VX2 liver tumor. *Radiology*, Vol. 229. pp. 126-131

5

Differences in the Development of the Small Intestine Between Gnotobiotic and Conventionally Bred Piglets

Soňa Gancarčíková
University of Veterinary Medicine and Pharmacy, Košice
Slovakia

1. Introduction

The health quality of human population is strongly connected to the decrease of environmental burden and increase of quality and safety of food. The production of high-quality and safe food and materials of animal origin is conditioned by the good health of raised animals. Diseases of the gastrointestinal tract can be considered the most important health and economic problem of rearing young animals, since they may cause extremely high losses due to morbidity, mortality, cost of treatment and weight loss. At an early age, diseases debilitate the animal organism and cause delays in development which can subsequently become evident as health problems and decreased productivity. For this reason, it is extremely important to ensure optimum development of the digestive tract in young animals. These relations are determined by digestive juice and enzyme secretion, morphological development and microbial colonization of the digestive tract as well as by absorption capacity of the latter. The pig gut is exposed to a variety of stress factors particularly in the early postnatal period and just after weaning. This is the period of significant growth, morphological changes and maturation of the gastrointestinal tract (Godlewski et al., 2005; Trahair & Sanglid, 2002; Xu, 1996). Prior to birth, the alimentary tract is exposed to substances from the ingested amniotic fluid which seems to be of importance to its development (Trahair & Sanglid, 2002). The colostrum, however, differs from the amniotic fluid by the density of nutrients and high immunoglobulin, enzyme, hormone, growth factor and neuroendocrine peptide levels. Widdowson & Crabb (1976) were the first to demonstrate the effect of the colostrum upon development of the alimentary tract by comparing the colostrums-suckling piglets with watered animals. Maternal colostrums contained high levels of several hormones and growth promoting peptides like insulin, epidermal growth factor (EGF), insulin-like growth factor-I and II (IGF-I and II), transforming growth factor-β (TGF-β), glucagon-like peptide-2 (GLP-2) and leptin. It was proved that colostral growth factors play an important role in the postnatal development of the digestive tract in newborn animals (Guilloteau et al., 2002; Xu, 1996). During the several initial days of life of newborns, their small intestine increases its weight by about 70%, length by approx. 20%, diameter by 15%. Its absorption area increases by about 50% during the first postnatal day and by 100% during the first 10 postnatal days (Marion et al., 2003; Xu, 1996). A large luminal surface area with optimal enterocyte functional maturity is important to young growing pigs so they may attain maximum digestive and absorptive capability. Consequently, suboptimal or adverse environmental factors, influencing the morphological development of intestinal tissue, may have critical functional consequences for the young growing pig. The marked and abrupt morphological responses to weaning in the small intestine, characterized by the transformation from a dense finger-like villi population to a smooth, compact, tongue-shaped luminal villi surface may indicate critical consequences for the young pig digestive capacity and subsequent use of nutrients during the starter phase (Skrzypek et al., 2005). The changes at weaning which include shortening of villi, hyperplasia of crypts, decrease in absorption capacity and certain loss of carbohydrate activity may, in combination with changes in the number and type of enterobacteria, induce various degree of post-weaning diarrhoea (Pluske et al., 1997). By now, the prevention and therapy of diseases of sucklings and weanlings was implemented by means of synthetic substances, which enormously burden not only the organisms, but also the living environment as a whole. The extensive use of antibiotics has increased the risk of development of resistance in human and animal pathogens and chemical residues in meat of animals. In progress is the research and development of new methods of biotechnological and natural character that with their complex influence will maximally make efficient the prevention of diseases of animals by the stabilisation of physiological function of biological barriers of the gastrointestinal tract ecosystem. Biological barriers of digestive tract represent the prime and basal protection of organism from negative impacts of external and internal environment, and therefore it is possible to decrease a health risk by its sophisticated modulation. The indigenous microbiota suppresses colonization of incoming bacteria by a process named colonization resistance that is a first line of defence against invasion by exogenous, potential pathogenic organisms or indigenous opportunists. Beneficial microbiota prevent bacterial colonization by competing for epithelium receptors and enteric nutrients, producing antimicrobial compounds such as bacteriocins and metabolizing nutrients to create a restrictive environment which is generally unfavourable for the growth of many enteric pathogens (Bomba et al., 2002; Marinho et al., 2007). Probiotics as natural bioregulators assist the maintenance of the homeostasis of the gastrointestinal tract ecosystem and, during the critical periods of animal life, can play an important role in prevention of diarrhoeic diseases of dietetic and bacterial origin (Bomba et al., 2002; Marinho et al., 2007). Gastrointestinal microflora may be affected by adding probiotic micro-organisms of genera *Lactobacillus*, *Bifidobacterium* (Bomba et al., 2002), *Bacillus*, *Enterococcus* and *Streptococcus* (Scharek et al., 2005) to feed or by their combinations (Bomba et al., 2002; Mathew et al., 1998). Enterococci belong to those lactic-acid bacteria which inhabit human and animal intestines (Devriese et al., 1991). It was observed that *Enterococcus faecium* prevents adherence of enterotoxigenic *Escherichia coli* K 88+ to the surface of intestinal mucosa of piglets (Scharek et al., 2005). In terms of exactitude and interpretability of results, gnotobiotic piglets are an ideal experimental model for the study of digestive processes and their development. The presence of normal microflora influences the structure of the host intestinal mucous membrane, its function and short-chain fatty acids (SCFAs) production. By means of gnotobiotic conditions, we excluded the influence of the normal microflora and sow's milk. The changes in the small intestine, observed under the specific controlled conditions, were compared to the development of the gut in conventionally bred piglets.

The aim of the study was to evaluate the effects of piglet´s age and diet (natural feeding, artificial feeding and gnotobiotic conditions) on the development of microflora, production of short-chain fatty acids (SCFAs), postnatal morphological development and disaccharidase enzymes activity in the small intestine in piglets reared under the sow, piglets fed on milk replacement, as well as in gnotobiotic piglets.

2. Materials and methods

The experiments on growing and weaned piglets were carried out at the Institute of Microbiology and Gnotobiology, University of Veterinary Medicine and Pharmacy, Košice, Slovakia. The State Veterinary and Food Administration of the Slovak Republic approved the experimental protocols and the animals were handled and sacrificed in a humane manner in accordance with the guidelines established by the relevant commission.

2.1 Animal, housing and diets

2.1.1 Gnotobiotic piglets - 1st experiment

The experiment was carried out in 4 gnotobiotic units, each consisting of reserve, waste and rearing isolator (Velaz s.r.o., Prague, Czech Republic). All experimental materials, including milk substitute, distilled water, saline solution and glass and metal materials were sterilised by autoclaving at 121°C and pressure 1.3 MPa for 30 minutes and cellulose wadding and other sanitary material was gamma-irradiated (Bioster, Veverská Bitýška, Czech Republic). The isolators were sterilized with a 2% solution of peracetic acid (36%, Merci s.r.o., Brno, Czech Republic), sealed for 24 hrs, and vented for a minimum of 72 hrs prior to placing pigs inside. Isolators were maintained under positive pressure, the filtering unit consisting of a fan with preliminary EU 3 filter and two-stage filtering chamber (Velaz s.r.o., Prague, Czech Republic). The first stage of filtration consisted of a frame filter type KS-W, filtration class F 7, the second stage used a KS MIKRO S filter, filtration class H 13, for removing of microparticles. The vented air passed through a frame filter KS W/48, filtration class F 5. The filtration unit assured a minimum of 10 exchanges of air per hour at overpressure of 50-70 kPa and air flow 8-30 m³.

The experiment was carried out on 18 gnotobiotic piglets of Slovak white × Landrace breed. Gnotobiotic sucklings were obtained using the method of open hysterotomy on day 112 of pregnancy. After opening the abdominal cavity and uterus the piglets were immediately transferred through a disinfectant bath containing 2% Incidur® (Ecolab GmbH & Co. OHG, Düsseldorf, Germany) into a hysterectomy box were they were subjected to preliminary treatment and then were placed into 1 of 4 gnotobotic rearing isolators. The floor of isolators was heated by electric underfloor heating system to ensure floor temperature of 34°C for new born piglets and 30°C for 7-14 days old piglets. The piglets were non-colostral and were fed autoclaved milk substitute (Sanolac Ferkel, Germany, in 1 kg dry matter: fat 18.0%, N-free extract 20.0%, lysine 1.7%, Ca 0.9%, P 0.7%, Na 1.0%, Mg 0.2%, fibre 1.5%, ash 10.0%, ME 17.5 MJ, vitamin A 50 000 IU, vitamin D_3 5 000 IU, vitamin E 100 mg, biotin 200 µg, Fe 100 mg, vitamin B_1 4 mg, vitamin B_2 4 mg, vitamin B_6 2 mg, vitamin B_{12} 20 µg, calcium pantothenate 10 mg, nicotinic acid 20 mg, folic acid 1 mg, vitamin C 100 mg, choline chloride 250 mg), diluted 1 : 5 with distilled water. The milk substitute was fed to piglets individually from a glass bottle six times daily (2, 6, 10, 14, 18, 22 h), ad libitum. A total of 18 gnotobiotic animals derived from 2 litters were divided into 4 isolators. From the first day of life, a probiotic strain of Enterococcus faecium isolated from non autoclaved milk substitute (Sanolac Ferkel, Germany) was administered continuously at a dose of 2 ml of inoculum;

1 ml contained 1×10^4 cfu (data analysed in the Laboratory of Gnotobiology). From the 5th day of life, autoclaved water was available to piglets *ad libitum* and they were fed irradiation-sterilized rations intended for early weaning of piglets. At the age of 28 days, the suckling piglets were weaned and fed irradiation-sterilized starter feedstuff *ad libitum* (OŠ-02®, Tajba Čaňa, Slovak Republic, in 1 kg dry matter: crude protein 180 g, fibre 45 g, lysine 11.5 g, methionine and cysteine 6.3 g, threonine 7.5 g, Ca 7 g, P 5.8 g, Na 1.5 g, Cu 10 mg, Zn 100 mg, Mn 30 mg, ME 13 MJ, vitamin A 8 000 IU, vitamin D_3 1 000 IU, vitamin E 20 mg, Fe 125 mg, vitamin B_2 3 mg, vitamin B_{12} 20 µg, choline 600 mg). A routine microbiological control of gnotobiotic isolators was performed throughout the experiment. Microbiological swabs were taken from isolator walls, surface of animals and from their rectum. The samples were cultivated in PYG medium (Imuna, Slovak Republic). The microbiological control was verified every day on TSA agar with 5% ram's blood (BBL, Microbiology systems, Cockeysville, USA).

2.1.2 Conventional suckled piglets - 2nd experiment

In the experiment, 24 piglets of both sexes (Large white breed x Landrace) from two litters were included. The pigs were housed in two pens, 12 piglets in each, equipped with automatic heating, forced ventilation and completely slatted floors. The suckling piglets had access to sows 6 times daily (2, 6, 10, 14, 18, 22 h.) and from day 5 onwards the animals were provided commercial mixed feed OŠ-01® (Tajba Čaňa, Slovak Republic, in 1 kg dry matter: crude protein 200 g, fibre 40 g, lysine 14 g, methionine and cysteine 6.3 g, threonine 9.1 g, Ca 8 g, P 6.7 g, Na 2 g, Cu 10 mg, Zn 100 mg, Mn 30 mg, ME 13.3 MJ, vitamin A 8 000 IU, vitamin D_3 1 000 IU, vitamin E 20 mg, Fe 125 mg, vitamin B_2 3 mg, vitamin B_{12} 20 µg, choline 300 mg) *ad libitum*. The piglets were weaned at 28 days of age, fed starter feedstuff *ad libitum* (OŠ-02®, Tajba Čaňa, Slovak Republic) and moved to 2 pens (375 x 165 cm) where three piglets were housed per pen. The temperature in the nursery was maintained at 32°C during the first week, and was gradually reduced to 25°C between weeks two and six. The animals had free access to water throughout the experiment (42 days).

2.1.3 Conventional replacer-fed piglets - 3rd experiment

The experiment included 26 piglets of both sexes (Large white breed x Landrace) from two litters. The experiment was carried out in two blocks, 13 piglets in each. The piglets were separated from the sow immediately after birth and had no contact with sow faeces. They were born naturally, were non-colostral, and were fed a commercial milk replacer diluted with distilled water 1:5 (Sanolac Ferkel, Germany), enriched by *Enterococcus faecium* 0.1×10^4 cfu/g of feed. Milk was given to piglets individually from a glass bottle 6 times daily (2, 6, 10, 14, 18, 22 h.), *ad libitum*. Starting from day 5, the suckling piglets were offered the same commercial mixed feed OŠ-01® (Tajba Čaňa, Slovak Republic) and were housed under the same hygiene conditions as those in the second experiment.

2.2 Experimental procedure

All pigs were sacrificed by intracardial euthanasia with 1 ml/kg BW T61® (Intervet International B.V. Boxmeer, The Netherlands). In the first experiment, three hours after birth and at the age of two and seven days, two piglets of each indicated age were sacrificed. Three piglets of each indicated age were sacrificed at the age of 14, 21, 28 and 35 days. In the course of conventional experiments, three piglets from each group were sacrificed at 3 hours post partum and at 2, 7, 14, 21, and 28 days of age. In the second experiment the piglets were slaughtered also on days 35 and 42 of age. The gastrointestinal tract was immediately removed and divided into six segments as follows: stomach, three equal segments of the small intestine, caecum and colon. The total content of each segment was weighed, pH was immediately measured. Intestinal tissue (1 cm^2) were taken from the duodenum (5 cm distal to the orifice of the pancreatic duct) and the medial part of both the jejunum and ileum. The samples were fixed in 4% formalin solution for microscopic assessment of mucosal morphology. Sections of jejunum, ileum and caecum (1 g) were collected and processed for microbial counting and short-chain fatty acids (SCFAs) determinations were carried out in the contents from jejunum, ileum and colon. The intestinal segments (duodenum, jejunum and ileum) were rinsed thoroughly with ice-cold saline solution, opened lengthwise and blotted dry. The mucosa was scraped using a glass slide and immediately frozen in liquid nitrogen. Samples of mucosa were then stored at -70°C until the analysis of digestive enzyme activities.

2.2.1 Microbiological analysis

For microbial analysis, about 1 g of samples (jejunum, ileum, caecum) was placed in a sterile polyethylene stomacher Lab Blender bag (Seward Medical Limited, London, UK) with 9 ml of sterile anaerobic diluent (0.4 g Na HCO$_3$, 0.05g L-cysteine HCl, 1 ml resazurine 0.1%), 7.5 ml mineral solution I (0.6% K$_2$HPO$_4$), 7.5 ml mineral solution II (1.2% NaCl, 1.2% (NH$_4$)$_2$SO$_4$, 0.6% KH$_2$PO$_4$, 0.12% CaCl$_2$, 0.25% MgSO$_4$ and 84 ml distilled water, pH 6.8) and stomached (Stomacher Lab Blender 80, Seward Medical Limited, London, UK) for 5 min under a CO$_2$ atmosphere. A series of 10-fold dilutions (10^{-2} to 10^{-8}) were made in the same diluents. From appropriate dilutions, 0.1 ml aliquots were spread onto one non-selective agar plate: trypticase soy blood agar with 10% sheep blood (BBL, Microbiology systems, Cockeysville, USA) for aerobes. Aliquots (0.1 ml) were also spread on 5 selective agar media as follows: Beerens medium (Beerens, 1990) for *Bifidobacterium,* Rogosa agar (Imuna, Šarišské Michaľany, Slovak Republic) for *Lactobacillus,* Enterococcosel agar (BBL) for *Enterococcus,* MacConkey agar (Imuna) for *Coliforms* and Endo agar (Imuna) for *Enterobacteriaceae.* Plates for the enumeration of *aerobic* bacteria were incubated for 2 days at 37°C. Colonies were counted and bacteria were Gram stained and visualized under a microscope for morphological characterization. The viable counts are expressed as the log 10 of colony forming units (cfu)g^{-1} of sample.

2.2.2 Biochemical analysis

After the collection, 1 g of digesta (jejunum, ileum, colon) was diluted in 50 ml of deionized H$_2$O and applied at a volume of 30 μl for analysis of SCFAs. The concentration of formic, acetoacetic, lactic, succinic, acetic, propionic, butyric and valeric acids in the intestinal content was determined by capillary isotachophoresis (ITP). The measurements were done on an „Isotachophoretic analyser ZKI 01" (SR). In the pre-separation capillary, a leading electrolyte of the following composition was used: 10^{-2} M HCl + 2.2. 10^{-2} M ε-aminocaproic acid + 0.1% methylhydroxyethylcellulosic acid, pH 4.3. As finishing electrolyte, a solution of 5.10^{-3} M caproic acid + histidine was used. This electrolytic system worked at 250μA in pre-separation and 50 μA in the analytic capillary. pH was measured by a pH meter (LP Prague, Czech Republic).

2.2.3 Disaccharidase activity

The lactase (EC 3.2.1.23), maltase (EC 3.2.1.20) and saccharase (EC 3.2.1.26) activities were measured according to Mir et al. (1997). Mucosa samples (200 mg) were homogenized for 3 min with 1 mL saline solution at 0°C. The homogenate was transferred to a test tube together with 2.5 mL (2 × aliquot) of saline solution. Three reaction tubes were filled with 100 µL of the homogenate and placed in a 37°C water bath, and then 400 µL of 56 mM lactose, maltose, saccharose in citrate buffer (pH 6.6, 0.01 mM) were added, respectively. After shaking and incubation for 30 min enzyme activity was stopped in boiling water. The reaction tubes were centrifuged at 2000 × g (30 min, 5°C). The individual enzymes were determined using enzymatic UV method (Boehringer Mannheim, Germany). Protein content in homogenate was started according to Bradford et al. (1976) and the results were expressed as µmol/ mg protein/ hour.

2.2.4 Small intestinal morphology

Fixed intestinal segments were rinsed with water, the samples were dehydrated in a graded series of absolute ethanol (30%, 50%, 70%, 90%), cleared with benzene, saturated with and embedded in paraffin. Sections of 7 µm thickness (10 slices of each sample) were stained with haematoxylin/eosin and observed under a light microscope. The length of 10 villi and depth of 10 crypts was determined by a computer operated Image C picture analysis system (Intronic GmbH, Berlin, Germany) and the IMES analysis software, using a colour video camera (Sony 3 CCD) and a light microscope (Axiolab, Carl Zeiss Jena, Germany).

2.2.5 Statistical analysis

Statistical analysis was performed using Statistic software PRIZMA (version 3.0). All the data were presented as means ± SEM. To estimate the effect of age and weaning on the concentration of SCFAs, bacterial count, disaccharidase activity and intestinal morphology, the data were evaluated statistically by one-way analysis of variance (ANOVA) followed by a multiple comparison Tukey´s test. Significant differences between the two groups of piglets were tested using analysis of variance and Student´s t-test. Probability values less than 0.05 were used as the criterion for statistical significance.

3. Results

3.1 Health status of animals

The deficit of colostral feeding on day 4 of life caused clinical symptoms of disease in 8 replacer-fed piglets (i.e. 30.8 % of the total number of 26 piglets). The other piglets from this group were healthy. The sick piglets were apathic and did not show any interest in feeding. The disease was peracute and proceeded with physiological temperature. Even though antibiotics were administered, the piglets died within 8 hrs of the first appearance of symptoms. Rectal smears and blood for hematological examination were taken from the piglets and both pathological and anatomical dissections were carried out. In the piglets, lymphocytic leukocytosis as well as hypochromic anaemia were diagnosed, and *E. coli* K88 was isolated from rectal swabs. The colonies from the final dilutions were verified by slide agglutination with K88ab antiserum (Imuna Šarišské Michaľany, Slovakia). The pathological and anatomical dissection for peracuteness of the course of the disease revealed only petechial bleeding on seroses and mucoses of the gastrointestinal tract. Transudate in the abdominal cavity was of a deep-red colour, and the blood was uncoagulated. In the groups of suckled piglets (natural feeding) and gnotobiotic piglets the health status was good.

3.2 Acidity

The actual acidity of stomach digesta in replacer-fed piglets ranged more widely - i.e. from pH 1.7 to 3.8. During the period of observation, only on day 2 of age the pH of stomach contents of these piglets was significantly lower ($p<0.01$, $p<0.05$) than in suckled piglets with pH ranging from 2.9 to 3.7 and gnotobiotic piglets with 2.7 - 4.1 pH range (Table 1). In the proximal segment of GIT (content of duodenum and jejunum) of gnotobiotic piglets we recorded between days 7 and 28 days of age the lowest levels of pH which differed significantly on day 14 of age ($p<0.001$) in duodenum and on day 21 of age ($p<0.01$) in jejunum in comparison with replacer-fed piglets. The pH level in the caudal segment of GIT (ileal content) of suckled piglets was lower in comparison with replacer-fed piglets and significantly lower on days 2 ($p<0.05$) and 21 ($p<0.01$) of age. The ileal and colonic pH were on average lower by 0.08 to 0.5 in the group of suckled piglets and the pH values ranged from 6.27 to 7.17 and from 6.50 to 7.21 compared to replacer-fed piglets in which the pH of the ileal content ranged from 6.93 to 7.64 and the pH of the colonic content ranged from 6.24 to 7.53.

3.3 Effect of age and weaning on production of SCFAs in the intestinal tract of gnotobiotic and conventionally bred piglets

3.3.1 Conventional suckled piglets (natural feeding)

Concentration of both acetoacetic and acetic acid in the jejunal content of suckled piglets (Table 2) within the period of milk nutrition was the highest at 7 days of age ($p < 0.001$ and $p < 0.01$, respectively). Subsequently the values declined at 2 weeks of age to 14.76 mmol/l of acetoacetic and to 28.02 mmol/l of acetic acid. This decline continued in acetoacetic acid by day 35 of age to 6.10 mmol/l and in acetic acid by week 4 of life to 7.71 mmol/l ($p < 0.01$). The concentration of lactic acid in jejunal contents was comparable to that of both acetoacetic and acetic acid, with a mean decline of 11.85 mmol lactic acid/l between day 2 and day 21. But a pronounced increase in the concentration of lactic acid was recorded at 1st week post-weaning - i.e. 53.91 mmol/l. The course of the concentration of both acetoacetic and lactic acid in the ileal content (Table 3) was largely similar to that recorded in the jejunal content. Under the influence of more diverse populations of microorganisms, the conditions in the colonic content changed. Propionic acid concentration (Table 4) increased gradually up to weaning (28 days) and then markedly after weaning (day 35: $p < 0.01$ and on day 42: $p < 0.05$). The most pronounced production of acids in the colonic content was observed in acetoacetic acid with highest concentrations at day 14 and 28 of age ($p < 0.001$ and $p < 0.001$) and a sudden 4-fold decline at 1st week post-weaning ($p < 0.01$). In acetic acid, a gradual increase in values was recorded from 7 days of age (11.91 mmol/l), with its highest concentration at 2 weeks post-weaning ($p < 0.001$).

3.3.2 Conventional replacer-fed piglets (artificial feeding)

In both acetoacetic and lactic acid, the highest levels in the jejunal content in replacer-fed piglets (Table 2) were recorded at 7 days of age (19.89 mmol/l and 24.92 mmol/l, $p < 0.01$,

	Segments of GIT						p - value	
	St	D	J	Ile	C	SEM	SC × RFP	GP × RFP
Day 2								
Suckled piglets	3.7	5.5	6.1	6.6a	7.2	0.27	p < 0.05	-
Replacer-fed piglets	1.7ba	5.7	6.8	7.4	7.4	0.12	p < 0.01	p < 0.05
Gnotobiotic piglets	4.1	ND	7.2	8.0	7.7	0.39	-	-
Day 7								
Suckled piglets	2.9	5.6	6.2	6.3	6.5	0.09	NS	-
Replacer-fed piglets	3.8	5.8	6.0	6.9	6.3b	0.22	NS	p < 0.01
Gnotobiotic piglets	4.1	4.5	5.9	7.4	7.0	0.56	-	-
Day 14								
Suckled piglets	3.4	5.4	6.1	7.2	6.7	0.09	NS	-
Replacer-fed piglets	2.5	5.5	5.9	7.1	7.5	0.18	NS	-
Gnotobiotic piglets	3.5	4.2c	5.4	7.0	6.4	0.23	-	p < 0.001
Day 21							p < 0.05	
Suckled piglets	3.3	5.2	6.2a	6.8b	7.4	0.15	p < 0.01	-
Replacer-fed piglets	3.4	5.4	6.7	7.5	7.5	0.23	-	-
Gnotobiotic piglets	3.1	4.2	5.9b	6.9	6.7	0.34	-	p < 0.01
Day 28								
Suckled piglets	3.2	5.8	5.9	6.6	6.5	0.18	NS	-
Replacer-fed piglets	2.9	6.0	6.7	7.6	6.2	0.25	NS	NS
Gnotobiotic piglets	2.7	4.4	5.8	6.7	6.6	0.34	-	NS

ND- not detectable, NS- not significant, SP- suckled piglets, GP- gnotobiotic piglets, RFP- replacer-fed piglets, St- stomach, D- duodenum, J- jejunum, Ile- ileum, C- colon, GIT- gastrointestinal tract
Significantly different (SP,GP vs RFP): a (p < 0.05), b (p < 0.01), c (p < 0.001)

Table 1. The pH along the gastrointestinal tract of gnotobiotic and conventionally bred piglets

respectively), with a slight decline in the concentration up to the end of observation. Concentrations of acetoacetic acid in the colonic content (Table 4) were similar to those in the jejunal content except on day 7 of age when a value of 24.09 mmol/l was recorded (p < 0.05). With lactic acid, the highest concentration was seen on day 7 of age (31.17 mmol/l), with a sudden 10-fold decline from day 14 of age (3.15 mmol/l) up to 28 days of life. Acetic acid concentration was relatively stable from 2 to 21 days of life. Thereafter, a marked increase in the concentration was observed at 4 weeks of life (p < 0.01).

3.3.3 Gnotobiotic piglets

The concentration of acetoacetic acid in the jejunal content of gnotobiotic piglets (Table 2) reached the highest level at the age of 7 days, in the period of milk nutrition (p < 0.05), in comparison with the concentration recorded three hours after birth (3.35 mmol/l). A more

	Age (days)									p - value					
	0	2	7	14	21	28	35	42	SEM	0 × 7	2 × 7	7 × 28	28 × 35	SC × RFP	GP × RFP
Formic acid															
Suckled piglets	ND	4.86	5.09	5.77	7.82	8.49	11.74	8.49	1.37	NS	NS	NS	NS	NS	-
Replacer-fed piglets	ND	7.00a	10.85a	11.50	7.21a	ND	ND	ND	1.82	NS	NS	-	-	p < 0.05	p < 0.05
Gnotobiotic piglets	1.00	6.64	7.54	4.46	3.62	10.67	4.58	ND	1.20	NS	NS	NS	NS	-	NS
Acetoacetic acid															
Suckled piglets	ND	18.12	28.69***	14.76	9.11	10.51	6.10	13.51	2.96	NS	p< 0.001	NS	NS	NS	-
Replacer-fed piglets	ND	9.11a	19.89	9.05	12.24	ND	ND	ND	1.81	NS	NS	-	-	NS	p< 0.05
Gnotobiotic piglets	3.35	6.47	17.78*	17.70	12.93	13.26	8.02*	ND	2.40	p < 0.05	NS	NS	p < 0.05	-	NS
Lactic acid															
Suckled piglets	ND	22.98	27.52*	18.18	11.13	17.89	53.91	30.26	8.17	NS	p < 0.05	NS	NS	NS	-
Replacer-fed piglets	ND	17.61	24.92**	23.75	21.98b	ND	ND	ND	1.10	NS	p < 0.01	-	-	p < 0.01	NS
Gnotobiotic piglets	14.22	16.57	23.59	19.96	21.94	21.38	31.25	ND	3.22	NS	NS	NS	NS	-	NS
Succinic acid															
Suckled piglets	ND	9.05	15.10	11.74c	5.36	4.24	5.92	11.74	1.77	NS	NS	NS	NS	p < 0.001	-
Replacer-fed piglets	ND	2.68	6.44	4.59	6.87	ND	ND	ND	0.89	NS	NS	-	-	NS	NS
Gnotobiotic piglets	2.01	2.01	2.67	4.09	5.79	6.03	4.40	ND	0.66	NS	NS	NS	NS	-	NS
Acetic acid															
Suckled piglets	8.50	21.14a	33.05**	28.02c	10.17	7.71**	11.45	11.69	2.99	NS	p < 0.01	p < 0.01	NS	p< 0.05, p< 0.001	-
Replacer-fed piglets	ND	6.71	21.43	13.49a	14.08	ND	ND	ND	2.49	NS	NS	-	(0×28) p < 0.01	NS	p < 0.05
Gnotobiotic piglets	6.57	5.20	8.18	5.80	12.86**	22.11**	15.95	ND	1.75	NS	NS	NS	p < 0.01	-	NS

Table 2. Effect of age, weaning and diets on production of SCFAs in the jejunum (mmol/l) of gnotobiotic and conventionally bred piglets. ND- not detectable, NS- not significant, SP- suckled piglets, GP- gnotobiotic piglets, RFP- replacer-fed piglets. Significantly different (SC,GP vs RFP): a (p < 0.05), b (p < 0.01), c (p < 0.001)

pronounced post-weaning decrease in the level of acetoacetic acid was recorded one week after weaning (p < 0.05). The proportion of lactic acid was relatively stable from day 7 to 28 of life and ranged between 19.96 and 23.59 mmol/l. Afterwards, in the 5th week of life, the lactic acid level increased to 31.25 mmol/l. Similarly, acetic acid level was relatively stable during the first two weeks of life of piglets, then increased significantly (p < 0.01) at the age of 28 days compared to the level at 3 hours after birth (6.57 mmol/l). The most important production of acids in the colon of gnotobiotic piglets (Table 4) was the production of acetic acid which remained relatively stable between days 7 and 35 of life and the difference between its concentration recorded at 3 hours after the birth (6.94 mmol/l) and that determined on day 7 of life (41.98 mmol/l) was significant (p < 0.05). A significant difference in concentration of lactic acid was recorded on day 28 of age (p < 0.001, p < 0.01) compared to the level on the second day (8.18 mmol/l) and 21st day (14.49 mmol/l). Subsequently, we recorded a non-significant, 3-fold increase in the level of this acid at 5 weeks of age (to 76.30 mmol/l). A similar tendency was recorded for acetoacetic and propionic acid in the colonal content with the exception of the level recorded at 3 hours after the birth. The level of acetoacetic acid was significantly higher on day 21 of age (16.22 mmol/l, p < 0.01) compared to the second day of life (6.71 mmol/l).

3.4 Effect of diets on production of SCFAs in the intestinal tract of gnotobiotic and conventionally bred piglets

The concentration of acetoacetic acid in the jejunal content (Table 2) was higher in suckled piglets at 7 days of life (28.69 mmol/l) compared to the replacer-fed animals in which the level of the above acid represented 19.89 mmol/l. In both groups of piglets observed, well-balanced levels of the above acid were recorded thereafter. The course of the concentration of lactic acid up to day 7 of age was the same in 3 groups of piglets with a subsequent increase in replacer-fed piglets at 21 days of age (p < 0.01) compared to suckled animals. In the acetic acid of suckled piglets, significantly higher levels were recorded at day 2 and 14 of age compared to the replacer-fed piglets (p < 0.05, p < 0.001). The proportion of acetic acid in gnotobiotic piglets was up to two weeks of life considerably lower in comparison with both investigated groups and the decrease on day 14 of life was significant (p < 0.05) in comparison with replacer-fed piglets. The course of the concentration of acetoacetic acid in the ileal content (Table 3) was the same in all 3 observed groups except at 3 weeks of age of replacer-fed piglets. While the content of acetoacetic acid represented 17.11 mmol/l in suckled piglets at 3 weeks of life, in the non-colostral group a decline to 8.78 mmol/l was observed. The level of acetic acid in the ileal contents of suckled piglets was higher throughout the period of investigation ranging from about 7 to 21.5 mmol/l compared with the replacer-fed piglets which showed the highest concentration on day 2 (p < 0.001) and 14 of life (p < 0.05). Insignificantly higher concentrations of acetic acid in the ileal content were observed also in gnotobiotic piglets (2.05 - 13.69 mmol/l) compared to replacer-fed piglets. A similar tendency was recorded in lactic acid, in the ileal content up to 14 days of age, with higher concentrations in suckled piglets as compared to the replacer-fed piglets in which the values later ranged about 8.2 till 21.4 mmol/l and a significantly higher level of the acid was recorded at 7 days of age (p < 0.001). Higher production of lactic acid by gnotobiotic piglets (0.6 - 10.14 mmol/l) was observed throughout the observation period in comparison with replacer-fed piglets with a significant increase on day 7 of age (p < 0.01).

	Age (days)								SEM	p - value		
	0	2	7	14	21	28	35	42		28 × 35	SC × RFP	GP × RFP
Formic acid												
Suckled piglets	ND	6.37	6.70	4.79	9.23	14.65	12.19	13.08	1.50	NS	NS	-
Replacer-fed piglets	ND	9.66	8.38	14.35a	8.55	7.41	ND	ND	1.20	-	p < 0.05	NS
Gnotobiotic piglets	3.28	9.02	26.17	22.82	20.84a	12.68	21.47	ND	3.57	NS	-	p < 0.05
Acetoacetic acid												
Suckled piglets	ND	9.06	26.17	13.58	17.11	14.16	4.18*	5.14	3.48	p < 0.05	NS	-
Replacer-fed piglets	ND	5.39	22.48	10.12a	8.78	9.13	ND	ND	2.75	-	NS	p < 0.05
Gnotobiotic piglets	6.37	6.84	13.42	6.14	13.08	7.68	6.17	ND	2.00	NS	-	NS
Lactic acid												
Suckled piglets	ND	25.63	26.91c	21.64	15.52	37.58	60.11	55.90	12.61	NS	p < 0.001	-
Replacer-fed piglets	ND	6.27	14.42	13.41	20.30	16.17	ND	ND	1.79	-	NS	NS
Gnotobiotic piglets	8.72	6.87	24.56b	12.25	24.40	20.67	23.73	ND	7.34	NS	-	p < 0.01
Succinic acid												
Suckled piglets	ND	7.24	23.62	11.07c	11.07	9.72	4.85	5.47	1.97	NS	p < 0.001	-
Replacer-fed piglets	ND	4.72	2.91	3.40	8.38	7.51	ND	ND	0.85	-	NS	NS
Gnotobiotic piglets	1.87	2.91	3.69	4.56	5.02	5.03	2.50	ND	0.79	NS	-	NS
Acetic acid												
Suckled piglets	ND	35.23c	21.81	27.18a	25.00	34.00	11.34	15.83	5.74	NS	p < 0.05, p < 0.001	-
Replacer-fed piglets	ND	15.10	10.47	20.13	19.86	13.43	ND	ND	2.03	-	NS	NS
Gnotobiotic piglets	7.71	11.14	24.16	22.18	32.08	21.58	25.41	ND	5.48	NS	-	NS
Propionic acid												
Suckled piglets	ND	ND	3.18	6.71	8.38	ND	ND	ND	1.06	-	NS	-
Replacer-fed piglets	ND	ND	5.30	4.57	5.03	7.24	ND	ND	1.36	-	NS	NS
Gnotobiotic piglets	ND	2.21	6.17	ND	1.84	3.52	1.17	ND	0.48	NS	-	NS
Butyric acid												
Suckled piglets	ND	2.68	ND	ND	1.67	ND	2.25	3.48	0.68	-	NS	-
Replacer-fed piglets	ND	2.51	ND	ND	ND	3.02	ND	ND	0.84	-	NS	NS
Gnotobiotic piglets	ND	2.01	ND	3.52	3.38	7.24	1.71	ND	1.03	NS	-	NS

Table 3. Effect of age, weaning and diets on production of SCFAs in the ileum (mmol/l) of gnotobiotic and conventionally bred piglets. ND - not detectable, NS- not significant, SP-suckled piglets, GP- gnotobiotic piglets, RFP- replacer-fed piglets. Significantly different (SP,GP vs RFP): a (p < 0.05), b (p < 0.01), c (p < 0.001)

The value of acetoacetic acid in the colonic content (Table 4) was significantly higher in the group of suckled piglets from day 14 to 28 of age (p < 0.01), compared to replacer-fed

	Age (days) 0	2	7	14	21	28	35	42	SEM	2 × 7	7 × 14	21 × 28	28 × 35	28 × 42	SC × RFP	GP × RFP
Formic acid																
Suckled piglets	9.22	3.85	4.12	5.03	6.59	6.04	9.29	8.04	0.67	NS	NS	NS	NS	NS	NS	-
Replacer-fed piglets	5.36	7.21b	10.77c	6.94	6.20b	5.36	ND	ND	0.83	NS	NS	NS	NS	-	p < 0.01, p < 0.001	p < 0.01
Gnotobiotic piglets	3.08	9.73	5.56	5.90	2.76	2.48	2.01	ND	1.43	NS	NS	NS	NS	-	-	NS
Acetoacetic acid																
Suckled piglets	3.18	7.55	12.91	71.3b***	54.58b	67.2b***	16.95**	18.00	4.39	NS	p<0.001	NS	p < 0.01	p<0.001	p < 0.01	-
Replacer-fed piglets	3.55	11.50a	24.09*	12.41	8.58	8.69	ND	ND	1.37	p < 0.05	NS	NS	-	-	p < 0.05	NS
Gnotobiotic piglets	9.09	6.71	10.57	22.85	16.22**	18.29	12.84	ND	3.12	NS	NS	NS	p < 0.01 (2×21)	-	-	p < 0.001
Lactic acid																
Suckled piglets	5.09	5.19	3.01	3.23	2.23	3.35	4.36	4.02	0.42	NS	NS	NS	NS	NS	NS	-
Replacer-fed piglets	6.94	4.96	31.17	3.15	4.19	4.69	ND	ND	2.96	NS	NS	NS	-	-	NS	NS
Gnotobiotic piglets	21.61	8.18a	19.09	19.39b	14.49b	26.34b ** ***	76.3	ND	6.42	NS	NS	p < 0.01	p < 0.001 (2×28)	-	-	p<0.05, p<0.01
Acetic acid																
Suckled piglets	27.17b	15.17	11.91	46.81***	57.22	71.14	89.99*	95.3 ***	2.39	NS	p<0.001	NS	p < 0.05	p<0.001	p < 0.01	-
Replacer-fed piglets	11.47	44.86bb	46.03	46.06	49.66	64.13a**	ND	ND	6.95	NS	NS	p < 0.01	NS	NS	p < 0.01	p<0.01, p<0.05
Gnotobiotic piglets	6.94	10.06	41.98*	44.96	44.20**	44.90	46.95	ND	8.05	p < 0.05	NS	NS	NS	NS	-	NS
Propionic acid																
Suckled piglets	8.72	ND	ND	16.27	13.08	22.59	59.63**	71.14*	4.46	NS	NS	NS	p < 0.01	p < 0.05	NS	-
Replacer-fed piglets	6.37	ND	11.07	14.76	18.28b	21.81b	ND	ND	4.18	NS	NS	NS	-	-	NS	p < 0.01
Gnotobiotic piglets	1.34	4.69	5.02	9.73	5.52	7.37	6.54	ND	1.28	NS	NS	NS	NS	-	-	NS
Butyric acid																
Suckled piglets	ND	3.39	2.01	11.74	14.76	14.43	11.40	14.65	3.74	NS	NS	NS	NS	NS	-	-
Replacer-fed piglets	2.55	11.12a	17.11	14.93	3.35	3.35	ND	ND	2.25	NS	NS	NS	-	-	p < 0.05	NS
Gnotobiotic piglets	3.02	ND	3.01	8.21	6.28	3.35	2.14	ND	1.27	-	NS	NS	NS	-	-	NS
Valeric acid																
Suckled piglets	ND	ND	ND	ND	5.53	3.91	6.71	5.20	0.68	-	-	NS	NS	NS	NS	-
Replacer-fed piglets	ND	5.03	2.01	2.14	ND	ND	ND	ND	0.60	NS	NS	-	-	-	NS	NS
Gnotobiotic piglets	ND	ND	ND	ND	ND	5.26	ND	2.93	1.57	-	-	-	-	-	-	-

Table 4. Effect of age, weaning and diets on production of SCFAs in the colon (mmol/l) of gnotobiotic and conventionally bred piglets. ND- not detectable, NS- not significant, SP-suckled piglets, GP- gnotobiotic piglets, RFP- replacer-fed piglets. Significantly different (SP,GP vs RFP): a (p < 0.05), b (p < 0.01), c (p < 0.001)

piglets. In the period between weeks 2 to 4 of life, production of this acid by gnotobiotic piglets was also higher in comparison with replacer-fed piglets with significant increase at 3 weeks of life (p < 0.001). While the dynamics of lactic acid in the colon of suckled and replacer-fed piglets was similar with the exception of week 1, and its levels were low and did not exceed 7 mmol/l, gnotobiotic piglets produced higher level of this acid with peaks at 2 days (p < 0.05) and 14, 21 and 28 days of age (p < 0.01) compared to the replacer-fed animals. Dynamics of acetic acid in colonal content of suckled piglets resembled that in jejunal and ileal contents and reached higher levels with the exception of days 2 and 7 of age. Significant difference (p < 0.01) was observed at 3 hours after the birth in comparison with replacer-fed piglets. Acetic acid in replacer-fed piglets showed an opposite trend in the proximal section of the intestinal tract where we recorded a gradual increase in concentrations up to the end of observation with highest levels at 2 days (p < 0.01) and 28 days of age (p < 0.05) compared to the gnotobiotic piglets. In the colon of replacer-fed piglets we recorded also higher production of propionic acid on days 21 and 28 of age (p < 0.01) compared to the gnotobiotic piglets and butyric acid at 2 days of age (p < 0.05) compared to suckled piglets.

3.5 Effect of diets on development of microflora in the digestive tract of suckling piglets and replacer-fed piglets

In suckled piglets, an increase in the followed microflora population was recorded towards the caudal part of the intestine. Bacterial populations ranged from 4 to 8 log cfu/g in the jejunum, from 4 to 9 log cfu/g in the ileum, and from 6 to 9 log cfu/g in the caecum. The lactobacilli in the ileum slightly increased within the period of observation ranging from 1 to 2 log. The cfu of E. coli and Enterobacteriaceae in the ileum remained more or less stable over time, while they declined in the caecum. The course of development of total aerobes was similar in the jejunum and ileum throughout the period of observation, in the colon, however, total aerobes populations maintained at a constant level of 9 log cfu/g.

Likewise, in conventional piglets fed on milk replacement, an increase in the microflora population was observed towards the caudal part of the intestine. Bacterial populations ranged from 4 to 8 log cfu/g in the jejunum, from 4 to 9 log cfu/g in the ileum and from 6 to 9 log cfu/g in the caecum. In all parts of the intestine, E. coli and Enterobacteriaceae increased by 1 to 3 log units between days 2 and 14, and decreased thereafter until day 28. In the jejunum and ileum lactobacilli and enterococci slightly increased throughout the period of observation, in the colon, however, lactobacilli populations persisted at a constant level of 9 log cfu/g. Enterococcus spp. in colon contents declined by about 2 log units until 28 days of age. The course of the development of total aerobes was the same throughout the period of observation in all parts of the intestine.

Total lactobacilli populations in the jejunal content were significantly higher in the group of conventional replacer-fed piglets with highest counts on days 21 and 28 of age (p < 0.001 and p < 0.001) compared to the group of suckled piglets (Figure 1). The course of E. coli development in the jejunal content was the same in both observed groups except at 2 weeks of age. Whereas total E. coli populations were lower in the group of suckled piglets at 2 weeks of life, i.e. 3.78 log cfu/g, a significant increase was observed in group of replacer-fed piglets (p < 0.001). In conventional piglets fed on milk replacement, an increase in enterococci populations (Table 5) in the jejunal content was seen throughout the period of

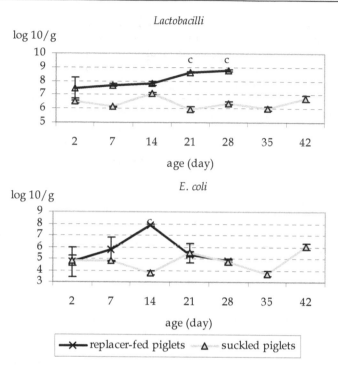

Each bar represents the mean ± SE of 3 piglets.
Significantly different (SP vs RFP): c (p < 0.001)

Fig. 1. Effect of diets on bacterial population (lactobacilli and *E.coli*) in the jejunum of suckling piglets and replacer-fed piglets

observation. In suckled piglets, on the other hand, total enterococci populations were by 0.5 - 2.5 log lower. The highest enterococci populations in the jejunal content of replacer-fed piglets were recorded at 21 and 28 d of age (p < 0.001 and p < 0.001, respectively). Total counts of *Enterobacteriaceae* in the jejunal content were the highest in replacer-fed piglets at 2 (6.95 log cfu/g) and 14 days of age (p < 0.001) compared to the group of suckled piglets in which lower numbers (by 3 logs) were seen at 2 days of life (4.00 log cfu/g) and at 14 days of age the populations were by 3.6 log lower (4.11 log cfu/g). The course of the development of total aerobes in the jejunal content was the same in both groups of piglets, however, with the difference that in replacer-fed piglets, the total numbers of observed bacteria were by 0.5 to 1.2 log higher with significantly higher numbers at 7 (p < 0.001), 14 (p < 0.05), and 21 days of age (p < 0.001).

In the ileal content of replacer-fed piglets we detected higher lactobacilli populations (Figure 2) compared to the suckled animals throughout the period of observation except at 14 days of age with significantly higher numbers at 7 and 21 days of age (p < 0.01 and p < 0.05). The course of development of *E. coli* was the same in both groups, however, with the difference that in the group of suckled piglets the total numbers were higher by 0.5 log except at 14 days of age when an increase in the total *E. coli* populations was recorded (p < 0.001). Total enterococci populations in the ileal content (Table 5) were higher by 1 to 3.5 log in replacer-

	Content						
	Jejunum		Ileum		Caecum		
	SP	RFP	SP	RFP	SP	RFP	SEM
Day 2							
Enterococci	6.36	6.83	6.10	7.70***	8.08	8.69*	0.31
Enterobacteiaceae	4.00	6.95	6.89***	4.55	8.95	7.92	0.25
Total aerobes	7.35	7.97	9.04	8.31	9.33	9.35	0.19
Day 7							
Enterococci	6.19	7.22	3.96	7.42***	7.49	8.73*	0.29
Enterobacteiaceae	4.43	4.02	7.24***	5.27	8.51	8.35	0.19
Total aerobes	6.56	8.15***	7.76	8.45**	9.24	9.57	0.14
Day 14							
Enterococci	5.12	6.80	5.06	7.49***	6.82	7.41	0.31
Enterobacteiaceae	4.11	7.72***	7.16***	8.17	7.37	9.42	0.26
Total aerobes	7.51	8.13*	7.46	8.83**	9.15	9.43	0.19
Day 21							
Enterococci	4.93	7.42***	6.01	6.93***	6.91	6.57	0.14
Enterobacteiaceae	5.38	4.69	6.69	6.57	7.10	8.13	0.19
Total aerobes	6.93	8.22***	8.77	9.35	9.13	9.12	0.29
Day 28							
Enterococci	5.52	7.46***	6.38	8.95***	7.17	6.94	0.16
Enterobacteiaceae	4.81	4.74	6.71**	5.96	6.07	6.53	0.28
Total aerobes	7.95	7.65	8.89	9.20	9.05	8.79	0.21
Day 35							
Enterococci	4.45	ND	5.15	ND	7.17	ND	0.39
Enterobacteiaceae	3.00	ND	5.79	ND	5.98	ND	0.19
Total aerobes	6.61	ND	9.26	ND	9.38	ND	0.14
Day 42							
Enterococci	6.75	ND	7.94	ND	8.91	ND	0.19
Enterobacteiaceae	5.38	ND	5.30	ND	5.36	ND	0.14
Total aerobes	7.80	ND	8.07	ND	9.13	ND	0.51

SP- suckled piglets (n=3), RFP- replacer-fed piglets (n=3), ND- not detectable
*p < 0.05, **p < 0.01, ***p < 0.001

Table 5. Effect of diets on bacterial population ($\log_{10}$ cfu/g of digesta) at various locations along the intestinal tract of suckling piglets and replacer-fed piglets

fed piglets than those in suckled piglets throughout the period of observation with significant difference between days 7 and 28 of age (p < 0.001). In suckled piglets, total *Enterobacteriaceae* populations were by 2 log higher by 1 week of life compared to the

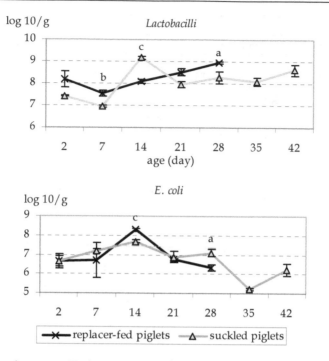

Each bar represents the mean ± SE of 3 piglets
Significantly different (SP vs RFP): a (p < 0.05), b (p < 0.01), c (p < 0.001)

Fig. 2. Effect of diets on bacterial population (lactobacilli and *E.coli*) in the ileum of suckling piglets and replacer-fed piglets

replacer-fed piglets. Thereafter, the populations of observed bacteria slightly declined up to the end of the period of observation. A significant increase in the *Enterobacteriaceae* populations in replacer-fed piglets was recorded at 14 days of age (p < 0.001). Numbers of total aerobes in the ileal content were by 0.5 - 1.5 log higher in replacer-fed piglets compared to colostral animals with significant difference on day 7 (p < 0.01) and 14 of age (p < 0.01).

In the caecum of suckled piglets, *E. coli* populations gradually declined throughout the period of observation (Figure 3) compared with replacer-fed piglets in which a significant increase in numbers was recorded at 14 and 21 days of age (p < 0.001 and p < 0.01, respectively). The course of the development of lactobacilli and total aerobes in the content of the caecum was the same. Total enterococci populations in replacer-fed piglets (Table 5) were by 0.6 - 1.2 log higher by day 14 of age, with significant enterococci populations at 2 and 7 days of age (p < 0.05 and p< 0.05). After day 14, the cfu of *Enterococcus* spp. in the caecum contents of replacer-fed piglets were about 0.3 log units lower than those of suckled piglets. A significant increase in the *Enterobacteriaceae* populations in replacer-fed piglets compared to the second group was recorded from day 14 of age (p < 0.001) to the end of the period of observation (p < 0.01) at 21 days of age and (p < 0.05) at 28 days of age.

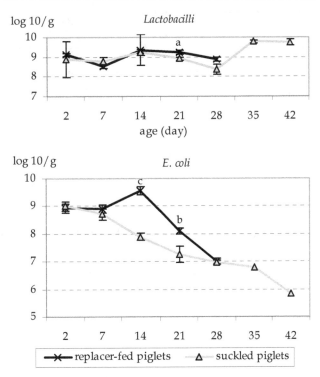

Each bar represents the mean ± SE of 3 piglets.
Significantly different (SP vs RFP): a (p < 0.05), b (p < 0.01), c (p < 0.001)

Fig. 3. Effect of diets on bacterial population (lactobacilli and *E.coli*) in the colon of suckling piglets and replacer-fed piglets

3.6 Effect of age, weaning and diets on development of intestinal morphology in gnotobiotic and conventionally bred piglets

From day 2 of age we recorded a gradual increase in body weight of gnotobiotic piglets from 0.75 kg up to 1.80 kg (p < 0.05) on day 14 of age and 3.90 kg (p < 0.01) on day 21 of age. On day 28 (day of weaning) and one week after weaning the body weight of piglets was decreased insignificantly (Table 6). The increase in relative weight of the small intestine resembled that of the large intestine throughout the period of investigation with the exception that the relative weight of the large intestine in comparison with the weight on day 2 of age was increased significantly on day 21 (p < 0.05), 28 (p < 0.05) and 35 of age (p < 0.001). Similar trend of body weight increase as that recorded in gnotobiotic piglets was observed also in conventional piglets, increasing from 1.41 kg at 2 days of age to 3.50 kg at 14 days of age (p < 0.05). The body weight of piglets increased gradually up to the end of observation with significant increase on day 35 of life (p < 0.01) in comparison with the day of weaning (Table 6).

The development of relative weight of the small and large intestine of suckled piglets was similar and the relative weights decreased gradually between days 2 and 21 of age. On day

	Age (day)						
	2	7	14	21	28	35	SEM
Suckled piglets							
Weight (kg)	1.41	2.05	3.50*a	4.30	5.35	8.55**a	0.39
Small intestinal weight (g/kg)	67.88	64.59	43.59	41.88	44.27	156.6***a	7.08
Large intestinal weight (g/kg)	25.52	24.65	15.68	15.53	23.38	125.4***a	2.38
Gnotobiotic piglets							
Weight (kg)	0.75	1.29	1.80*	3.90**	3.65	3.25	0.46
Small intestinal weight (g/kg)	42.47	52.59	53.02	64.68b	55.41	60.67	6.14
Large intestinal weight (g/kg)	13.89	18.31	20.07	47.41*b	42.1*	85.63***	4.07

Significantly different (SP vs GP): a ($p < 0.05$), b ($p < 0.01$)
*$p < 0.05$, **$p < 0.01$, ***$p < 0.001$

Table 6. Effect of age, weaning and diets on weight, gut weight of suckling piglets and gnotobiotic piglets

28 of age the relative weights showed an insignificant increase but in the first week post-weaning the relative weights of both small and large intestine increased significantly ($p < 0.001$) in comparison with all periods of investigation. The weight of conventional piglets was greater throughout the experiment and significant differences ($p < 0.05$) were recorded on days 14 and 35. Completely opposite trend was recorded for relative weights of small and large intestines of these piglets (Table 6). While relative weights of intestines of gnotobiotic piglets gradually increased throughout the experiment with the exception of day 28 of life, the weight of small and large intestine in suckled piglets decreased gradually between days 2 and 21 of life. Between days 2 and 28 of life the relative weight of the intestines of gnotobiotic piglets was higher compared to conventional piglets with significant difference on day 21 of life ($p < 0.01$). In the post-weaning period (one week post-weaning), the weight of small and large intestine of suckled piglets was significantly higher ($p < 0.05$) in comparison with gnotobiotic piglets in the same period of observation.

The development of the height of villi in individual segments of the small intestine of gnotobiotic piglets is shown in Table 7. On day 21, the height of villi in the duodenum was decreased significantly ($p < 0.01$). A decrease in their length was also recorded on day 28 but the difference was insignificant. In the duodenum of suckled piglets, the height of villi (Table 7) increased significantly ($p < 0.001$) in the period between birth and day 14 of age. Subsequently, their length decreased gradually up to the weaning ($p < 0.01$). Throughout the experiment, the willi in the duodenum of gnotobiotic piglets were higher and their height differed significantly from that of conventional piglets at 3 hours after birth, days 2 and 7 of age ($p < 0.01$) and day 14 of age ($p < 0.05$) (Figure 4).

The length of jejunal villi of gnotobiotic piglets (Table 7) increased from day 0 up to day 2 of age reaching maximum of 725.18 μm. In the subsequent 5 weeks, the length of villi decreased gradually down to 387.44 μm in the week after weaning and the decrease was significant on days 14 ($p < 0.05$) and 21 of age ($p < 0.001$). In the jejunum of suckled piglets we observed a gradual but insignificant increase in villi height in the period from birth up to day 7 of life. In the following period, from day 14 of age till one week post-weaning we recorded gradual decrease in the height of villi, significant on days 21 ($p < 0.001$) and 35 of

	Content						
	Duodenum		Jejunum		Ileum		
	SP	GP	SP	GP	SP	GB	SEM
Day 0							
Villus height, μm	253.67	371.29	689.68	679.43	574.80	587.37	47.11
Crypt depth, μm	129.13	81.63	53.67	67.12	48.14	79.43	1.96
Day 2							
Villus height, μm	308.42***	424.81	701.57	725.18	588.29	455.05	45.66
Crypt depth, μm	140.23	104.15	69.77	72.66	77.77	82.54	2.73
Day 7							
Villus height, μm	374.98***	502.63	718.21	691.74	401.54***	393.00	28.60
Crypt depth, μm	188.00	124.10	83.82	90.97	71.18	111.35	5.03
Day 14							
Villus height, μm	547.83***	605.14	661.59	581.23*	369.52	424.16	29.03
Crypt depth, μm	151.79	119.27	92.53	103.47	178.96	118.22	3.96
Day 21							
Villus height, μm	454.48**	478.43**	492.42***	442.86***	351.01	423.29	34.21
Crypt depth, μm	168.54	162.33*	129.44	136.17	134.26	176.15*	3.60
Day 28							
Villus height, μm	351.81**	349.21	447.67	401.93	361.69	358.57	31.64
Crypt depth, μm	220.94	197.82	164.80	145.50	165.94	157.69	3.70
Day 35							
Villus height, μm	364.13	396.07	324.23**	387.44	310.00	336.54	25.33
Crypt depth, μm	343.56***	205.10	230.11**	164.23	206.80*	166.91	5.83
Day 42							
Villus height, μm	379.44	ND	440.08	ND	358.65	ND	18.32
Crypt depth, μm	322.66	ND	223.39	ND	174.81	ND	4.22

SP- suckled piglets, GP- gnotobiotic piglets, ND- not detectable
*p < 0.05, **p < 0.01, ***p < 0.001

Table 7. Effect of age and weaning on small intestinal morphology at various locations along the intestinal tract of suckling piglets and gnotobiotic piglets

age ($p < 0.01$). Comparison of both animal groups showed that villi in the jejunum of conventional piglets were higher between days 14 and 28 of age, the difference being significant on day 14 ($p < 0.05$). In the post-weaning period, villi were significantly higher ($p < 0.05$) in gnotobiotic piglets on day 35 (Figure 4).

When comparing both mentioned groups, higher villi were observed in ileum of gnotobiotic piglets, resembling the situation in duodenum, with significant difference ($p < 0.05$) on days

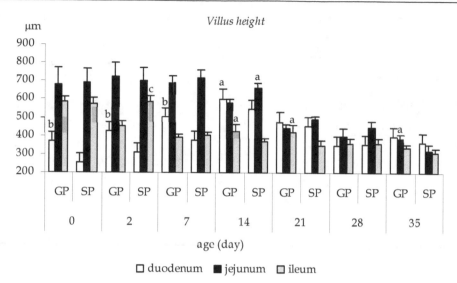

☐ duodenum   ■ jejunum   ☐ ileum

SP- suckled piglets, GP- gnotobiotic piglets
Significantly different (SP vs GP): a (p < 0.05), b (p < 0.01), c (p < 0.001)

Fig. 4. Effect of diets on small intestinal morphology at various locations along the intestinal tract of suckling and gnotobiotic piglets

14 and 21 of age with the exception of day 2 of life when ileal villi were significantly higher (p < 0.001) in conventional piglets (Figure 4).

The postnatal changes in the depth of crypts (Table 7) were the same in all small intestinal segments of gnotobiotic piglets. From the birth up to day 35 of life the crypts in the jejunal segment gradually deepened and reached 164.23 µm on day 35 of life. Similar development was observed also in the duodenal segment of the small intestine, where, with the exception of slight decrease on day 14 of age, the depth of crypts gradually increased throughout the observation period with significant difference on day 21 of age (p < 0.05). One week after weaning the depth of crypts in the duodenum reached 205.1 µm. A significant increase in the depth of crypts (p < 0.05) was recorded on day 21 of age also in the ileal segment of gnotobiotic piglets. Also dynamics of development of the depth of crypts was similar in all small intestine segments of colostral piglets. In the first post-weaning week we recorded a significant deepening of crypts in duodenal (p < 0.001), jejunal (p < 0.01) and ileal (p < 0.05) segments.

Staining with haematoxylin/eosin showed that the small intestinal mucosa of gnotobiotic piglets and suckled piglets at 3 h after birth (Figure 5/a,b) and on day 2 of age (Figure 5/c,d) was covered by population of dense, finger-like villi of the same height. While on the surface of villi of gnotobiotic piglets we were able to observe enterocytes with apically located nucleus, in suckled piglets the enterocytes had apically to medially located nucleus. The fibrous base of intestinal villi was poorly differentiated and the intestinal crypts were small. By day 7 of age of gnotobiotic piglets (Figure 5/e) the height of villi decreased but their diameter increased. In the same period the villi in suckled piglets preserved their finger-like shape with medially to basally located nucleus in enterocytes (Figure 5/f). At the

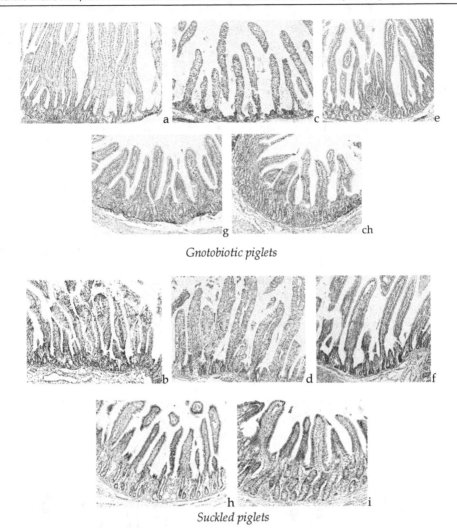

Gnotobiotic piglets

Suckled piglets

(a, b) 3 hours after birth, (c, d) 2 days of age, (e, f) 7 days of age, (g, h) 28 days of age, (ch) 35days of age of GP, (i) 42 days of age of SP, SP- suckled piglets, GP- gnotobiotic piglets, Magnification x 125.

Fig. 5. Light micrograph of hematoxylin and eosin-stained jejunal mucosa of gnotobiotic and suckling piglets

time of weaning (day 28 of age) the differentiated basis of intestinal villi in both observed groups of piglets consisted of thin fibrous tissue containing fascicles of smooth muscle cells. On the surface of the villi we were able to observe goblet cells interspersed among enterocytes (Figure 5/g, h). The enterocyte nuclei were located in the medial part of the cytoplasm. The villi stroma was infiltrated with small number of lymphocytes and plasmatic cells. By day 35 of life, the jejunal villi acquired tongue-like shape (Figure 5/ch). On day 42 of age intestinal crypts of suckled piglets (Figure 5/i) almost completely filled up *lamina propria* of the small intestine and their bases almost reached *lamina muscularis mucosae*.

Intestinal villi were shorter and acquired tongue-like shape. Such characteristic development was observed in all investigated segments of the small intestine which, however, differed by morphometric parameters of villi height.

3.7 Effect of age, weaning and diets on development of specific activity of disaccharidases in the small intestine of gnotobiotic and conventionally bred piglets

In our study we registered that development of lactase activity of gnotobiotic piglets was similar in the duodenum and jejunum in the period from day 0 to 35 of age. The specific activity of lactase (Figure 6) in the duodenum reached at birth the level of 3.4 μmol/mg protein/hour. From the 2nd day of life the increasing enzyme activity was noticed with a measured maximum on day 7 of life (p < 0.001). High enzyme levels were observed until the 21th day of life (5.80 μmol/mg protein/hour), after which the enzyme activity decreased in the weeks 4 (p < 0.001) and 5 (p < 0.001) to levels similar to those noticed at birth. In terms of lactase activity distribution throughout the small intestine, higher activity in the duodenum and jejunum were noticed than in distal parts of the small intestine, where the incidence of enzyme was 4 times lower. The specific activity of lactase in the duodenum of conventional piglets (Figure 6) reached at birth 3.6 μmol/mg protein/hour. The course of activity of this enzyme during our observations resembled that of gnotobiotic piglets with maximum recorded on day 7 of age (p < 0.001), gradual decrease from day 14 of life and significant decrease (p < 0.001) on the day of weaning and in the 1st post-weaning weak. As far as the distribution of lactase in the small intestine was concerned, the highest activity of lactase

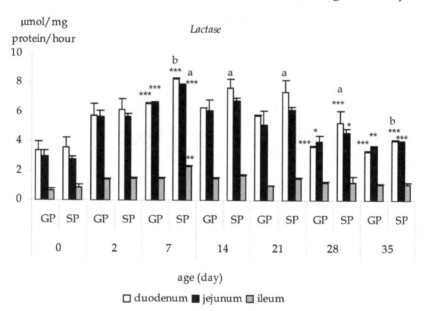

Significantly different (SP vs GP): a (p < 0.05), b (p < 0.01), *p < 0.05, **p < 0.01, ***p < 0.001

Fig. 6. Effect of age, weaning and diets on specific activity of lactase at various locations along the intestinal tract of suckling and gnotobiotic piglets, SP- suckled piglets, GP- gnotobiotic piglets

was recorded in duodenum and the lowest in ileum where lactase levels were 4-fold lower compared to proximal small intestine segments. Significant increase in the activity of enzyme was observed in jejunum ($p < 0.001$) and ileum ($p < 0.01$) of conventional piglets on day 7 of age. Comparison of both animal groups (Figure 6) showed that specific activity of lactase in the intestinal tract was higher in conventional piglets throughout the experiment with significantly higher lactase activity in duodenum from day 7 to 35 of age ($p < 0.05$, $p < 0.01$) and significantly higher level in the jejunum ($p < 0.05$) on day 7 of age.

The post-natal dynamics of maltase (Figure 7) and saccharase (Figure 8) in gnotobiotic piglets took a completely different course. Very low levels of maltase in the jejunum detected at birth (0.3 µmol/mg protein/hour) and during the 1st week of life slightly increased in the following period and on the 14th day reached 1.2 µmol/mg protein/hour. The slightly increased specific activity of maltase persisted also in the following period. Maltase distribution (Figure 7) throughout the small intestine changed depending on the age with a predominant concentration of maltase activity in the jejunum at the age of 1-2 weeks, through a higher activity in the duodenal part at the age of 21 days, until a balanced distribution in the proximal and medial part of the small intestine was achieved at the age of 4-5 weeks. Similarly also very low specific saccharase activity in the jejunum (Figure 8) recorded until the 1st week of life (1.12 µmol/mg protein/hour) progressively increased with a maximum on the 21st day of life ($p < 0.001$), sustained values were reached in the 4th and 5th week of the life of piglets. Saccharase activity distribution throughout the small intestine of gnotobiotic piglets was higher in the jejunum during the entire period of observation. Specific activities of maltase (Figure 7) and saccharase (Figure 8) in newborn

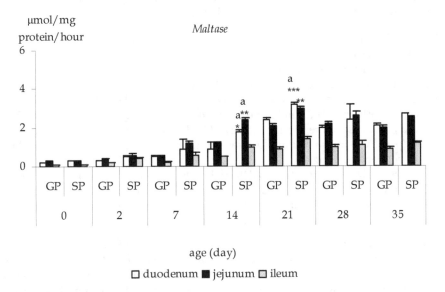

Significantly different (SP vs GP): a ($p < 0.05$), *$p < 0.05$, **$p < 0.01$, ***$p < 0.001$

Fig. 7. Effect of age, weaning and diets on specific activity of maltase at various locations along the intestinal tract of suckling and gnotobiotic piglets, SP- suckled piglets, GP- gnotobiotic piglets.

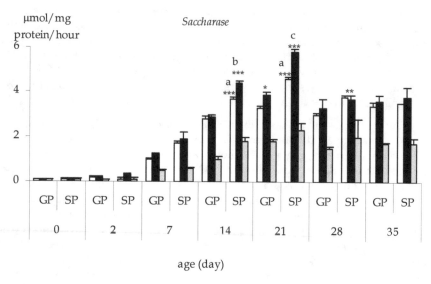

Fig. 8. Effect of age, weaning and diets on specific activity of saccharase at various locations along the intestinal tract of suckling and gnotobiotic piglets

and 2-day old conventional piglets were very low and did not exceed 0.6 µmol/mg protein/hour. After one week of age of piglets, activities of both enzymes increased. The maximum specific activity of maltase peaked on days 14 and 21 (p < 0.05, p < 0.001) in the duodenum and significant difference was observed (p < 0.05) in the jejunal segment. Similarly, activity of saccharase reached highest values on days 14 and 21 of age and differed significantly (p < 0.001) in both the duodenal and jejunal segment. On day 28 of age we observed a decrease in the specific activity of both enzymes with significant difference in saccharase (p < 0.01) in the jejunum. Observation of distribution of maltase in the small intestine of conventional piglets showed that in the direction of terminal ileum, up to the age of 2 weeks the highest activity was detected in the jejunum and the lowest in the ileum. In the following period activity of this enzyme was higher in proximal to medial segments of the intestine than in the distal ones. Throughout the experiment saccharase reached the highest activity in the jejunum and the lowest in the ileum.

The postnatal development of specific activity of enzymes maltase and saccharase showed a similar trend with higher activities of both enzymes in suckled piglets in all digestive tract segments throughout the observation. The highest activity of the enzymes in comparison with gnotobiotic piglets was recorded on days 14 and 21 of age with significant differences in the level of maltase (p < 0.05, p < 0.001) in the duodenum and significantly different activity of the enzyme (p < 0.05) in jejunum. Significantly different activities of saccharase compared to the other group of piglets were observed in the same period (days 14 and 21) in duodenum (p < 0.05) and jejunum (p < 0.01, p < 0.001).

4. Discussion

4.1 Effect of age and diets on development of the small intestine – Intestinal microflora

At birth, a young pig which is axenic during its uterine life is suddenly confronted with a complex bacterial environment. Beginning with birth, the young are in contact with several microbial ecosystems - i.e. faeces, contaminated vagina and perineum, but also from the skin and teats of the sow which are usually contaminated as well. It could be assumed that each of these ecosystems contributes to constituting the gut flora of the newborn (Siggers et al., 2007). However, in the following days, simplified microbiota profiles have been characterized, which will become more complex with time, increasing its diversity as the animal grows (Inoue at al., 2005). The population level of the microbiota in various parts of the gastrointestinal tract of monogastric animals depends on the attachment ability, replication period of the microorganism under the physicochemical tract conditions and the emptying rhythm in the part of the gastrointestinal tract under investigation. Swords et al. (1993) studied pig faecal microbiota evolution within the first four months of life, and concluded that the establishment of the adult faecal flora is a large and complex process with three different marked phases in the bacterial succession. The first phase corresponds with the first week of life, the second one, from the end of the first week to conclusion of suckling, and the third phase from weaning to final adaptation to dry food. In this first phase, aerobes and facultative anaerobes from the sow and the environment become the predominant bacterial groups, comprising 80% of the total flora by three hours after birth. The gut colonization is extremely fast, only twelve hours after birth, total bacteria in distal colon reaches counts of 10^9 cfu/g colonic content (Jensen et al., 1998; Swords et al., 1993). First colonizers modify the gastrointestinal environment (by consumption of molecular oxygen and reduction of the redox potential), making it more favourable for the following colonization by anaerobes. As a result, aerotolerant bacteria are gradually supplanted by strict anaerobes, and 48h after birth, piglets already show 90% of anaerobic bacteria (Swords et al., 1993). Of these bacterial groups, lactobacilli and streptococci become the dominant bacteria at the end of the first week of life and will be maintained for the whole suckling period with counts of around 10^7-10^9 cfu/g digesta (Swords et al., 1993). Microbiota remains fairly stable in terms of species composition during the second phase when the piglets receive milk from their mother (Mathew et al., 1996). The diversity of anaerobic bacteria increases in this period (Inoue et al., 2005) and supplantation of aerobic and facultative anaerobic bacteria by anaerobic bacteria become almost completed in this phase. As has been mentioned before, lactobacilli and streptococci continue being dominant bacteria, which are well adapted to utilize substrate from the milk diet. *Clostridium, Bacteroides, bifidobacteria,* and low densities *Eubacterium, Fusobacterium, Propionibacterium* and *Streptococcus* spp. are also usually found in this second phase (Swords et al., 1993). In our experiment with piglets fed maternal milk, the gut flora developed very quickly post partum. As early as within 48 hrs post partum, *Escherichia coli,* enterococci and lactobacilli were detected in the content of digesta in suckled piglets, the populations of which represented 10^5 - 10^9 bacteria/g per sample. The gut flora of piglets in the proximal part (jejunum) consisted of facultatively anaerobic bacteria (enterococci, *E. coli*) and aerotolerant anaerobes (lactobacilli) counting 10^4 - 10^6 bacteria/g per sample. These numbers increased progressively in the ileum and the dominant flora in the posterior portions of the digestive tract (caecum) was facultatively anaerobic bacteria (*E. coli,* enterococci, *Enterobacteriaceae* and lactobacilli) counting 10^8 - 10^9 bacteria/g per sample. As the piglets grew, the flora progressively changed. The replacement of maternal milk by a milk replacement diet in our third experiment resulted at 2 and 14 days of age in increased numbers of bacterial flora, of the family *Enterobacteriaceae* in the proximal small intestine (jejunum) by 3 log compared to suckled piglets. At the same time a gradual increase in the numbers of coliform bacteria (p < 0.001) in the proximal (jejunum) and terminal (caecum) part of the intestine occurred reaching numbers as much as by 4 log higher in the jejunum at 14 d of age compared to colostral piglets. Similar findings were obtained by (Franklin et al. 2002; Jensen et al., 1998; Pluske et al., 1997) which observed, in addition to higher populations of anaerobic and coliform bacteria, a significant decline in lactobacilli populations in piglets fed replacement milk. The mechanism of the selection has not yet been determined, although feeding may be a primary factor. According to different authors it is almost impossible to prevent neonatal *E. coli* diarrhoea in piglets which do not receive maternal colostrum (Pluske et al., 1997; Xu et al., 1996). Colostrum and also maternal milk contain highly digestible nutrients and components such as immunoglobulins and lysozymes and have both bacteriostatic and antiadhesive properties towards the pathogen *E. coli* (Xu et al., 1996). This protective effect, however, does not seem to be accompanied by an elimination of *E. coli* from the digestive tract. In addition, in both the jejunal and ileal part (p < 0.001) of the small intestine of replacer-fed piglets, high numbers of enterococci were recorded, being by 1-3.5 log higher compared to the colostrum-fed piglets throughout the period of observation. It is likely, however, that this result was influenced by the milk replacement having been enriched by *Enterococcus faecium* counting 10^4 cfu/g of feed. The human intestinal microbiota is a complex ecosystem, consisting of several hundred (more than 800) different bacterial species. This microbiota plays an important role in human health and nutrition by producing nutrients, preventing colonization of the gut by potential pathogenic microorganisms (Guarner & Malagelada, 2003), and preserving the health of the host through interactions with the developing immune system. The microbiota in early life has been linked to allergy risk (Penders et al., 2007). Major changes in the intestinal microbial composition occur in early life. Sterile *in utero*, the gastrointestinal tract of the newborn infant is rapidly colonized at birth by a myriad of maternal vaginal and faecal bacteria and other sources from its environment. The first few weeks after birth correspond to critical stages of gut colonization. Bacterial colonization of the gastrointestinal tract is influenced by numerous factors including diet, environment, antibiotic treatment, mucosal maturation, and age. Naturally delivered babies experienced a period of 2-3 days in which, as a consequence of the low selective potential of their stomach and small bowel, bacteria invading and reproducing within the gut belong to aerobic species as *Enterobacteriaceae*, streptococci, and staphylococci. These bacteria, arriving from the external environment, belong to species with a pathogenic potential, and therefore, it might seem that they would not be the best choice for the health of neonates. However, the metabolisms of these bacteria are believed to be positive factors in preparing the path to a beneficial enteric flora. In the study of Fallani et al. (2010) they confirmed previously published work (Hopkins et al., 2005; Penders et al., 2007) that bifidobacteria are the predominant group detected in the faeces of pre-weaned infants, followed by *Bacteroides* and enterobacteria.

4.2 Production of SCFAs and pH

Organic acids are the main metabolites of intestinal fermentation. The degree of their concentration in the digesta reflects the level of intestinal fermentation (Piva et al., 2002). It is well known that organic acids exhibit antibacterial activity (Piva et al., 2002), increase intestinal absorption of minerals and improve ileal digestion of proteins and amino acids. Their relative levels vary depending on location (stomach, small intestine, large intestine) and diet composition (dietary lactose level, fibre level, etc). Lactic acid is in the greatest concentration in the stomach and small intestine while other organic acids, acetic along with propionic and butyric, are predominant in the large intestine. In our study, in suckled piglets we recorded higher level of acetic acid in the ileal contents in comparison with the replacer-fed piglets throughout the observation, ranging from about 7 to 21.5 mmol/l. Higher concentrations of this acid were observed in the same segment also in gnotobiotic piglets compared to replacer-fed piglets, ranging from 2.05 to 13.69 mmol/l. A similar tendency was recorded in lactic acid, in the ileal content, with higher concentrations in suckled piglets compared to the replacer-fed piglets in which the values later ranged from about 8.2 to 21.4 mmol/l. Higher production of lactic acid in gnotobiotic piglets in comparison with replacer-fed piglets was recorded throughout the observation and ranged from 0.6 to 10.14 mmol/l. Increasing concentrations of lactate in ileal digesta should therefore reflect an increased population and activity of lactic acid bacteria (Pluske et al., 2002). These findings are of importance relative to the management of growing pigs, because lactate has been shown to have antibacterial effects on E. coli and Salmonella species, and lactobacilli have been shown to inhibit adhesion of enterotoxigenic E. coli to the ileal epithelium (Pluske et al., 2002). The ability to generate organic acids, particularly lactic and acetic acid, present one of the mechanisms by which lactobacilli perform their inhibitory effect upon pathogens. With decreasing pH values, the inhibitory activity of the above acids increases, their molecular form being toxic for bacteria. The increased toxicity of acetic acid is attributed to its higher pKa in comparison to lactic acid. Increased lactic acid levels intensify the toxicity of acetic acid. Comparison of lactic acid levels in the jejunal and ileal contents of one week old gnotobiotic piglets (Bomba et al., 1998) and conventional suckling piglets (Zitnan et al., 2001) revealed that the highest levels were found in conventional animals (29.30 and 27.90 mmol/l, resp.) and in Lactobacillus plantarum inoculated gnotobiotic piglets (26.60 and 14.20 mmol/l, resp.). High levels of lactic acid were recorded in our study in jejunal and ileal contents of conventional suckling piglets (27.52 and 26.91 mmol/l, resp.) and piglets inoculated with Enterococus faecium at the age of 1 week (23.59 and 24.56 mmol/l, resp.). Lower concentrations of this acid were found in replacer-fed piglets (24.92 and 14.42) and the lowest levels of lactic acid in the jejunal and ileal contents (Bomba et al., 1998) were seen in germ-free piglets (4.40 and 6.45 mmol/l, resp.). At the age of 3 weeks, the level of lactic acid in the jejunum of piglets inoculated with Enterococcus faecium was lower in comparison with that in the jejunum of piglets inoculated with Lactobacillus plantarum (21.94 and 33.15 mmol/l, resp.) but in the ileum of Enterococcus faecium inoculated piglets we found the highest level of this acid (24.40 mmol/l) in comparison with all other groups of piglets. The mentioned authors presented different results also with regard to acetic acid, as the highest concentrations of acetic acid in the jejunum and ileum (30.05 and 23.61 mmol/l, resp.) were observed in conventional piglets by Zitnan et al. (2001) and in conventional suckling piglets investigated in our study (33.05 and 21.81 mmol/l, resp.). Lower levels were observed in replacer-fed piglets (21.43 and 10.47 mmol/l, resp.) and in gnotobiotic piglets (Bomba et al. 1998) inoculated with lactobacilli (11.80 and 11.85 mmol/l, resp.) and in those inoculated with Enterococcus faecium (8.18 and 24.16 mmol/l, resp.). Similarly low levels were detected also in germ-free piglets (13.15 and 3.9 mmol/l, resp.). On the contrary, at the age of 3 weeks, we recorded higher levels of acetic acid in the jejunal and ileal content of gnotobiotic piglets inoculated with *Enterococcus faecium* (12.86 and 32.08 mmol/l, resp.) in comparison with all other groups of piglets (10.7 and 25.9 mmol/l, resp.) of conventional suckling piglets (Zitnan, 2001), (5.36 and 25.00 mmol/l, resp.) of conventional suckling piglets in our study, (6.87 and 19.86 mmol/l, resp.) of replacer-fed piglets and gnotobiotic piglets inoculated with *Lactobacillus plantarum* (11.85 and 14.2 mmol/l, resp.). Under the influence of more diverse populations of microorganisms the conditions in the colonic content changed with gradual occurrences of propionic, butyric, and valeric acids. Organic acids and ammonia concentrating in the colon were according to Kiare et al. (2007) 5-10-fold bigger than those in the ileum and their increased concentrations resulted in additional fermentation activity of short-chain organic acids. This indicates higher microbial activity and considerable N-metabolism in the caudal segment of the intestine. The most significant increase in production of organic acids in the colonic segment observed in our study involved acetoacetic, acetic, propionic and butyric acids in the group of suckled piglets compared to replacer-fed piglets, at important concentrations of acetoacetic acid from 14 to 28 days of age (p < 0.01). Significant increase was observed also in production of lactic acid in gnotobiotic piglets compared to the replacer-fed animals throughout the observation period with the highest concentrations reached on days 2 (p < 0.05), 14, 21 and 28 of age (p < 0.01). Decreased pH of the gut content and increased production of lactic and acetic acids affects positively optimisation of digestive processes. Bomba et al. (1998) investigated intestinal metabolism of gnotobiotic piglets and recorded significantly lower pH (p<0.05) in the jejunal content in piglets inoculated with *Lactobacillus plantarum* in the 1st week of life in comparison with germ-free piglets. Zitnan et al. (2001) observed pH in the jejunal and ileal content of conventional piglets of the same age. When comparing the actual acidity in individual segments of the small intestine, pH of the jejunum content of germ-free piglets was higher in the first week of life (7.49) in comparison with pH of conventional piglets (6.23) of the same age. Contrary to that, pH of the jejunal content of gnotobiotic piglets inoculated with *Lactobacillus plantarum* was considerably lower (5.63). Similar low pH was recorded in our study in gnotobiotic piglets of the same age inoculated with *Enterococcus faecium* (6.02). Bomba et al. (1998) conducted two experiments to investigate the influence of short-term and continuous preventive administration of *Lactobacillus casei* subs.casei against *E.coli* on actual acidity, production of organic acids and colonisation of jejunum with *E.coli* O8:K88 in gnotobiotic piglets. After the short-term administration of *L.casei* they recorded lower pH in the jejunal content of experimental piglets (L-E) while pH of the ileal content of these piglets increased significantly (7.63) in comparison with the control (7.03). After continuous administration, the authors recorded lower pH in the experimental group L-E (6.1) in comparison with the control group (6.28). In our experiment we observed a positive influence of *Enterococcus faecium* on intestinal metabolism in replacer-fed piglets in terms of increased production of organic acids (formic acid, acetoacetic, propionic and butyric acid). However, production of lactic acid responsible for decrease in pH was lower in our observations and their concentrations ranged between 6.27 and 20.30 mmol/l in the ileal segment of replacer-fed piglets in comparison with suckled piglets (15.52 to 60.11mmol/l) and failed to induce the corresponding pH reduction. pH in the ileum of non-colostral piglets ranged from 6.9 to 7.6. Although acetic acid reached higher levels in the colon segment, it could become toxic only at low pH of the environment dependent on sufficient concentration of lactic acid in the gut. According to Mufandaedza et al. (2006), decreased active acidity, pH < 5.0, limits even stops growth and multiplication of *E. coli*. Similar conclusions were drawn from our study. Production of organic acids by replacer-fed piglets was low and resulted in their low concentrations which did not decrease pH so effectively as it was observed in gnotobiotic piglets inoculated with *Enterococcus faecium*. Deficit of colostral nutrition in these piglets resulted in worsened health in 8 out of total 26 piglets. The disease was peracute and proceeded with physiological temperature. Even though antibiotics were administered, the piglets died within 8 hrs of appearing of the first symptoms. In the piglets, lymphocytic leukocytosis as well as hypochromic anemia were diagnosed, and *E. coli* K88 was isolated from rectal swabs.

4.3 Intestinal morphology and disaccharidase activity

Due to numerous similarities of the physiology and anatomy of the gastrointestinal tract of man and pigs, the pig model is a very attractive model for human nutritional studies (Miller & Ullrey, 1987). Investigations performed in humans and pigs showed that the portions of total life required to reach chemical maturity for both these species are nearly identical, 4.4% and 4.6, respectively. Even though there are species-specific differences of the placenta and immunological system of pigs and human, the piglets are optimum experimental model for investigations concerning physiology and pathology of the gastrointestinal tract of human newborn (Miller & Ullrey, 1987). The postnatal development of the gastrointestinal (GI) system is a very dynamic process. In the neonatal pig with the mean birth body weight of 1.45kg, the small intestine and pancreas weight contribute to 3.1% and 0.14% of the total body weight, respectively (Zabielski et al., 2008). Within the first four postnatal weeks weight of the piglet is increased >5-fold, with the GI organs growing faster than many other organs of the body (Zabielski et al., 2008). Can we suspect the same changes in human neonates? Presumably yes, but the intensity of the remodelling is not as dramatic. The development in humans is slower, and the growth rate is slower in comparison to pigs. In humans the birth weight is doubled within ca. 170 days. Nevertheless, a number of similarities pig and human in the process of the development can be seen. In the study of Len et al. (2009), similar to our investigations of conventional piglets, the absolute weight of visceral organs and GI tract increased with piglet age. However, when expressed as g/kg empty body weight, the weight of visceral organs decreased with age (Len et al., 2009), which is in agreement with Pluske et al. (2002), who found that the relative weight of the visceral organs of piglets had a tendency to decrease between 14 and 28 days of age. In our study we observed a gradual decrease in the weight of small and large intestine between days 2 and 21 of age in suckled piglets while in gnotobiotic piglets the relative weight of intestines increased gradually throughout the period of observation. In germ-free and monoassociated pigs (Shirkey et al., 2006), the relative small intestine length was reduced compared with conventional pigs. The mechanisms affecting intestinal length are unknown, however, it can be hypothesized that increased small intestine length in conventionalized pigs is a compensatory response to the decreased absorptive capacity associated with decreased surface area (decreased villi length) and/or to direct competition with the microbiota for dietary nutrients. Shirkey et al. (2006) observed that in the proximal region of the small intestine, the relative weights for segments from conventional pigs tended to be higher than those from germ-free and monoassociated pigs. This is consistent with our study, as well as with the previous reports indicating that compared with germ-free animals, conventionally reared animals experience intestinal "thickening" associated primarily with increased *lamina propria* cellularity (Miniats & Valli, 1973) as well as thickening of the submucosa and muscular layers (Furuse & Okumura, 1994). On the contrary, higher relative weight of the distal part of the intestine was reported in germ-free piglets (Shirkey et al., 2006). Similar results were obtained in our study which showed higher relative weight of the large intestine in gnotobiotic piglets inoculated with *Enterococcus faecium* in comparison with conventional piglets starting from the second week of age up to the weaning (day 28 of age). In addition to an intensive growth of the GI system, during the first month of life an intense rebuilding of the tissues takes place. The most intensive processes are observed in the epithelium of the small intestine (Zabielski et al., 2008). The weight of small intestinal mucosa doubles during the first postnatal day due to a complex of processes involving, accumulation of colostrum proteins in the enterocytes as a result of an open „gut barrier", increase of local blood flow concurrently with a reduction in basal vascular resistance (Nankervis et al., 2001), and finally changes in epithelial cell turnover, namely, increased mitosis accompanied by the inhibition of apoptosis which result in a 2-fold increase in the mitosis/apoptosis ratio within the first 2 postnatal days (Zabielski et al., 2008). The regulation of small intestine development (especially the tissue growth) is in a positive feed-back to colostrum and milk intake (Marion et al., 2003). Currently none artificial feeding system (milk, artificial milk formula, nor feeding with any other compositions like lactose, glucose solutions) could reproduce the developmental characteristics obtained with maternal colostrum feeding (Zabielski et al., 2008). Furthermore, high specificity of colostrum, especially concerning the composition of hormones and bioactive compounds prevents utilization of colostrum of other species as the replacement. In the study of Meslin et al. (1973), the overall mass of the small intestine in germ-free species was decreased, and its surface area was smaller, whereas the villi of the small intestine were unusually uniform in shape and appear slender, with crypts, which were shorter and less populated than in the respective conventional control animals. Our study showed that the jejunal part of the intestinal tract in gnotobiotic pigs was characterized up to 14 days of life by relatively short crypts, extremely long villi and narrow *lamina propria* containing few cells. Reduced crypt depth and increased villus length agree with the previous observations in germ-free pigs (Shirkey et al., 2006; Shurson et al., 1990). In the present study in gnotobiotic piglets villi were the longest in the jejunum and shortest in the duodenum and ileum, whereas crypt depth was shortest in the jejunum and deepest in the duodenum throughout the observation period. These morphological characteristics suggested that the rates of enterocyte proliferation and exfoliation were the highest in the proximal small intestine, as indicated by deep crypts and shorter villi, respectively, with rates decreasing distally along the small intestine (Hampson & Kidder, 1986). In agreement with our morphological findings, Miniats & Valli (1973) reported longer jejunal villi in germ-free pigs but did not measure villi in other regions. Shurson et al. (1990) reported that germ-free pigs had longer ileal and duodenal villi but shorter jejunal villi compared to their conventional counterparts. Similar results were obtained also in our study as the villi in the duodenum and ileum of gnotobiotic piglets were higher in comparison with conventional piglets throughout the experiment. The difference was significant at 3 hours after birth, on days 2 and 7 of age (p < 0.01) and day 14 of age (p < 0.05) in the duodenum and on days 14 and 21 in the ileum (p < 0.05). Shirkey et al. (2006) suggested that regional variation in morphology, especially in the proximal small intestine, is not entirely dependent on microbial colonization but is also influenced by such non-microbial factors as bile salts, pancreatic secretions, and compounds of dietary origin which would be expected to be in higher concentration and have more contact with mucosal surface in the duodenum.

The gastrointestinal tract goes through substantial structural and functional changes in the early postnatal period (Walthall et al., 2005). As the piglets grow, functional changes occur in the expression and kinetics (Fan et al., 2002) of brush border digestive enzymes. Each brush border enzyme shows a specific developmental pattern as the animal ages, which have been associated with the maturation of enterocytes (Walthall et al., 2005). Specifically, changing disaccharidasae activities have been used as an indicator of intestinal maturation. Measurable lactase levels were detected in bush border homogenates and membrane vesicles of the small intestine in the 7th week of pregnancy (Buddington & Malo, 1996). For comparison, activity of lactase in human foetuses was confirmed only later and only in the 34th week of gravidity (Menard & Basque, 2001). Aumaitre & Corring (1978) measured lactase in small intestine homogenates from pig foetuses at 105th day of gravidity and observed that the total activity of lactase in the intestine amounted to only 10% of the activity determined at birth. It was stated that specific activities of lactase in homogenates or membrane vesicles of the small intestine brush border were high at birth and stayed at this level during the first 7-10 days of postnatal life (Torp et al., 1993). In suckling pigs, lactase activity was observed to undergo an initial marked decrease sometime during the second to fifth week of age which was followed by a period when it remained relatively constant or continued to decrease gradually up to 8 weeks of age (Kelly et al., 1991). In terms of enzyme distribution throughout the intestine, neonatal and 1-day old piglets show the highest specific lactase activity in the proximal part of the small intestine and the lowest in the distal part, but at the age of 6-10 days its distribution throughout the intestine was more regular (Buddington & Malo, 1996). The intestinal microbiota has been shown to affect brush border enzyme expression, as the intestine of a germ-free mouse has a different pattern of brush border enzymes than a conventional mouse (Kozakova et al., 2001). The mechanism by which bacteria induce changes in brush border enzyme activities or which bacteria are responsible has not been elucidated. According to (Willing & Kessel, 2009), conventionalization in pigs reduced enterocyte brush border enzyme activity compared with germ-free without a concomitant reduction in gene expression in the case of lactase phlorizin hydrolase. Because of the reduced villus height and increased enterocyte replacement rate observed in conventional as compared with germ-free animals (Furuse & Okumura, 1994), it has been postulated that the higher disaccharidase activity in the small intestine of germ-free as compared with conventional rats is because of an increased number of mature enterocytes (Willing & Kessel, 2009). These reports were confirmed by Reddy & Wostmann (1966) who observed that disaccharidase activity was higer in the small intestine of the germ-free as compared with conventional rats. However, in our study, contrary to previous studies, specific activities of lactase along the entire intestinal tract were higher in conventional piglets throughout the experiment. Kozakova et al. (2001) concluded that individual bacteria can stimulate a similar response, as monoassociation of gnotobiotic mice with *Bifidobacteria bifidum* induces a shift in enzyme activity to a pattern similar to that of a conventional mouse. Aumaitre & Corring (1978) reported that the intestinal tract of foetal (105th day of gravidity) and newborn piglets contained maltase but saccharase was present in one week old piglets. Similar observations for saccharase were presented by Buddington & Malo (1996). However, the studies by James et al. (1987) and Sangild et al. (1991) revealed low activities of saccharase and maltase in the small intestine of newborn piglets. Starting from 1 week of age specific activities of maltase and saccharase abruptly increased reaching maximum at the age of 10 - 16 days and sustained values at the age of approximately 3 weeks (James et al., 1987; Sangild et al., 1991). Similar tendencies of specific activity of maltase and saccharase were observed also in our study. When comparing the postnatal development of specific activities of enzymes maltase and saccharase in gnotobiotic and conventional piglets we observed a similar trend but higher activities of both enzymes in all segments of digestive tract of conventional piglets throughout the observation period. In 6 - 7 days old piglets, the distribution of activities of saccharase and maltase was similar along the small intestine but the activities of both enzymes were higher in the proximal to medial parts of the jejunum compared to distal part of the small intestine (Aumaitre & Corring, 1978; Buddington & Malo, 1996). In our study, saccharase activity distribution throughout the small intestine of gnotobiotic and conventional piglets was higher in the jejunum during the entire period of observation. Distribution of maltase along the small intestine changed depending on age, from predominant concentration of the activity in the proximal half of the small intestine at the age of 1-2 weeks (Aumaitre & Corring, 1978) through uniform distribution along the small intestine at the age of 2-3 weeks (Kelly et al., 1991) up to higher activity in the range of 10-15% along 80-90% of the intestine length at the age of 5 - 8 weeks (Hampson & Kidder, 1986). Similar distribution of maltase along the small intestine was observed also in our study in both gnotobiotic and conventional piglets. Transition from milk nutrition to definitive nutrition in children is accompanied with induction of maltase and decreasing activity of lactase as an adaptation of GIT to changes in nutrition with age (Menard & Basque, 2001). Other factors besides age which affect development of disaccharidases activities in the small intestine include: feed offered to piglets in the period of suckling (Hampson & Kidder, 1986), weaning to dry or liquid feed, growth factors, for example epidermal growth factor (James et al., 1987) and hormones, for example insulin (Shulman, 1990), corticosteroids (Kreikemeier et al., 1990), ACTH - adrenocorticotropin (Sangild et al.,1991). Willing & Kessel (2009) concluded that enterocyte upregulation of brush border enzyme expression occurs as either a direct response to microbial colonization or as a feedback mechanisms in response to reduced enzyme activity through microbial degradation. This mechanism may play a role in ensuring effective competition of the host with the intestinal microbiota for available nutrients.

4.4 Effect of weaning on development of the small intestine of conventionally and gnotobiotic bred piglets

Another critical phase in the gastrointestinal tract development of young animals is the weaning period. The weaning of piglets usually takes place between 3 and 4 week of life, when the majority of nutrients are ingested with milk. Weaning for farm animals occurs in an early age, when the gastrointestinal system motility, digestive and absorptive functions are not yet matured and prepared for food other than milk. In a wild boar, domestic pig ancestor, the offspring is weaned in much older age and change of the diet is gradual, therefore weaning disorders are nearly nonexistent. In intensive livestock production shorter suckling period benefits in increased number of piglets born per year, but at the negative side is an increased number of weaning disorders (Zabielski et al., 2008). Weaning is associated with mixing of piglets from different litters and sometimes also with the transport of animals from the place of birth to specialized nursery units. This results in profound social and environmental stress which is a caused also by the changes in the diet. The gastrointestinal tract has to adapt to the new type of feed, which leads to changes in myenteron motility, enzymes secretion and activity, and the composition of bacterial flora (Barszcz & Skomial, 2011). According to Lalles et al. (2007) weaning is a critical phase for piglets, it is associated with a variable period of anorexia during the first days after weaning, the deterioration of the digestive function and accumulation of undigested feed as a result of inefficient digestion. During this period, piglets are more susceptible to suffer from post-weaning diarrhoea with the proliferation and attachment to the intestinal mucosa of β-haemolytic strains of E. coli (Fairbrother et al., 2005). Nabuurs (1998) and Pluske et al. (1997) stated that predisposition to infections with eneterotoxigenic bacteria depends on a number of factors. Miller et al. (1986) concluded that the problems induced by weaning were caused rather by the changes in the structure of the intestines and specific loss of digestive enzymes than by any great changes in absorption function despite the fact that the data of Nabuurs et al. (1998) were contradictory. Nabuurs (1998) concluded that piglets suffering from post-weaning diarrhoea excreted enterotoxigenic E. coli strains and rotavirus, and that these piglets developed a hyperregenerative villus atrophy, and subsequently a severe loss of net absorption of fluid and electrolytes in the small intestine. A simulated halving of the absorption in the large intestine of weaned piglets aggravates the adverse effects of an enterotoxigenic E. coli in the small intestine (Nabuurs, 1998). Franklin et al. (2002) recorded no post-weaning increase in E.coli in pigs weaned at 17 days of age, in agreement with the studies of Etheridge et al. (1984) and Mathew et al. (1998), but in contrast with others (Mathew et al., 1996) who reported increase in E.coli populations after weaning. We have observed changes during the first week post-weaning in the jejunal part of the digestive tract of colostral piglets that pointed to a decrease in all observed groups of bacteria with the highest decrease by 1-1.8 log for enterococci, E. coli and Enterobacteriaceae. Mathew et al. (1998) postulated the absence of an E.coli increase may be due to weaning pigs into a highly sanitized, environmentally controlled room with limited contact among pigs. Franklin et al. (2002) also observed E.coli populations to be lower in pigs remaining on the sow, as have other investigators (Etheridge et al., 1984; Mathew et al., 1996). Jensen (1998) reported that lactobacilli are inversely proportionate to coliform bacteria during 1 week post-weaning. This is also confirmed by the results of Risley et al. (1992), but however, has not been confirmed in our experiments. In the study by Franklin et al. (2002) faecal populations of lactobacilli and E.coli followed patterns typical of those observed in the more anterior portions of the gastrointestinal tract. However, faecal bifidobacteria populations increased post-weaning, possibly due to the decrease in lactobacilli and E.coli in the posterior gastrointestinal tract. The loss of direct competition may benefit other bacterial populations, including bifidobacteria. The infant's microbiota initially shows low diversity and instability, but evolves into a more stable adult-type microbiota over the first 24 months of life (Zoetendal et al., 1998). Bifidobacterium populations are dominant in the first months of life, especially in breast-fed infants due to the bifinogenic effect of breast milk, while a more diverse microbiota is found in formula-fed infants, weaning children and adults (Gueimonde et al., 2006). In adults and weaned children the major constituents of the colonic microbiota are Bacteroides, followed by several genera belonging to the division Firmicutes, such as Eubacterium, Ruminococcus and Clostridium, and the genus Bifidobacterium. By contrast, in infants the genus Bifidobacterium is predominant and also a few genera from the family Enterobacteriaceae, as a Escherichia, Raoultella, and Klebsiella (Kurokawa et al., 2007). It is well know that weaning has a dramatic negative impact on the intestinal mucosal morphology of piglets. Significant post-weaning reduction in villus height has been observed by study (Berkeveld et al., 2007). In study of Hedemann et al. (2003) villus height decreased to a minimum during the first 3 days post-weaning and this is in accordance with the other studies showing that villous height is minimal 2-5 days post-weaning (Hampson & Kidder, 1986; Kelly et al., 1991). In the jejunum and ileum of conventional piglets, investigated in our study, we observed a post-weaning decrease in the height of villi significant on day 35 of age in the jejunum (p < 0.01). Elongation of the crypts post-weaning has been observed in several studies (Hampson & Kidder, 1986; Hedemann et al., 2003) and was confirmed in the present experiment. In our study, in the first week after weaning, conventional piglets showed significant deepening of crypts in duodenal (p < 0.001), jejunal (p < 0.01) and ileal (p < 0.05) segments. Villous atrophy may result both from increased rate of cell loss leading to higher rate of mitosis in crypts and their hyperplasia and from slower rate of cell renewal resulting from the reduction of cell division, i.e. in case of underfeeding. During the time of weaning villous shape also undergoes modifications. The marked and abrupt morphological response to weaning in the small intestine, characterized by transformation from a dense finger-like villi population to a smooth, compact, tongue-shaped luminal villi was observed in previous study (Skrzypek et al., 2005) and in the present study. The morphological changes observed in the small intestine around weaning are closely related to changes in the mucosal enzyme activity observed at the same time. When shortening of the villi is associated with cell loss, loss of mature enterocytes where digestive enzymes are located also occurs. The disaccharidases have been the most commonly investigated mucosal enzymes in relation to weaning of piglets (Kelly et al., 1991). Morphological changes in the small intestine of piglets after weaning are accompanied by smaller activity of brush border enzymes, lactase and sucrase (Pacha, 2000). In our study we registered that of lactase activity of gnotobiotic piglets decreased in the weeks 4 (p < 0.001) and 5 (p < 0.001) to levels similar to those noticed at birth. Similarly, we recorded a post-weaning decrease in lactase specific activity also in conventional piglets. The results of these studies have been used to interpret the digestive and absorptive capacity of the small intestine as well as the maturity of the enterocytes.

5. Conclusion

Gnotobiotic animals are a very useful model in studying the physiology of the digestive tract. The gnotobiotic model allowed us to carry out systematic examination of the effect of a defined microbial population on postnatal intestinal development. We characterized regional variations in morphological and functional responses of the small intestine. We also identified that morphological and functional responses were affected differently by respective bacterial species, supporting the assumption that postnatal bacterial colonization patterns play an important role in neonatal intestinal development. Very good application of gnotobiotic animals is anticipated in the field of study of mutual interaction of natural microflora and pathogens in the digestive tract, mechanisms of probiotic effects of micro-organisms. We can conclude that the development of the intestinal mucosa membrane is in direct junction to breeding conditions. In connection with postnatal differentiation and the development of the small intestine in piglets, currently there is increasingly high interest in the explanation of the important role that can be played by colostrum and by milk containing growth factors, hormones and other bio-active compounds. It is likely that removal of milk will have a profound influence upon the processes regulating the growth of cells in the small intestine, their differentiation and function.

6. Acknowledgments

This study was supported by the project SK0021, co-financed through the EEA financial mechanism, the Norwegian financial mechanism and the state budget of the Slovak

Republic and by the project from the Research and Development Support Agency APVV-20-062505.

7. References

Aumaitre, A. & Corring, T. (1978). Development of digestive enzymes in the piglet from birth to 8 weeks. II. Intestine and intestinal disaccharidases. *Nutrition and Metabolism*, Vol.22, No.4, (July-August 1978), pp.244-255, ISSN 0029-6678

Barszcz, M. & Skomial, J. (2011). The development of the small intestine of piglets-chosen aspects. *Journal of Animal and Feed Sciences*, Vol.20, No.1, (January 2011), pp.3-15, ISSN 1230-1388

Beerens, H. (1990). An elective and selective isolation medium for *Bifidobacterium spp. Letters in Applied Microbiology*, Vol.11, No.3, (September 1990), pp. 155-157, ISSN 1472-765X

Berkeveld, M.; Langendijk, P.; van Beers-Schreurs, H.M.G.; Koets, A.P.; Taverne, M.A.M.; Verheijden, J.H.M. (2007). Intermittent suckling during an extended lactation period: Effects on piglet behavior. *Journal of Animal Science*, Vol.85, No.12, (December 2007), pp.3415-3424, ISSN 0021-8812

Bomba, A.; Gancarcikova, S.; Nemcova, R.; Herich, R.; Kastel, R.; Depta, A.; Demeterova, M.; Ledecky, V.; Zitnan, R. (1998). The effect of lactic acid bacteria on intestinal metabolism and metabolic profile of gnotobiotic pigs. *Deutsche Tierarztliche Wochenschrift*, Vol.105, No.10, (October 1998), pp. 384-389, ISSN 0341-6593

Bomba, A.; Nemcova, R.; Gancarcikova, S.; Herich, R.; Guba, P.; Mudronova, D. (2002). Improvement of the probiotic effect of microorganisms by their combination with maltodextrins, fructo-oligosacharides and polyunsaturated acids. *British Journal of Nutrition*, Vol.88, No.1, (September 2002), pp. 95-99, ISSN 0007-1145

Buddington, R. K. & Malo, CH. (1996). Intestinal brush-border membrane enzyme activities and transport functions during prenatal development of pigs. *Journal of Pediatric Gastroenterology and Nutrition*, Vol.23, No.1, (July 1996), pp.51-64, ISSN 0277-2116

Bradford, M.M. (1976). A rapid and sensitive method for the quantitation of microgram quantities of protein utilizing the principle of protein-dye binding. *Analytical Biochemistry*, Vol.72, No.7, (May 1976), pp. 248-254, ISSN 003-2697

Devriese, L.A.; Hommez, J.; Wijfels, R.; Haesebrouck, F. (1991). Composition of the enterococcal and streptococcal intestinal flora of poultry. *Journal of Applied Bacteriology*, Vol.71, No.1, (July 1991), pp. 46-50, ISSN 0021-8847

Etheridge, R.D.; Seerley, R.W. & Wyatt, R.D. (1984). The effect of diet on performance, digestibility, blood composition and intestinal microflora of weaned pigs. *Journal of Animal Science*, Vol.58, No.6, (June 1984), pp.1396-1402, ISSN 0021-8812

Fairbrother, J.M.; Nadeau, E. & Gyles, C.I. (2005). *Escherichia coli* in postweaning diarrhea in pigs: an update on bacterial types, pathogenesis, and prevention strategies. *Animal Health Research Reviews*, Vol.6, No.1, (June 2005), pp.17-39, ISSN 1466-2523

Fallani, M.; Young, D.; Scott, J.; Norin, E.; Amarri, S.; Adam, R.; Aguilera, M.; Khanna, S.; Gil, A.; Edwards, C.A.; Dore, J. (2010). Intestinal microbiota of 6-week-old infants across Europe: geographic influence beyond delivery mode, breast-feeding, and antibiotics. *Journal of Pediatric Gastroenterology and Nutrition*, Vol.51, No.1, (July 2010), pp.77-84, ISSN 0277-2116

Franklin, M.A.; Mathew, A.G.; Vickers, J.R.; Clift, R.A. (2002). Characterization of microbial populations and volatile fatty acid concentrations in the jejunum, ileum and cecum, of pigs weaned at 17 vs. 24 days of age. *Journal of Animal Science*, Vol.80, No.11, (November 2002), pp. 2904-2910, ISSN 0021-8812

Furuse, M. & Okumura, J. (1994). Nutritional and physiological characteristics in germ-free chickens. *Comparative Biochemistry and Physiology A - Physiology*, Vol.109, No.3, (November 1994), pp. 547-556, ISSN 1096-4940

Godlewski, M.M.; Slupecka, M.; Wolinski, J.; Skrzypek, T.; Skrzypek, H.; Motyl, T.; Zabielski, R. (2005). Into the unknown - the death pathways in the neonatal gut epithelium. *Journal of Physiology and Pharmacology*, Vol.56, No.3, (June 2005), pp. 7-24, ISSN 0867-5910

Guarner, F. & Malagelada, J.R. (2003). Gut flora in health and disease. *Lancet*, Vol.361, No.9356, (February 2003), pp. 512-519, ISSN 0140-6736

Gueimonde, M.; Salminen, S. & Isolauri, E. (2006). Presence of specific antibiotic (tet) resistance genes in infant faecal microbiota. *FEMS Immunology and Medical Microbiology*, Vol.48, No.1, (October 2006), pp.21-25, ISSN 0928-8244

Guilloteau, P.; Biernat, M.; Wolinski, J.; Zabielski, R. (2002). Gut regulatory peptides and hormones of the small intestine, In: *Biology of the Intestine in Growing Animals*, R. Zabielski; P.C. Gregory & B. Westrom, (Eds.), 325-362, Elsevier, ISBN 978-044-4509-28-4, Amsterdam, The Netherlands

Hampson, D.J. & Kidder, D.E. (1986). Alteration in piglet small intestinal structure at weaning. *Research in Veterinary Science*, Vol.40, (1986), pp.32-40, ISSN 0034-5288

Hedemann, M.S.; Hojsgaard, S. & Jensen, J.J. (2003). Small intestinal morphology and activity of intestinal peptidases in piglets aroun weaning. *Journal of Animal Physiology and Animal Nutrition*, Vol.87, No.1-2, (February 2003), pp.32-41, ISSN 0931-2439

Hopkins, M.J.; Macfarlane, G.T.; Furrie, E.; Fite, A.; Macfarlane, S. (2005). Characterisation of intestinal bacteria in infant stools using real-time PCR and northern hybridisation analyses. *FEMS Microbiology Ecology*, Vol.54, No.1, (September 2005), pp. 77-85, ISSN 1574-6941

Inoue, R.; Tsukahara, T.; Nakanishi, N.; Ushida, K. (2005). Development of the intestinal microbiota in the piglet. *Journal of General and Applied Microbiology*, Vol.51, No.1, (August 2005), pp. 257-265, ISSN 0022-1260

James, P.S.; Smith, M.W.; Tivey, D.R. & Wilson, T.J.G. (1987). Epidermal growth factor selectively increases maltase and sucrase activities in neonatal piglet intestine. *Journal of Physiology*, Vol.393, (December 1987), pp.583-594, ISSN 0022-3751

Jensen, B.B. (1998). The impact of feed additives on the microbial ecology of the gut in young pigs. *Journal of Animal and Feed Sciences*, Vol.7, No.1, (1998), pp. 45-64, ISSN 1230-1388

Kelly. D.; Smyth, J.A. & McCracken, K.J. (1991). Digestive development in the earlyweaned pig. I. Effect of continuous nutrient supply on the development of the digestive tract and on changes in digestive enzyme activity during the first week post-weaning. *British Journal of Nutrition*, Vol.65, No.2, (March 1991), pp. 169-180, ISSN 0007-1145

Kiarie, E.; Nyachoti, C.M.; Slominski, B.A.; Blank, G. (2007). Growth performance, gastrointestinal microbial activity and nutrient digestibility in early-weaned pigs fed diets containing flaxseed and carbohydrase enzyme. *Journal of Animal Science*, Vol.85, No.11, (November 2007), pp. 2982-2993, ISSN 0021-8812

Kozakova, H.; Rehakova, Z. & Kolinska, J. (2001). *Bifidobacterium bifidum* monoassociation of gnotobiotic mice: effect on enterocyte brush-border enzymes. *Folia Microbiologica (Praha)*, Vol.46, No.6, (November-December 2001), pp.573-576, ISSN 0015-5632

Kreikemeier, K.K.; Harmon, D.L. & Nelssen, J.L. (1990). Influence of hydrocortisone acetate on pancreas and mucosal weight, amylase and disaccharidase activities in 14-day-old pigs. *Comparative Biochemistry and Physiology*, Vol.97, No.1, (January 1990), pp.45-50, ISSN 0300-9629

Kurokawa, K.; Itoh, T.; Kuwahara, T.; Oshima, K.; Toh, H.; Toyoda, A.; Takami, H.; Morita, H.; Sharma, V.K.; Srivastava, T.P.; Taylo, T.D.; Noguchi, H.; Mori, H.; Ogura, Y.; Ehrlich, D.; Itoh, K.; Takag, T.; Sakaki, Y.; Hayashi, T.; Hattori, M. (2007). Comparative metagenomics revealed commonly enriched gene sets in human gut microbiomes. *DNA Research*, Vol.14, No.4, (October 2007), pp. 169-181, ISSN 1340-2838

Lalles, J.P.; Bosi, P.; Smidt, H.; Stokes, C.R. (2007). Weaning-a challenge to gut physiologists. *Livestock Science*, Vol.108, No.1-3, (May 2007), pp.82-93, ISSN 1871-1413

Len, N.T.; Hong, T.T.T.; Ogle, B.; Lindberg, J.E. (2009). Comparison of total tract digestibility, development of visceral organs and digestive tract of Mong cai and Yorkshire × Landrace piglets fed diets with different fibre sources. *Journal of Animal Physiology and Animal Nutrition*, Vol.93, No.2, (April 2009), pp.181-191, ISSN 0931-2439

Marinho, M.C.; Lordelo, M.M.; Cunha, L.F.; Freire, J.P.B. (2007). Microbial activity in the gut of piglets: I. Effect of prebiotic and probiotic supplementation. *Livestock Science*, Vol. 108, No.1, (May 2007), pp. 236-9, ISSN 1871-1413

Marion, J.; Rome,V.; Savary, G.; Thomas, F.; Le Dividich, J.; Le Huerou-Luron, I. (2003). Weaning and feed intake alter pancreatic enzyme activities and coresponding mRNA levels in 7-d-old piglets. *Journal of Nutrition*, Vol.133, (February 2003), pp. 362-368, ISSN 0022-3166

Mathew, A.G.; Franklin, M.A.; Upchurch, W.G.; Chattin, S.E. (1996). Effect of weaning on ileal short-chain fatty acid concentrations in pigs. *Nutrition Research*, Vol.16, No.10, (October 1996), pp.1689-1698, ISSN 0271-5317

Mathew, A.G.; Chattin, S.E.; Robbins, C.M.; Golden, D.A. (1998). Effects of a direct-fed yeast culture on enteric microbial populations, fermentations acids, and performance of weanling pigs. *Journal of Animal Science*, Vol.76, No.8, (August 1998), pp. 2138-2145, ISSN 0021-8812

Menard, D. & Basque, J.R. (2001). Gastric digestive function, In: *Nestle' Nutrition Workshop Series. Gastrointestinal Functions*, E.E. Delvin & M.J. Lentze, (Eds.), 147-164, Lippincott Williams & Wilkins, ISBN 0-7817-3208-5, Philadelphia, USA

Meslin, J.C.; Sacquet, E.; Guenet, J.L. (1973). Action of bacterial flora on the morphology and surface mucus of the small intestine of the rat. *Annales de Biologie Animale Biochimie Biophysique*, Vol.13, No.2, (April-June 1973), pp. 334-335, ISSN 0003-388X

Miller, B.G.; James, P.S.; Smith, M.W.; Bourne, F.J. (1986). Effect of weaning on the capacity of pig intestinal villi to digest and absorb nutrients. *Journal of Agricultural Science*, Vol.107, No.3, (April 1986), pp.579-589, ISSN 0021-8596

Miller E.R. & Ullrey, D.E.(1987). The pig as a model for human nutrition. *Annual Review of Nutrition*, Vol.7, (1987), pp. 361-382, ISSN 0199-9885

Miniats, O.P. & Valli, V.E. (1973). The gastrointestinal tract of gnotobiotic pigs, In: *Germfree Research: Biological Effects of Gnotobiotic Environments*, J.B. Henegan, (Ed.), 575-588, Academic Press, ISBN 978-012-3406-50-7, New York, USA

Mir, P.S.; Bailey, D.R.C.; Mir, Z.; Morgan Jones, S.D.; Douwes, H.; Mc Allister, T.A.; Weselake, R.J.; Lozeman, F.J. (1997). Activity of intestinal mucosal membrane carbohydrases in cattle of different breeds. *Canadian Journal of Animal Science*, Vol.77, No.3, (May 1997), pp. 441-444, ISSN 0008-3984

Mufandaedza, J.; Viljoen, B.C.; Feresu, S.B.; Gadaga, T.H. (2006). Antimicrobial properties of lactic acid bacteria and yeast-LAB cultures isolated from traditional fermented milk against pathogenic *Escherichia coli* and *Salmonella enteritidis* strains. *International Journal of Food Microbiology*, Vol.108, No.1, (April 2006), pp.147-152, ISSN 0168-1705

Nabuurs, M.J.A. (1998). Weaning piglets as a model for studying pathophysiology of diarrhoea. *The Veterinary Quarterly*, Vol.20, No.3, (1998), pp.42-45, ISSN 0165-2176

Nankervis, C.A.; Reber, K.M. & Nowicki, P.T. (2001). Age-dependent changes in the postnatal intestinal microcirculation. *Microcirculation*, Vol.8, No.6, (December 2001), pp. 377-387, ISSN 1073-9688

Pacha, J. (2000). Development of intestinal transport function in mammals. *Physiological Reviews*, Vol.80, No.4, (October 2000), pp.1633-1667, ISSN 0031-9333

Penders, J.; Thijs, C.; van de Brandt, P.A.; Kummeling, I.; Snijders, B.; Stelma, F.; Adams, H.; van Ree, R.; Stobberingh, E.E. (2007). Gut microflora composition and development of atopic manifestations in infancy: the KOALA birth cohort study. *Gut*, Vol.56, No.5, (May 2007), pp. 661-667, ISSN 0017-5749

Piva, A.; Prandini, A.; Fiorentini, L.; Morlacchini, M.; Galvano, F.; Luchansky, J.B. (2002). Tributyrin and lactitol synergistically enhanced the trophic status of the intestinal mucosa and reduced histamine levels in the gut of nursery pigs. *Journal of Animal Science*, Vol.80, No.3, (March 2002), pp. 670-680, ISSN 0021-8812

Pluske, J.R.; Hampson, D.J. & Williams, I.H. (1997). Factors influencing the structure and function of the small intestine in the weaned pig. *Livestock Production Science*, Vol.51, No.1-3, (November 1997), pp. 215-236, ISSN 0301-6226

Pluske, J.R.; Pethick, D.W.; Hopwood, D.E. & Hampson, D.J. (2002). Nutritional influences on some major enteric bacterial diseases of pigs. *Nutrition Research Reviews*, Vol.15, No.2, (December 2002), pp. 333-371, ISSN 0954-4224

Reddy, B.S. & Wostmann, B.S. (1966). Intestinal disaccharidase activities in the growing germfree and conventional rats. *Archives of Biochemistry and Biophysics*, Vol.113, No.3, (March 1966), pp.609-616, ISSN 0003-9861

Risley, C.R.; Kornegay, E.T.; Lindemann, H.D.; Wood, C.M.; Eigel, W.N. (1992). Effect of feeding organic acids on selected intestinal content measurements at varying times postweaning in pigs. *Journal of Animal Science*, Vol.70, No.1, (January 1992), pp.196-206, ISSN 0021-8812

Sangild, P.T.; Cranwell, P.D.; Sorensen, H.; Mortensen, K.; Noren, O.; Wetteberg, L. & Sjostrom, H. (1991). Development of intestinal disaccharidases, intestinal peptidases and pancreatic proteases in sucking pigs. The effects of age and ACTH treatment, In: *Digestive Physiology in Pigs*, M.W.A. Verstegen; J. Huisman & L.A. den Hartog, (Eds.), 73-78, Pudoc, ISBN 978-902-2010-40-2, Wageningen, The Netherlands

Scharek, L.; Guth, J.; Reiter, K.; Weyrauch, K.D.; Tara, D.; Schwerk, P.; Schierack, P.; Schmidt, M.F.; Wieler, L.H.; Tedin, K. (2005). Influence of a probiotic *Enterococcus faecium* strain on development of the immune system of sows and piglets. *Veterinary Immunology and Immunopathology*, Vol.105, No.1-5, (May 2005), pp. 151-161, ISSN 0165-2427

Shirkey, T.W.; Siggers, R.H.; Goldade, B.G.; Marshall, J.K.; Drew, M.D.; Laarveld, B.; Van Kessel, A.G. (2006). Effects of commensal bacteria on intestinal morphology and expression of proinflammatory cytokines in the gnotobiotic pig. *Experimental Biology and Medicine*, Vol.231, No.8, (September 2006), pp.1333-1345, ISSN 1535-3702

Shulman, R.J. (1990). Oral insulin increases small intestinal mass and disaccharidase activity in the newborn miniature pig. *Pediatric Research*, Vol.28, No.2, (August 1990), pp.171-175, ISSN 0031-3998

Shurson, G.C.; Ku, P.K.; Waxler, G.L.; Yokoyama, M.T.; Miller, E.R. (1990). Physiological relationships between microbiological status and dietary copper levels in the pig. *Journal of Animal Science*, Vol.68, No.4, (April 1990), pp.1061-1071, ISSN 0021-8812

Siggers, R.H.; Thymann, T.; Siggers, J.L.; Schmidt, M.; Sangild, P.T. (2007). Bacterial colonization affects early organ and gastrointestinal growth in the neonate. *Livestock Science*, Vol.109, No.1-2, (May 2007), pp. 14-18, ISSN 1871-1413

Skrzypek, T.; Valverde Piedra, J.L.; Skrzypek, H.; Wolinski, J.; Kazimierczak, W.; Szymanczyk, S.; Pawlowska, M.; Zabielski, R. (2005). Light and scanning electron microscopy evaluation of the postnatal small intestinall mucosa development in pigs. *Journal of Physiology and Pharmacology*, Vol.56, No.3, (June 2005), pp.71-87, ISSN 0867-5910

Swords, W.E.; Wu, C.C.; Champlin, F.R.; Buddington, R.K. (1993). Postnatal changes in selected bacterial groups of the pig colonic microflora. *Biology of the Neonate*, Vol.63, No.3, (March 1993), pp. 191-200, ISSN 0006-3126

Torp, N.; Rossi, M.; Troelsen, J.T.; Olsen, J. & Danielsen, E.M. (1993). Lactase - phlorizin hydrolase and aminopeptidase N are differentially regulated in the small intestine of the pig. *Biochemical Journal*, Vol.295, No.1, (October 1993), pp.177-182, ISSN 0264-6021

Trahair, J.F. & Sanglid, P.T. (2002). Studying the development of the small intestine: Philosophical and anatomical perspectives, In: *Biology of the Intestine in Growing Animals*, R. Zabielski; P.C. Gregory & B. Westrom, (Eds.), 1-54, Elsevier, ISBN 978-044-4509-28-4, Amsterdam, The Netherlands

Walthall, K.; Cappon, G.D.; Hurt, M.E.; Zoetis, T. (2005). Postnatal development of the gastrointestinal system: a species comparison. *Birth Defects Research Part B, Developmental and Reproductive Toxicology*, Vol.74, No.2, (April 2005), pp.132-156, ISSN 1542-9733

Widdowson, E.M. & Crabb, D.E. (1976). Changes in the organs of pigs in response to feeding for the first 24 h after birth. *Biology of the Neonate*, Vol.28, No.5-6, (1976), pp.261-271, ISSN 1661-7800

Willing, B.P. & Van Kessel, A.G. (2009). Intestinal microbiota differentially affect brush border enzyme activity and gene expression in the neonatal gnotobiotic pig. *Journal of Animal Physiology and Animal Nutrition*, Vol.93, No.5, (October 2009), pp.586-595, ISSN 0931-2439

Xu, R.J. (1996). Development of the Newborn GI tract and its relation to colostrum/milk intake. A rewiev. *Reproduction, Fertility and Development*, Vol.8, No.1, (1996), pp. 35-48, ISSN 1031-3613

Zabielski, R.; Godlewski, M.M. & Guilloteau, P. (2008). Control of development of gastrointestinal system in neonates. *Journal of Physiology and Pharmacology*, Vol.59, No.1, (July 2008), pp. 35-54, ISSN 0867-5910

Zitnan, R.; Gancarcikova, S.; Nemcova, R.; Sommer, A.; Bomba, A.(2001). Some aspects of the morphological and functional development of the intestinal tract in piglets during milk feeding and weaning, *Proceedings of the Society of Nutrition Physiology*, p.116, ISBN 3-7690-4094-5, Frankfurt, Germany, May 2-3, 2001

Zoetendal, E.G.; Akkermans, A.D. & De Vos, W.M. (1998). Temperature gradient gel electrophoresis analysis of 16S rRNA from human fecal samples reveals stable and host-specific communities of active bacteria. *Applied and Environmental Microbiology*, Vol.64, No.10, (October 1998), pp.3854-3859, ISSN 0099-2240

6

Superior Mesenteric Artery Syndrome

Rani Sophia and Waseem Ahmad Bashir
Yeovil Hospital NHS Foundation Trust, Yeovil, Somerset
United Kingdom

1. Introduction

Superior mesenteric artery syndrome (SMAS) mostly occurs in adolescent or young adults and is a rare disorder. The syndrome was first described by the Von Rokitansky in 1842 and since then about 400 cases has been reported in literature but SMAS is not well recognised and often diagnosed late till the patients are far advanced with their symptoms (Geer 1990, Raissi et al1996). In general population the incidence with the help of upper gastrointestinal barium studies were reported to be around 0.013-0.3 %(Ylinen et al 1989). However after the scoliosis surgery the prevalence was reported to be in range of 0.5-4.7 %(Tsirikos, Jeans 2005). Geer (1990) reported that 75% of the cases occurred in patients aged between 10-30 years. In a large series of 75 patients it was reported that two third of the cases were women and one third men and the average age was around 40 years (Wilkie 1927). The morbidity caused by this syndrome and the difficulty in diagnosing it prompted this review, and at the same time it will also act as a fresh reminder for the clinicians.

2. Anatomy and pathology

The superior mesenteric artery (SMA) originates behind the neck of the pancreas at the level of the first lumbar vertebra and leaves the aorta at an acute angle. It forms an angle of approximately 45° with the abdominal aorta. The third part duodenum crosses caudal to the origin of superior mesenteric artery (SMA), coursing between SMA and aorta just inferior to the left renal vein from right to left (Fig 1). Any factor that sharply narrows the aortomesenteric angle from approximately 45° (range between 38-56°) to 6-25° will thus reduce the aortomesenteric distance to about 2-8mm (Hines et al 1984, Neri et al 2005). The mean radiographic aortomesenteric distance is 10–28 mm (Neri et al 2005).This can cause entrapment and compression of the third part of duodenum. Thus conditions such as loss of mesenteric and retroperitoneal fat and subsequent decrease of the aortomesenteric distance can cause SMAS.

3. Causes

- In elderly patients heavily calcified or tortuous aorta can cause SMAS.
- Other causes reducing the aortomesenteric angle are:
- Severe cachexia or catabolic states such as weight loss due to neoplasia, anorexia nervosa
- Severe head injuries or prolonged bed rest or severe burns
- Bariatric surgery or Nissan fundoplication, spinal scoliosis surgery
- Spinal deformities or trauma

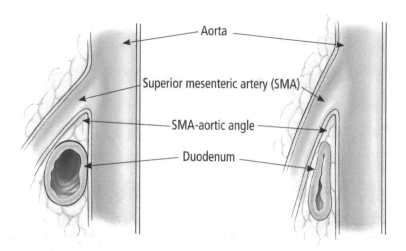

Fig. 1. Left, the normal angle between the superior mesenteric artery (SMA) and the aorta is 25 to 60 degrees. Right, in SMA syndrome, the SMA-aortic angle is more acute, and the duodenum is compressed between the aorta and the SMA (Reproduced with permission from Pasumarthy et al (2010) Cleveland Clinic Journal of Medicine. 77:45-50)

- Anatomic or congenital anomalies as high insertion of the ligament of Treitz, Intestinal malrotation, peritoneal adhesions and low origin of the superior mesenteric artery

4. Symptoms and signs

The most common symptom in these patients is intermittent abdominal pain and copious vomiting. The abdominal pain can be postprandial and the nausea, vomiting can lead to anorexia and weight loss. Early satiety, eructations, and at times sub-acute small bowel obstruction can develop. The symptoms are relieved when patient lies in left lateral decubitus, prone or knee-to-chest position (Geer 1990, Wilkie 1927, Raissi et al 1996). They are often aggravated by in an asthenic patient in supine position. Examination of the abdomen may reveal a succussion splash. Peptic ulcer disease is found in 25-45% of the patients and hyperchlohydria in 50 %(Geer 1990, Ylinen et al 1989). Dilated duodenum and stomach could predispose a patient to aspiration pneumonia and acute gastric rupture.

5. Diagnosis

To diagnose a patient with SMAS traditionally barium meal studies with hypotonic duodenography is being used. A positive diagnosis will include duodenal dilatation, retention of barium with in duodenum, the classical vertical linear impression caused by extrinsic pressure in the third part of duodenum and frequent relief of obstruction in left lateral or decubitus position (Tsirikos , Jeans 2005, Raissi et al 1996). In the past angiographic measurement of the aortomesenteric angle was thought to be a gold standard. An aortomesenteric angle of < 22–25° and a distance of <8 mm correlated well with symptoms of SMAS (Hines et al 1984). Because of its invasive nature, Computed tomography (CT) scan or CT angiogram/MR angiogram have taken over as a gold standard (Tsirikos , Jeans 2005,

Lee, Mangla 1978). CT or CT angiogram is also superior to ultrasound because it can measure the reduced aortomesenteric angle and show the gastric and duodenal dilatation at the same time. CT scan will also be helpful in finding the cause of SMAS e.g high insertion of ligament of Trietz or a neoplasia in that region. Upper gastrointestinal endoscopy is essential to rule out mechanical outlet obstruction of stomach or an ulcer (Ylinen et al 1989, Raissi et al 1996).

6. Treatment

If there is a neoplasm causing SMAS, anatomic or congenital abnormality then the treatment is surgical, otherwise this condition is treated conservatively. Patients are fed frequent small meals orally or if it is not possible then through enteral jejunal tube. After feeding the patient, he/she should be placed in either prone or lateral decubitus position. If patient cannot tolerate tube feeding because of excessive vomiting then he/she needs to be fed parentally. Both ways of feeding have shown to be effective (Barnes, Lee 1996).This conservative treatment should aim to correct the fluid and electrolyte balance and increase the body weight in an attempt to increase the retroperitoneal fat so that the aortomesenteric angle is corrected.

Surgical treatment is indicated if conservative treatment fails or if there is severe progressive weight loss, pronounced duodenal dilatation with stasis and complicating peptic ulcer disease. Several surgical procedures have been tried and tested in the management of SMAS. Gastrojejunostomy, dudenojejunostomy, Strong's operation (duodenal mobilisation for lowering the duodenojejunal flexure) have been performed to treat this condition. Gastrojejunostomy and lysis of the ligament of Treitz provided adequate decompression of the stomach but was not helpful in overcoming the duodenal obstruction and at times leading to blind loop syndrome with reflux of bile necessitating duodenojejunostomy (Lee, Mangla 1978). A review of 146 cases showed that duodenojejunostomy was the treatment of the choice (Lee, Mangla 1978) and success rate was 90 %(Raissi et al 1996). Recently laparoscopic dudenojejunostomy has become treatment of choice. Massoud (1995) reported his experience of laparoscopic division of the ligament of Treitz in 4 cases. It was successful in 3 cases. Gerson and Heniford (1998) reported first laparoscopic duodenojejunostomy and then further cases were reported in the literature (Richardson, Surowiec 2001). Minimally invasive surgery with less operative time, quick post operative recovery and relief of the symptoms were the advantages over traditional duodenojejunostomy.

7. Conclusion

SMAS is a rare disorder and is under-diagnosed in our practice of medicine. It should be ruled out in the patients with postprandial abdominal pain, vomiting and weight loss. It is caused by compression of the third part of duodenum by the narrowed aortomesenteric angle. There are different predisposing factors but severe weight loss and cachexia, spinal deformities and congenital anomalies are some of them. SMAS is treated initially conservatively but laparoscopic duodenojejunostomy has high success rate as well.

8. References

Barnes JB, Lee M (1996) Superior mesenteric artery syndrome in an intravenous drug abuser after rapid weight loss. *South Med J.* 89: 331–334.

Geer D (1990) Superior mesenteric artery syndrome. *Mil Med.* 155:321-3

Gersin KS, Heniford BT (1998) Laparoscopic duodenojejunostomy for treatment of superior mesenteric artery syndrome. *JSLS.* 2: 281–284.

Hines JR, Gore RM, Ballantyne GH (1984) Superior mesenteric artery syndrome. Diagnostic criteria and therapeutic approaches. *Am J Surg.* 148: 630–632.

Lee CS, Mangla JC (1978) Superior mesenteric artery compression syndrome. *Am J Gastroenterol* .70: 141–150.

Massoud WZ (1995) Laparoscopic management of superior mesenteric artery syndrome. *Int Surg.* 80: 322– 27.

Neri S, Signorelli SS, Mondati E, Pulvirenti D, Campanile E, Di Pino L, Scuderi M, Giustolisi N, Di Prima P, Mauceri B, Abate G,Cilio D, Misseri M, Scuderi R: (2005) Ultrasound imaging in diagnosis of superior mesenteric artery syndrome. *J intern Med.* 257: 346–351.

Raissi B, Taylor B, Traves D (1996) Recurrent mesenteric artery (Wilkie's) syndrome: a case report. *Can J Surg.* 39: 410-6.

Richardson WS, Surowiec WJ (2001) Laparoscopic repair of superior mesenteric artery syndrome. *Am J Surg.* 181: 377–78.

Tsirikos AI, Jeans LA (2005) Superior mesenteric artery syndrome in children and adolescents with spine deformities undergoing corrective surgery. *J Spinal Disord Tec.* 18:263–271.

Wilkie DPD (1927) Chronic duodenal ileus. *Am J Med Sci.* 173: 643-9

Ylinen P, Kinnunen J, Hockerstedt K (1989) Superior mesenteric artery syndrome. *J Clinn Gastroenterol.* 11: 386-91

7

The Surgical Management
of Chronic Pancreatitis

S. Burmeister, P.C. Bornman, J.E.J. Krige and S.R. Thomson
University of Cape Town
South Africa

1. Introduction

Chronic pancreatitis (CP) has been defined as a continuing inflammatory disease of the pancreas characterized by irreversible morphological changes, often associated with pain and with the loss of exocrine and endocrine function which may be clinically relevant (Clain JE Surg Clin North Am 1999). Pain is the principal cause of intractability and together with pancreatic insufficiency may have a significantly deleterious effect on a patient's quality of life as well as their ability to work and contribute to society, often leading to loss of their' social support network (Lankisch PG Digestion 1993). Progressive disease may culminate in severe and disabling symptoms requiring narcotic analgesia and frequent hospital admission with a consequent impact on health resources (Bornman PC W J Surg 2003; Braganza JM The Lancet 2011). The incidence and prevalence of disease has not been well documented however it is considered uncommon in Europe and the USA. This is in contrast to data available from South India where a prevalence of 114-200/100 000 people has been documented. Alcohol is the leading cause in western developed countries and some developing countries such as Brazil, Mexico and South Africa while idiopathic disease predominates in Asia and the subcontinent (Braganza JM The Lancet 2011; Garg PK J Gastroenterol Hepatol 2004).

Despite extensive study, the pathogenesis of chronic pancreatitis and the mechanisms which result in the development of pain remain poorly understood. As a result, treatment strategies have been largely empirical and based on symptoms, management of clinically evident exocrine and endocrine dysfunction and gross morphological abnormalities. Modalities employed have included medical support (with analgesics, anti-diabetic medication, pancreatic enzyme replacement, nutrient support and steroids in autoimmune disease), interventional endoscopy and surgery. The role of surgery has been primarily to relieve pain refractory to medical therapy, to address complications and to resect suspected or confirmed neoplastic disease (Bornman PC S Afr Med J 2010). The causes of pain in CP are likely multifactorial and proposed factors include excessive oxygen-derived free radicals, tissue hypoxia and acidosis, inflammatory infiltration accompanied by an influx of pain transmitted substances into damaged nerve ends and the development of pancreatic ductal and tissue fluid hypertension (Bornman PC W J Surg 2003). Surgical intervention for the relief of pain focuses primarily on the latter two proposed mechanisms. Two distinct principles have been applied in the development of procedures to address these mechanisms. Resection of diseased pancreatic tissue, in particular inflamed tissue within the head of the pancreas containing altered neural tissue and diseased ducts, considered the "pacemaker of disease" (Beger HG World J Surg 1990) and drainage of the pancreatic ductal system, in order to relieve ductal and parenchymal tissue hypertension. Removal of sufficient pancreatic tissue as to result in effective and durable relief of symptoms must however be balanced against the desire to avoid surgically related morbidity and mortality as well as to prevent post-operative pancreatic functional insufficiency. This has led to the development of less extensive resections and hybrid procedures which attempt to combine the advantages while avoiding the disadvantages of each approach.

This chapter will describe the theories around the pathophysiology of pain in chronic pancreatitis, discuss the rationale and indications for surgical intervention and detail the procedures currently available. It will also review the literature guiding the choice of these procedures for the relief of pain.

2. Pathophysiology of pain in chronic pancreatitis

The pathophysiology of CP is complex and remains poorly understood, with a number of theories having been put forward. Together with this, understanding of the mechanisms leading to the development of pain has also remained largely theoretical, confounded to a large extent by small and to some degree poorly designed studies, which have at times been contradictory. Furthermore, it is likely that the cause of pain is multi-factorial and may vary during the course of the disease (Bornman PC W J Surg 2003). To date, the most predominant theories regarding genesis of pain in CP have included:

2.1 Morphological pancreatic ductal changes resulting in obstruction and pancreatic ductal and tissue hypertension

In large duct chronic pancreatitis, changes in the composition of pancreatic fluid occur including an increase in free oxygen radicals and secretion of enzymes and calcium but a concomitant decrease in serine protease inhibitor Kazal type 1 (SPINK1), bicarbonate and citrate. (Sarles H Dig Dis Sci 1986). These changes are followed by precipitation of proteins such as lactoferrin and altered levels of pancreas related secretory stress proteins (including pancreatitis associated protein and pancreatic stone protein) (Singh SM W J Surg 1990; Graf R J Surg Res 2006). Glycoprotein plugs are formed which later become calcified leading to calcific disease with associated parenchymal fibrosis. Calcified protein plugs or calculi damage the ductal epithelium further and contribute to stasis thereby facilitating further stone formation. These changes are believed to begin in the side ducts but progress to involve the main pancreatic duct (PD) with the development of pancreatic duct strictures and obstruction (PDSO) as a consequence of fibrosis or calculi. Ductal hypertension follows with associated dilatation (Nagata A Gatroenteology 1981). Together with ductal hypertension, pancreatic tissue pressure may become elevated, particularly in areas of calcification (Okazaki K Gastroenterology 1986; Manes G Int J Pancreatol 1994; Jalleh RPBr J Surg 1991). The exact mechanism of elevated PTP in CP has not been proven, however it has been speculated that it may be a reflection of obstructed pancreatic side ducts rather than main PD obstruction. This situation may be aggravated by the development of perilobular fibrosis and a fibrotic peripancreatic capsule, resulting in a compartment syndrome like scenario with consequent tissue ischaemia and acidosis. (Karanjia ND Br J Surg 1994). While PDSO with ductal and tissue hypertension have not been consistently demonstrated in CP, nor a definite correlation shown with the development of pain (Novis BH Dig Dis Sc 1985; Manes G Int J Pancreatol 1994; Ugljesic M Int J Pancreatol. 1996; Bornman PC W J Surg 2003), surgical drainage procedures have been documented to reduce pancreatic tissue pressures (PTP), while a significant association between recurrence of pain and subsequent elevation of PTP has been shown. (Ebbehøj N Scand J Gastroenterol. 1990). On the other hand, ductal dilatation has been observed in the absence of ductal obstruction giving rise to the suggestion that dilatation may also be related to parenchymal destruction; this is supported by the association between duct dilatation and pancreatic insufficiency (Jensen AR Scand J Gastroent 1984). Thus, while PDSO is likely an important factor in generating pain, there are likely factors other than main pancreatic duct abnormalities that can also be implicated (Bornman PC W J Surg 2003). Furthermore, the role of side duct obstruction in the genesis of pain has not yet been clearly defined; it may be that side branch disease contributes to the development of an inflammatory mass in the pancreatic head which is recognised as important in driving the disease process (the so called "pacemaker" of disease) (Beger HG World J Surg 1990).

2.2 Interaction between the processes of inflammation and damaged neural structures

Histological studies have shown that there is invasion of neural tissue by inflammatory cells associated with chronic pancreatitis. This is accompanied by disruptions in the perineural sheaths which expose the internal neural compartments to the inflammatory response (Bockman DE Gastroenterol 1988). In addition, there are increased amounts of pain transmitted substances, pain modulators and nerve growth factors and receptors in enlarged / damaged pancreatic nerve structures, which appear to correlate with the intensity and frequency of pain (Büchler M Pancreas 1992, Zhu ZW Dig Dis Sci 2001,McMahon SP Nat Med 1995,Friess H Ann Surg 1999). Surgical resection of a pancreatic inflammatory mass effectively removes the pain stimulus together with the altered / damaged neural structures.

2.3 Toxin metabolism and generation of excessive oxygen derived free radicals resulting in electrophilic stress and inflammation

Acinar cells and proliferated islets of Langerhans are known to express cytochrome P450 (CYP) mono-oxygenases which metabolise xenobiotics (substances foreign to a living organism), often utilizing glutathione & catalysed by glutathione transferases. (Foster JR J Pathol 1993). There may however be adverse consequences to these metabolic reactions with the generation of reactive oxygen species (ROS) and toxic xenobiotic metabolites. Prevention of cellular injury relies on defences against ROS and xenobiotic metabolites; these defences include: selenium dependant glutathione peroxidase, glutathione transferases, glutathione and ascorbic acid. These varied properties make the pancreas a versatile yet vulnerable xenobiotic metabolizing organ (Braganza JM JOP 2010; Foster JR. Toxicology of the exocrine pancreas. In: General and applied toxicology 2009). Inhaled xenobiotics (such as cigarette smoke, occupational volatile hydrocarbons and petrochemicals) that pass through the pulmonary circulation represent the biggest threat by striking the pancreas through its rich arterial supply (Braganza JM Lancet 2011). When the acinar cell's defence mechanisms are insufficient to meet the increased oxidant load from ROS and xenobiotic metabolites, eletrophilic stress results (Braganza JM Digestion 1998; Braganza JM JOP 2010; Foster JR. Toxicology of the exocrine pancreas. In: General and applied toxicology 2009). Dietary insufficiency of micronutrients and ascorbic acid may predispose to this (Braganza JM Digestion 1998). Electrophilic stress in turn results in pancreastasis, the failure of apical exocytosis in the acinar cell (Sanfey H Ann Surg 1984; Leung P Antioxid Redox Signal 2009). Enzymes (both newly synthesised & those stored in zymogen granules) not able to be released apically, are released via the basolateral memebrane into the interstitium, lymphatics and bloodstream (Cook LJ Scand J Gastroenterol 1996). Entrance of enzymes and free radical oxidation products into the interstitium causes mast cell degranulation, resulting in local inflammation, activation of nociceptive axon reflexes and fibrosis. (Cook LJ Scand J Gastroenterol 1996; Braganza JM Digestion 1998). This inflammatory response is potentiated by cytokines produced by the damaged acinar cell as a result of activated signaling cascades caused by the release of ROS. (Leung P Antioxid Redox Signal 2009).

2.4 Fibrosis as a result of pancreatic stellate cell activation in the necrosis-inflammation-fibrosis sequence and sentinel acute pancreatitis events

Pancreatic stellate cells play a central role in the fibrotic process associated with chronic pancreatitis (Stevens T Am J Gastroenterol 2004). This is particularly relevant in the necrosis-inflammation-fibrosis sequence, the most widely accepted hypothesis in the pathogenesis of chronic pancreatitis (Bornman PC in Chronic pancreatitis. Hepatobiliary and pancreatic surgery – a companion to specialist surgical practice. 2009). Initially this hypothesis held that fibrosis developed as a stepwise progressive process from recurrent bouts of acute pancreatitis (Comfort MW Gastroenterology 1946; Kloppel G Hepatogastroenterol 1991). An alternative theory suggested that alcohol might be directly toxic to the acinar cell through a change in cellular metabolism (toxic-metabolic theory). Alcohol was purported to produce cytoplasmic lipid accumulation within the acinar cell, leading to fatty degeneration, cellular necrosis and eventual fibrosis (Bordalo O Am J Gastroenterol 1977). More recently the theory of a sentinel acute pancreatitis event (SAPE) has been proposed. This theory hypothesizes that stimulation of the pancreatic acinar cell by alcohol or oxidative stress activates trypsin which results in a sentinel acute pancreatitis event. This is followed by a dual phase chronic inflammatory response, with the early phase characterised by a pro-inflammatory cell infiltrate including macrophages and lymphocytes. Cytokines released during the early phase also attract a later anti-inflammatory cellular infiltrate comprising pro-fibrotic cells, including stellate cells. These cells, once attracted, are activated by lipid peroxidation products (caused by excess ROS) and mast cell degranulation products, and are considered "primed"; continued stimulation by cytokines (in particular TGF-β1) produced by acinar cells, inflammatory cells or the stellate cells themselves as a result of oxidative stress, alcohol or recurrent acute pancreatitis, cause these activated stellate cells to deposit collagen, resulting in fibrosis and the features of chronic pancreatitis (Whitcomb DC Best Pract Res Clin Gastroenterol 2002). The transient formation of fatty acid ethanol esters and the role of macrophages and lymphocytes in pancreatic tissue destruction are also thought to be integral to this process (Pandol SJ Pancreatology 2007). It is suggested that the contractive potential and perivascular location of the stellate cells results in fibrosis that leads to microvascular ischaemia and pain (Wells RG Gastroenterol 1998).

2.5 Primary duct hypothesis

This theory suggests a primary immunological attack on ductal epithelium leading to inflammation and scarring of ductal architecture. This may have specific relevance in autoimmune pancreatitis. (Cavallini G. Ital J Gastroenterol 1993).

Once inflammation becomes established in CP, patients may enter a phase of stable disease with the histological features of acinar loss, mononuclear cell infiltrate and fibrosis (Shrikhande SV Br J Surg 2003). Subsequent progression to end stage disease is characterised by loss of all secretory tissue, disappearance of inflammatory cells and intense fibrosis. This may be accompanied by loss of pancreatic function together with diminished pain, the so-called "pancreatic burn-out syndrome"; this phenomenon is however not a universal outcome in patients with CP, thereby confounding potential treatment strategies (Girdwood AH J Clin Gastroenterol 1981; Amman RW Gastroenterol 1984; Lankisch PG Digestion 1993).

Complications of CP related to inflammation and fibrosis may develop which can alter the course of disease as well as clinical presentation. These include

1.   Biliary obstruction

This is common in advanced disease, particularly when there calcification and an inflammatory mass in the head. Obstruction may be transient when related to oedema during acute flaring of disease or more permanent when occurring as a result of a fibrotic stricture or mass effect from an adjacent pseudocyst. .

2.   Duodenal obstruction

This may be the result of peri-duodenal fibrosis or from the mass effect provided by a pseudocyst.

3.   Development of a pseudocyst / pancreatic ascites

Pancreas related fluid collections or pseudocysts occur in 30-40% of patients with CP and are thought to be the consequence of either ductal obstruction or pancreatic necrosis with ductal disruption (D'Egidio A BJS 1991). Typically cysts communicate with the pancreatic ductal system which shows gross morphological abnormalities. Postnecrotic peripancreatic collections occur only rarely, usually as a consequence of an acute on chronic attack of pancreatitis. Pseudocysts in CP are usually located either near the head when they are mostly intra-pancreatic or in the lesser sac. Pseudocysts in CP are less likely to spontaneously resolve than those associated with acute disease as they have usually matured by the time of presentation and typically communicate with the pancreatic ductal system. Pancreatic ascites occurs when there is rupture of a pseudocyst or duct into the peritoneal cavity (Bornman PC in Hepatobiliary and pancreatic surgery – a companion to specialist surgical practice. 2009).

4.   Gastro-intestinal bleeding, related to
a.   Portal hypertension

Portal hypertension may develop in up to 10% of patients as a result of venous compression or thrombosis. Splenic vein thrombosis may result in segmental portal hypertension giving rise to gastric and oesophageal varices, although frank variceal bleeding in this setting is uncommon (Bornman PC in Hepatobiliary and pancreatic surgery – a companion to specialist surgical practice. 2009).

b.   Pseudoaneurysms

Enzyme rich fluid collections may erode into vascular structures resulting in false aneurysms with bleeding into the cyst and pancreatic duct, peritoneum or retroperitoneum.

3. Rationale and indications for surgical intervention

Surgery is indicated in chronic pancreatitis for the relief of pain, to manage complications and to resect confirmed or suspected neoplastic disease (Bornman PC S Afr Med J 2010). Two theoretical principles underlie the rationale for surgery to alleviate pain in CP. The first utilises the ductal / parenchymal tissue hypertension and inflammatory-neural theories on the pathogenesis of pain in CP. It postulates that surgical decompression of the main pancreatic duct will alleviate interstitial hypertension thereby improving parenchymal perfusion and acidosis (Patel AG Gastroent 1995) with consequent reduction of inflammatory stimulation and influx of mediators into damaged nerves (Salim AS HPB Surg 1997). The second principle focuses on removal of pathologically inflamed parenchyma together with altered neural tissue in particular that within the head, which is considered the "pacemaker" of disease. Emphasis has also been placed on the importance of addressing diseased side ducts, thereby limiting the possibility of recurrence (Beger HG World J Surg 1990).

The objectives of surgery for pain in CP are effective and durable relief of symptoms while preserving endocrine and exocrine function, thereby restoring the patient's quality of life. The potential for morbidity and mortality as well as recurrence should be low. Based on these objectives and the principles outlined above, a number of procedures have been developed. Essentially, these procedures fall into a spectrum covering three broad categories. At one end of the spectrum are drainage procedures which focus on decompressing the main pancreatic duct by establishing a new pancreatic-enteric communication which bypasses any native obstruction to pancreatic outflow. At the other end of the spectrum are resectional procedures which aim to remove diseased ductal and neural tissue within chronically inflamed parenchyma. Over time, a number of modified and hybrid procedures have evolved which attempt to retain the advantages while limiting the disadvantages of both the former 2 categories.

Little data exists to guide decision making regarding the optimal timing of surgery to alleviate pain in CP. There are two schools of thought. The first suggests that conservative non-surgical management should be pursued for as long as possible in order to avoid morbidity and side effects that may be associated with surgical intervention, in particular pancreatic insufficiency. They argue that the long term outcome of surgery is no different from medical management, and that the "pancreatic burn-out syndrome" is likely responsible for pain relief observed after surgery (Amman RW gastroenterol 1984). In contrast to this, others have argued that pain relief is better when surgical drainage is carried out earlier rather than later (Nealon WH Ann Surg 1993). It also remains controversial whether surgery can delay the natural course of the disease in terms of deterioration in pancreatic function (Warshaw AL Gastroenterol 1980; Nealon WH Ann Surg 1993; Jalleh RP Ann Surg 1992). Both arguments appear to have merit. While it seems foolhardy to offer surgical intervention with it's attached risk of morbidity and even mortality in patients whose symptoms might be controlled by medical means, it seems equally unreasonable to persist with a conservative approach in anticipation of pain relief, delaying surgery until narcotic addiction has developed and the outcomes from surgery may be worse (Warshaw AL gastroenterol 1984). In the absence of good evidence to guide decision making, it seems most appropriate that the decision regarding timing of surgery be individualized on a patient to patient basis. Surgical intervention should be performed only once an adequate trial of medical therapy has failed to control symptoms and the patient has been counseled regarding the risks and benefits of both modalities.

Patients referred for surgery for relief of intractable symptoms of CP should be evaluated by experienced clinicians working in a high volume, multi-disciplinary environment. All other treatment options should have been exhausted or considered not appropriate. Cross sectional imaging should be conducted to clearly delineate pancreatic morphology and detect local complications or features suggestive of neoplastic disease. The presence of portal hypertension, particularly as a result of portal or superior mesenteric vein thrombosis should be noted, as this may preclude surgical intervention (Bornman PC S Afr Med J 2010). With careful patient selection and modern surgical strategies, surgery may offer effective pain relief in over 90% of patients at 5 year follow up (Beger HG Ann Surg 1989).

In considering intervention for complications of CP, the clinical picture is paramount in decision making. Biliary obstruction may be asymptomatic, detected only biochemically or during imaging for other indications. In addition, there may be transient jaundice as a result of oedema during acute flares of the disease. The above are not indications for intervention. It must be remembered that once the biliary system has been entered, either percutaneously, endoscopically or surgically, this once sterile system should be considered contaminated with the risk of sepsis developing should obstruction recur in the future. On the other hand, persistent biliary obstruction of sufficient duration may result in secondary biliary cirrhosis, atrophy and deterioration in hepatic function. (Abdallah A HPB 2007). Obstruction longer than 4 weeks should arouse concern and warrants intervention. Decompression by means of endoscopic stenting should only be considered as a temporary bridge to surgery, in acute cholangitis or where patient factors preclude surgery (Bornman PC S Afr Med J 2010). Duodenal obstruction on the other hand typically represents either advanced fibrosis or a clinically significant pseudocyst, neither of which are likely to resolve before progression or further complications develop. Intervention is therefore indicated. Pseudocysts in CP are less likely to resolve than their acute counterparts and thus more often require drainage. The indications for drainage are the presence of symptoms or complications. Although size alone is not a criterion for intervention, cysts larger than 6cm are more likely to be symptomatic and require treatment (Bornman PC S Afr Med J 2010). Percutaneous procedures are generally not favoured for these lesions due to an increased risk of failure, introducing sepsis or creating an external fistula. Endoscopic drainage is associated with a success rate of 65-95% and a low complication rate and is preferred to surgery due to its less invasive nature. (Beckingham IJ Br J Surg 1997). Strict morphological criteria are required however, relating to cyst maturity, intra-luminal bulging, wall thickness (less than 10mm) and vascularity, particularly in the presence of portal hypertension. To this end, careful cross sectional imaging and endoscopic ultrasound are important adjuncts in assessing patients for this modality of treatment. Transmural drainage may be transduodenal or transgastric depending on the best route into the cyst while transpapillary drainage is an alternative option when communication with the pancreatic duct can be demonstrated. Surgery is indicated when endoscopic intervention fails or is not appropriate due to cyst morphology or patient factors. Surgical drainage of a pseudocyst may also be employed as part of an intervention planned for treatment of pain or additional complications. Pancreatic ascites is an uncommon but serious complication of CP which is managed in the first instance with paracentesis, nutritional support and endoscopic stenting of the pancreatic duct (Kozarek RA Gastrointest Endosc Clin North Am 1998; Bornman PC in Hepatobiliary and pancreatic surgery – a companion to specialist surgical practice 2009). Use of a somatostatin analogue remains controversial. Surgery is reserved for failures of conservative treatment. Bleeding from gastric varices related to segmental portal vein thrombosis is uncommon, thus the authors recommend intervention only once there is proven bleeding from gastric varices. Haemorrhage related to a pseudoaneurysm is best dealt with via selective angiography and embolisation due to the hazards of surgery in this setting. Surgery is reserved for failure of angiographic treatment.

4. Surgery for chronic pancreatitis – Drainage procedures

For many years longitudinal pancreaticojejunostomy (LPJ) as described by Partington and Rochelle in 1960 was the favoured surgical option in the treatment of chronic pancreatitis. This involves entering and laying open of the pancreatic duct followed by a splenic preserving pancreaticojejunostomy without resection of the pancreatic tail (Partington PF, Rochelle REL. Ann Surg 1960). This procedure is relatively simple in comparison to many of the other available operations and has a low mortality and morbidity with maximal pancreatic tissue preserved. Pain relief in the short term approximates 75% but there is frequently recurrence in the long term (Bachmann K Best Pract and res Clin Gastro 2010). This is thought to be due to incomplete decompression of the main pancreatic duct, particularly in the head. There remains a residual inflammatory mass containing altered nerve fibres (Pessaux P Pancreas 2006) as well as obstructed second and third order ducts causing ongoing intraductal hypertension (Markowitz JS Arch Surg 1994). Current indications for this procedure are isolated dilatation of the pancreatic duct greater than 7mm or where the duct has a "chain of lakes" appearance without an inflammatory mass in the head (Yekebas EF Ann Surg 2006). Where the duct is undilated (less than 3mm) a longitudinal V-shaped excision of the ventral pancreas combined with a longitudinal pancreatico-jejunostomy has been described (Izbicki JR Ann Surg 1998, 227). This may be particularly useful when a sclerosing form of chronic pancreatitis results in so called small duct disease (Bachmann K Best Pract and res Clin Gastro 2010). Good results with pain relief in 89% of patients and comparable morbidity of 19.6% have been reported (Yekebas EF Ann Surg 2006).

5. Surgery for chronic pancreatitis – Resectional procedures

With recognition that inflamed, fibrotic tissue containing damaged neural structures within the pancreatic head is critical in the generation of symptoms, pancreaticoduodenectomy became the gold standard in surgical treatment against which other procedures were measured. It has been assumed that outcomes concerning pain and quality of life are better than simple drainage procedures performed in isolation, however clear evidence of this is in randomized trials is lacking.

In the modern era, pylorus preservation as in a Pylorus Preserving Pancreaticoduodenectomy (PPPD) has been shown to result in less pain and nausea and improved quality of life when compared with the traditional Whipples pancreaticoduodenectomy (Mobius C Langenbecks Arch Surg 2007). This procedure can be performed with a mortality of 5-10% and morbidity of 20-40% and improves pain and quality of life in both the short and long term in up to 90% of patients (Bachmann K Best Pract and res Clin Gastro 2010). There are however a number of disadvantages relating to the sacrifice of functional pancreatic parenchyma and the non-diseased duodenum and common bile duct. The loss of natural bowel continuity and reduced endocrine and exocrine function result in side effects and reduced quality of life (Izbicki JR Ann Surg 1998 (228); Koninger J Surgery 2008). In order to allow organ preservation and reduce adverse effects, duodenum preserving resections of the pancreatic head (DPPHR) were developed. The Beger procedure was introduced in 1980 and was the first to include these principles (Beger HG Chirurg 1980). It consists of a subtotal resection of the head following transection of the pancreas above the portal vein. The Pancreas is then drained by an end-to-side or end-to-end pancreaticojejunostomy using a Roux-en-Y loop. Physiological gastroduodenal passage and CBD continuity are therefore preserved. This procedure could be performed with low mortality (0-3%) and morbidity (15-32%) and long term pain relief in 75-95% of patients (Izbicki JR Ann Surg 1995, Buechler MW J Gastrointest Surg 1997Frey CF Ann Surg 1994). The Frey procedure (Frey CF Pancreas 1987) subsequently combined an LPJ (as described by Partington and Rochelle) with a limited duodenum preserving excision of the head. Following exploration of the main pancreatic duct well into both the head and the tail, the head is cored out leaving a small cuff of parenchyma along the duodenal wall. This results in a lesser resection of the head than that described by Beger. In further contrast to the Beger operation, the pancreas is not divided over the SMV/portal vein complex making it an easier operation to perform. Care is taken not to enter the CBD. Drainage of the resection cavity within the head and from the opened main pancreatic duct within the body and tail is obtained with an LPJ using a Roux-en-Y loop (Frey CF Pancreas 1987). Good results have been obtained with substantial pain relief in more than 85% of patients while mortality is less than 1% and morbidity 9-39% (Izbicki JR Ann Surg 1995, Izbicki JR Ann Surg 1998, Beger HG Ann Surg 1989). Endocrine & exocrine function are well preserved and the operation may control complications such as CBD stenosis, duodenal stenosis and internal pancreatic fistulas. The Frey operation is currently the most widely performed operation for patients with an inflammatory mass in the head together with pancreatic duct dilatation while the Beger procedure is reserved for patients where the main pancreatic duct is not dilated (Bornman PC S Afr Med J 2010).

Two further modifications of the above procedures have been described. The Hamburg operation employs subtotal excision of the pancreatic head including the uncinate process(a more extensive resection than the Frey operation but comparable to Beger's procedure) together with a V-shaped excision of the ventral aspect of pancreas into the pancreatic duct. Pancreatic-enteric continuity is re-established with an LPJ using a Roux-en-Y loop (comparable to the Partington-Rochelle and Frey reconstructions).This operation combines aspects of the Frey and Beger procedures, without transection of gland over SMV/portal vein. The extent of resection is customized to pancreatic morphology while the V-shaped excicion creates a trough-like new ductal system allowing better drainage of ductal side branches (Izbicki JR Ann Surg 1998, 227, Bachmann K Med Sci Monit 2008). In the Berne operation, an extensive duodenum-preserving resection of the head is performed (as in the

Beger procedure), but without division of pancreas anterior to superior mesenteric / portal vein complex and without laying open the pancreatic duct in the FU in the body and tail. In biliary obstruction a longitudinal opening may be made in the CBD within the cavity created in the pancreatic head. Drainage of the cavity is achieved with a pancreatic-enteric anastomosis to small bowel in a Roux-en-Y reconstruction similar to the reconstructions described above. Results of the Berne procedure are comparable to the other duodenum preserving resections (Gloor B Dig Surg 2001).

Little comparative data is available to guide choice between the various available procedures in CP. Four randomized controlled trials have been conducted comparing PPPD with DPPHR, with 2 providing long term follow up (table 1). In the short to medium term,

Study	Follow up	Procedure	Mortality	Morbidity	Pain free	Pain relief	Better QOL	Endocrine function	Exocrine function	Weight gain
Buchler 1995	6 months							Glucose tolerance at 150min	Pancreolauryl test: pre- vs post-op	
		PPPD (n=20; FU 15)	0	4	6	4	8	130mg/dL	2.05µg/mL (0.48-6.6) vs 1.13µg/mL (0-4.37)	1.9+/-1.2kg
		Beger (n=20; FU 16)	0	3	12	3	12	88mg/dL	2.7µg/mL (0-8.25) vs 1.4µg/mL (0-4.41)	4.1+/-10.9kg
		P value	NS	NS	<0.05	Not stated	NS	<0.01	NS	<0.05
Klempa 1995	36 to 60 months							New onset IDDM	Steatorrhea; enzyme substitution	
		PPPD (n=21; FU 20)	1	5		14		6	20/20	
		Beger (n=22; FU 20)	0	4		20		2	3/4	
		P value	NS	NS		<0.05		Not stated	<0.05	
Izbicki 1998	12 - 36 months					Pan relief; median pain score (range)	Median post-op global QOL score; prof rehab	Insulin dose or Glucose tolerance: improved vs worsened	Abnormal faecal chymotrpsin, pancreolauryl test	Median (range)
		PPPD (n=30; FU 30)	0	16 (53%)		28; 18.1 (0-37.5)	85.7 (71.4-100); 13	0 vs 6	7	6.7kg (3.1-9.2)
		Frey (n=31; FU 31)	1	6 (19%)		26; 6.1 (0-40)	57.1 (33.3-100); 21	3 vs 2	1	1.9kg (0-6.3)
		P value	NS	<0.05		NS; not stated	<0.05; <0.05	Not stated	Not stated	Not stated
Farkas 2006	12 months						Prof rehab	New onset DM	Stool elastase; pre- vs post op	

	Follow up	Procedure	Mortality	Morbidity	Pain free	Pain relief	Better QOL	Endocrine function	Exocrine function	Weight gain
Muller 2008 (FU of Buchler 1995)	14 years	PPPD (n=20; FU 20)	0	8	13	2	11/17	3	128 +/- 29µg/g vs 122.2 +/- 23 µg/g	7.8+/- 0.9kg
		Berne (n=20; FU 20)	0	0	17	3	14/18	0	124.3 +/- 33µg/g vs 132.7 +/- 39µg/g	3.2+/- 0.3kg
		P value	NS	<0.05	NS	NS	NS	NS	NS	<0.05
Izbicki 1998			NS - Mortality unrelated to surgery	N		Median pain score	EORTC QLQ 30 – global health status (s.d.)	Presence of IDDM; new onset DM	Enzyme substitution	
		PPPD (n=20; FU=14)	5			0	58.3 (34.2)	11; 6/9	8/14	
		Beger (n=20; FU= 15)	5			0	65.0 (22.3)	7; 4/11	8/15	
		P value				S N	S, apart from greater appetite loss in PPPD group	0.128; 0.327	NS	
Strate 2008 (FU of Izbicki 1998)	median of 7 years					Pain score	EORTC Global quality of life	Presence of DM or abnormal glucose tolerance test	Abnormal faecal chymotrpsin	
		PPPD (n=30; FU 23)	4			18.75 (0-75)	50 (0-100)	15/23	22/23	
		Frey (n=30; FU 24)	6			17.5 (0-100)	58.35 (0-83.4)	13/23	18/21	
		P value				0.821	0.974	0.672	0.335	
		3 patients lost to FU							3 patients did not attend for assessment	

QOL= quality of life; pre-op= pre-operative; post-op= post-operative; FU= follow up; PPPD= pylorus preserving pancreatico-duodenectomy; NS= not significant; IDDM= insulin dependant diabetes mellitus; DM= diabetes mellitus: Prof rehab= professional rehabilitation; EORTC= European Organisation for Research and Treatment of Cancer; QLQ= Quality of Life Questionnaire; s.d= standard deviation

Buchler MW Am J Surg 1995
Klempa I Chirurg 1995
Izbicki JR Ann Surg 1998; 228
Farkas G Langenbecks Arch Surg 2006
Muller MW Br J Surg 2008
Strate T Gastroenterology 2008

Table 1. Outcomes of Pylorus preserving pancreaticoduodenectomy (PPPD) vs duodenum preserving pancreatic head resection (DPPHR)

	Follow up	Procedure	Mortality	morbidity	Pain relief	QOL	Endocrine function	Exocrine function	Weight gain
Izbicki 1995	Mean 1.5 yrs (6-24 months)				Pre-op vs post-op pain score	Prof rehab; post-op global QOL score	worsened DM control; new onset DM; newly abnormal Oral GTT	New faecal chymotrypsin/ Pancreolauryl test abnormality on post-operative FU	
		Beger (n=20)	0	6	62.25; 3	14; 28.6	2; 0; 1	2	6.7 +/- 2.1kg
		Frey (n=22)	0	2	61.50; 4	15; 28.6	0; 0; 1	2	6.4 +/- 2.5kg
		P value	NS	<0.05	NS	NS; NS	Not stated	NS	Not stated
						Less fatigue with Beger			
Strate 2005 (FU of Izbicki 1995)	Median 8.5 yrs (72-144 months)			Pancreas related repeat surgery	Pain score	global QOL score; Prof rehab	Presence of DM	Abnormal faecal pancreatic elastase	
		Beger (n=38; FU= 26)	8	3	11.25 (0 - 75)	66.7 (0-100); 16	14/25	22/25	
		Frey (n=36; FU=25)	8	0	11.25 (0 - 99.75)	58.35 (0-83.4); 11	15/25	18/23	
		P value	NS	0.08	0.679	0.476; NS	0.774	0.157	
		7 patients lost to FU (Beger 4, Frey 3)					1 patient declined testing	3 patients declined testing	
Köninger 2008	6 months and 2 years					EORTC QLQ-C30, QLQ-PAN26 scores			

Follow up	Procedure	Mortality	morbidity	Pain relief	QOL	Endocrine function	Exocrine function	Weight gain
	Beger (n=32; FU=30 and 26)		6		65.6 +/- 24.8, 63.9 +/- 23.7			
	Berne (n=33; FU=32 and 29)		7		71.3 +/- 21.6, 75.8 +/- 15.7			
	P value		>9,9		0.371, 0.037			
	Patients analysed on intention to treat; but 8 in Beger and 6 in Berne groups had technique converted							

QOL= quality of life; pre-op= pre-operative; post-op= post-operative; GTT= glucose tolerance test; FU= follow up; NS= not significant; DM= diabetes mellitus: Prof rehab= professional rehabilitation; EORTC= European Organisation for Research and Treatment of Cancer; QLQ= Quality of Life Questionnaire

Izbicki JR Ann Surg 1995

Strate T Ann Surg 2005

Koninger J Surgery 2008

Table 2. Comparisons of duodenum preserving resections of the pancreatic head.

there was evidence for significant benefit of DPPHR over PPPD in terms of morbidity (2 trials), pain relief (2 trials), quality of life (1 trial), endocrine function (1 trial), exocrine function (1 trial) and weight gain (2 trials). In addition, 2 trials showed a benefit for DPPHR in terms of operating time while hospital stay and requirement for blood transfusion were improved in 1 trial each. A Cochrane review on short term outcomes concluded that there was benefit for DPPHR in respect of quality of life and professional rehabilitation, exocrine insufficiency, weight gain, hospital stay and intra-operative blood replacement. There was also a trend towards reduced post-operative diabetes (Diener MK Ann Surg 2008). However, in the 2 studies examining long term outcomes, it was seen that many of the short term clinical benefits described above were not maintained. Proposed reasons for this were study error related to the small population sizes studied and that pancreatic gland burn-out might be delayed by DPPHR (Muller MW Br J Surg 2008). Nevertheless, at 14 year follow up there remained a trend towards better endocrine function, while there was significant benefit in terms of appetite, subjective feeling of well being and mean period of employment after surgery for patients undergoing DPPHR(Muller MW Br J Surg 2008). Thus, while short term results favour DPPHR over PPPD in CP, long term results appear equivalent and probably reflect the natural course of the disease.

Only 2 randomized trials have compared different DPPHR procedures, with 1 trial undergoing long term follow up (table 2). The first trial compared the Beger and Frey procedures with no significant differences being found in the short term apart from a benefit for the Frey operation in terms of morbidity. After a median of 8.5 years, all variables had comparable outcomes while almost all patients were noted to be exocrine insufficient (Izbicki JR Ann Surg 1995; Strate T Ann Surg 2005). The second study compared the Beger and Berne procedures, suggesting a benefit for the Berne operation in terms of operation time and hospital stay. Results were analysed on intention to treat basis however, including 8 out of 32 (Beger procedure) and 6 out of 33 (Berne procedure) patients who had their operations altered for technical reasons. When patients were analysed per protocol ie only those who underwent their assigned procedure, only the difference in operating times remained significant.

More extensive pancreatic resections such as total or near total distal pancreatectomy offer only short term relief and are associated with significant mortality and morbidity, often as a result of markedly reduced pancreatic function. They have largely been abandoned with their main role being as salvage procedures for complications relating to previous surgical interventions (including anastamotic leakage, pancreatic fistula and intractable pain following previous adequate resection or drainage surgery).

6. Surgery for the complications of chronic pancreatitis

Surgery for the complications of CP should be individualized to cater to a patient's specific morphology and clinical presentation.

6.1 Biliary obstruction

Choledocho-duodenostomy or hepatico-jejunostomy using a Roux-en-Y loop are the preferred procedures to resolve isolated biliary obstruction although the former may result in enteric refux and a sump-like syndrome. Cholecysto-enterostomy has been associated with poor results and has fallen into disfavour. A Hepatico-jejunostomy may be included in the Roux loop used to drain the pancreatic duct in dedicated drainage, resection or hybrid procedures performed to relieve pain. Alternatively, the CBD may opened within the surgically created cavity in the pancreatic head during the Berne procedure.

6.2 Duodenal obstruction

Surgical relief of obstruction related to a fibrotic stricture involves duodenal mobilization by Kocher's maneouvre with division of all fibrotic tissue. Should this be insufficient to restore patency, duodeno-duodenostomy or a gastro-jejunostomy may be considered, although the latter may be associated with biliary reflux. Where biliary obstruction co-exists in the presence of duodenal obstruction together with an inflammatory mass in the head, two options exist: PPPD or gastric bypass with a gastro-jejunostomy as part of the Roux drainage limb in a DPPHR.

6.3 Development of a pseudocyst

The choice of surgical procedure is dictated by the location of the pseudocyst and its proximity to a section of bowel suitable for drainage. Cyst-gastrostomy, cyst-duodenostomy and cyst-jejunostomy may all be employed depending on individual patient characteristics. Distal pancreatectomy may be employed for segmental disease within the body/tail together with an associated pseudocyst (Bornman PC S Afr Med J 2010). Surgery for pancreatic fistulae / ascites entails either a roux-en-Y jejunostomy to the fistula tract or an appropriate resection.

6.4 Gastro-intestinal bleeding, related to

a. Portal hypertension

Patients who have bled from gastric varices related to segmental portal hypertension as a consequence of splenic vein thrombosis can usually be managed with distal pancreatectomy.

b. Pseudoaneurysms

Where angiographic embolisation has failed to control a bleeding pseudoaneurysm vascular control may be achieved using a Frey-type procedure in preference to a more extensive resection which may be hazardous under these circumstances, while bleeding from the tail can usually be dealt with safely by means of a distal pancreatectomy (Bornman PC S Afr Med J 2010).

Surgery for suspected malignancy should utilize either a pancreatico-duodenectomy or distal pancreatectomy depending on tumour location and should be performed in keeping with the oncological principle of clear resection margins.

7. Conclusion

The pathophysiology of chronic pancreatitis is complex and as yet incompletely understood, confounding attempts at effective management strategies. The clinical picture is dominated by progressive pain which may become intractable and pancreatic endocrine and exocrine dysfunction which may severely impact on a patient's quality of life. Surgery aims to relieve ductal and tissue hypertension related to obstruction in the main and side branch ducts while also removing inflamed and fibrotic parenchymal tissue containing diseased nerve fibres. Duodenal preserving pancreatic head resections, usually combined with drainage of the main pancreatic duct, achieve both objectives with short and long term relief of pain in approximately 90% of patients at 5 year follow up. By preserving some parenchymal tissue these procedures attempt to limit pancreatic functional insufficiency. With acceptable morbidity and mortality figures, they have evolved as the surgical procedure of choice for the majority of patients with pain refractory to medical treatment. Surgery for complications of CP should be individualized while resection for neoplastic disease should be performed according to oncological principles, ensuring a clear margin of resection. More extensive resections should generally only be performed as salvage procedures for complications of previous surgery. Patients requiring surgery for chronic pancreatitis should be evaluated and treated by experienced surgeons in high volume centres utilizing a multi-disciplinary approach. Prior to undergoing surgery for pain, patients should have completed an adequate trial of medical therapy and been thoroughly counseled regarding the risks of surgery and its likely outcomes.

8. References

[1] Abdallah AA, Krige JEJ, Bornman PC. Biliary tract obstruction in chronic pancreatitis. HPB 2007; 9: 421-428

[2] Amman RW, Akovbiantz A, Largiader F et al. Course and outcome of chronic pancreatitis. Longitudinal study of a mixed medical-surgical series of 245 patients. Gastroenterol 1984; 86: 820-828

[3] Bachmann K, Izbicki JR, Yekebas EF. Chronic pancreatitis: modern surgical management Langenbecks Arch Surg. 2011 Feb; 396(2):139-49.

[4] Bachmann K, Kutup A, Mann O et al. Surgical treatment in chronic pancreatitis timing and type of procedure. Best Pract and res Clin Gastro 2010; 24: 299-310

[5] Bachmann K, Mann O, Izbicki JR et al. Chronic pancreatitis – a surgeons' view. Med Sci Monit 2008; 14:RA 198-205

[6] Beckingham IJ, Krige JEJ, Bornman PC et al. Endoscopic management of pancreatic pseudocysts. Br J Surg 1997; 84: 1638-1645

[7] Beger HG, Büchler M. Duodenum preserving resection of the head of the pancreas in chronic pancreatitis with inflammatory mass in the head. World J Surg 1990; 14: 83-87

[8] Beger HG, Buechler M, Bittner R et al: Duodenum preserving resection of the head of the pancreas in severe chronic pancreatitis. Ann Surg 1989: 209: 273-278

[9] Beger HG, Witte C, Krautzberger W et al. [Experiences with duodenum-sparing pancreas head resection in chronic pancreatitis]. Chirurg 1980; 51: 303-307

[10] Bockman DE, Büchler M, Malfertheiner P et al. Analysis of nerves in chronic pancreatitis. Gastroenterol 1988; 94: 1459-146

[11] Bordalo O, Goncalves D, Noronha M et al. Newer concept for the pathogenesis of chronic alcoholic pancreatitis. Am J Gastroenterol 1977; 68:278-285

[12] Bornman PC (Eds) O James Garden 4th edition. Chronic pancreatitis. Hepatobiliary and pancreatic surgery – a companion to specialist surgical practice. WB Saunders Co Ltd, London, Edinburgh, New York 2009: 259-283

[13] Bornman PC, Botha JF, Ramos JM et al. Guidelines for the diagnosis and treatment of chronic pancreatitis. S Afr Med J 2010; 100(12): 845-860

[14] Bornman PC, Marks IN, Girdwood AW et al. Pathogenesis of Pain in Chronic Pancreatitis: Ongoing Enigma. W J Surg 2003; 27: 1175-1182

[15] Bornman PC, Marks IN, Girdwood AW et al. Is pancreatic duct obstruction or stricture a major cause of pain in calcific pancreatitis. Br J Surg 1980; 67: 425-428

[16] Braganza JM. A framework for the aetiogenesis of chronic pancreatitis Digestion 1998; 58(suppl 4): 1-12

[17] Braganza JM, Dormandy TL. Micronutrient therapy for chronic pancreatitis: rationale and impact. JOP 2010; 11: 99-112

[18] Braganza JM, Lee SH, McCloy RF et al. Chronic pancreatitis. The Lancet 2011; 377, April 2: 1184 – 1197

[19] Buchler MW, Friess H, Muller MW et al. Randomised trial of duodenum-preserving pancreatic head resection versus pylorus-preserving Whipple in chronic pancreatitis. Am J Surg 1995; 169: 65-69

[20] Büchler M, Weihe E, Friess H et al. Changes in peptidergic innervations in chronic pancreatitis. Pancreas 1992; 7: 182-192

[21] Buechler MW, Friess H, Bittner R et al. Duodenum-preserving pancreatic head resection: long term results. J Gastrointest Surg 1997; 1: 13-19

[22] Cavallini G. Is chronic pancreatitis a primary disease of the pancreatic ducts. A new pathogenetic hypothesis. Ital J Gastroenterol 1993; 25:400-407

[23] Clain JE, Pearson RK. Diagnosis of chronic pancreatitis: is a gold standard necessary? Surg Clin North Am 1999; 79: 829-845

[24] Comfort MW, Gaubill EE, Baggenstos AM. Chronic pancreatitis: a study of 29 cases without associated disease of the biliary or gastro-intestinal tract. Gastroenterology 1946; 6:239

[25] Cook LJ, Musa OA, Case RM. Intracellular transport of pancreatic enzymes. Scand J Gastroenterol 1996; 219(suppl): 1-5

[26] D'Egidio A, Schein M. Pancreatic pseudocysts: a proposed classification and its management implications. BJS 1991; 78(8): 981-984

[27] Diener MK, Rahbari NN, Fisher L et al. Duodenum-preserving pancreatic head resection versus pancreaticoduodenectomy for surgical treatment of chronic pancreatitis: a systemic review and meta-analysis. Ann Surg 2008; 247: 950-961

[28] Ebbehøj N, Borly L, Bülow J et al. Evaluation of pancreatic tissue fluidpressure and pain in chronic pancreatitis. A longitudinal study. Scand J Gastroenterol. 1990; 25: 462-466

[29] Farkas G, Leindler L, Daroczi M et al. Long term follow-up after organ preserving pancreatic head resection in patients with chronic pancreatitis. J Gastrointest Surg 2008; 12: 308-312

[30] Farkas G, Leindler L, Daroczi M et al. Prospective randomised comparison of organ preserving pancreatic head resection with pylorus-preserving pancreaticoduodenectomy. Langenbecks Arch Surg 2006; 391: 338-342

[31] Foster JR. Toxicology of the exocrine pancreas. In: Ballantyne B, Marrs T, Syversen T eds. General and applied toxicology, 3rd edition. Chichester: John Wiley and sons, 2009: 1411-1455

[32] Foster JR, Idle JR, Hardwick JP et al. Induction of drug metabolisingenzymes in in human pancreatic cancer and chronic pancreatitis. J Pathol 1993; 169: 457-463

[33] Friess H, Zhu ZW, di Mola FF et al. Nerve growth factor and its high affinity receptor in chronic pancreatitis. Ann Surg 1999; 230: 615-624

[34] Frey CF, Amikura K. Local resection of the head of the pancreas combined with longitudinal pancreaticojejunostomy in the management of patients with chronic pancreatitis. Ann Surg 1994; 220: 492-507

[35] Frey CF, Smith GJ. Description and rationale of a new operation for chronic pancreatitis. Pancreas 1987; 2: 701-707

[36] Garg PK, Tandon RK. Survey on chronic pancreatitis in the Asia-Pacific region. J Gastroenterol Hepatol 2004; 19: 998-1004

[37] Graf R, Scheisser M, Reding T. Exocrine meets endocrine: pancreatic stone protein and regenerating protein – two sides of the same coin. J Surg Res 2006; 133: 113-120

[38] Girdwood AH, Marks IN, Bornman PC et al. Does progressive pancreatic insufficiency limit pain in calcific pancreatitis with duct stricture or continued alcohol insult. J Clin Gastroenterol 1981; 3:241-245

[39] Gloor B, Friess H, Uhl W et al. A modified technique of the Beger and Frey procedure in patients with chronic pancreatitis. Dig Surg 2001; 18: 21-25

[40] Izbicki JR, Bloechle C, Broering DC et al. Extended drainage versus resection in surgery for chronic pancreatitis – prospective randomized trial comparing the longitudinal pancreaticojejunostomy combined with local pancreatic head excision with the pylorus preserving pancreaticoduodenectomy. Ann Surg 1998; 228: 771-779

[41] Izbicki JR, Bloechle C, Broering DC et al. Longitudinal V-shaped excision of the ventral pancreas for small duct disease in severe chronic pancreatitis. Ann Surg 1998; 227: 213-219

[42] Izbicki JR, Bloechle C, Knoefel WT et al. Complications of adjacent organs in chronic pancreatitis managed by duodenum preserving resection of the head of the pancreas. Br J Surg 1994; 81: 1351-1355

[43] Izbicki JR, Bloechle C, Knoefel WT et al. Duodenum preserving resections of the head of the pancreas in chronic pancreatitis – a prospective randomized trial. Ann Surg 1995; 221: 350-358

[44] Jalleh RP, Aslam M, Williamson RCN. Pancreatic tissue and ductal pressures in chronic pancreatitis. Br J Surg 1991; 78: 1235-1237

[45] Jensen AR, Matzen P, Malchow-Møller A et al. Pattern of pain, duct morphology and pancreatic function in chronic pancreatitis. A comparative study. Scand J Gastroent 1984; 9: 334-338

[46] Karanjia ND, Widdison AL, Leung F et al. Compartment syndrome in experimental chronic obstructive pancreatitis: effects of decompressing the main pancreatic duct. Br J Surg 1994; 81: 259-264

[47] Klempa I, Spatny M, Menzel J et al. Pankreasfunktion und lebensqualität nach pankreaskopfresektion bei der chronischen pankreatitis. Chirurg 1995; 66: 350-359

[48] Kloppel G, Maillet B. Chronic pancreatitis: evolution of the disease. Hepatogastroenterol 1991; 38: 408-412

[49] Koninger J, Seiler CM, Sauerland S et al. Duodenum-preserving pancreatic head resection – a randomised controlled trial comparing the original Beger procedure with the Berne modification. Surgery 2008; 143: 490-498

[50] Kozarek RA. Endoscopic therapy of complete and partial pancreatic duct disruption. Gastrointest Endosc Clin North Am 1998; 8: 39-53

[51] Lankisch PG, Löhr-Happe A, Otto J et al. Natural course in chronic pancreatitis. Pain, exocrine and endocrine pancreatic insufficiency and prognosis of the disease. Digestion 1993; 54: 148-155

[52] Leung P, Chan YC. Role of oxidative stress in pancreatic inflammation. Antioxid Redox Signal 2009; 11: 135-165

[53] McMahon SP, Bennett DL, Priestly JV et al. The biological effects of endogenous nerve growth factor on adult sensory nerves revealed by a tryA-IgG fusion molecule. Nat Med 1995; 1: 774-780

[54] Manes G, Büchler M, Pieramico O et al. Is increased pancreatic pressure related to pain in chronic pancreatitis? Int J Pancreatol 1994; 15: 113-117

[55] Markowitz JS, Rattner DW, Warshaw AL. Failure of symptomatic relief after pancreaticojejunal decompression for chronic pancreatitis. Strategies for salvage. Arch Surg 1994; 129: 374-379

[56] Mobius C, Max D, Uhlmann D et al. Five-year follow -up of a prospective non-randomized study comparing duodenum-preserving pancreatic head resection with classic Whipple procedure in the treatment of chronic pancreatitis. Langenbecks Arch Surg 2007; 392: 359-364

[57] Muller MW, Friess H, Martin DJ et al. Long term follow-up of a randomized clinical trial comparing Beger with pylorus-preserving Whipple procedure for chronic pancreatitis. Br J Surg 2008; 95: 350-356

[58] Nagata A, Homma T, Tamai K et al. A study of chronic pancreatitis by serial endoscopic pancreatography. Gatroenteology 1981; 81: 884-891

[59] Nealon WH, Thompson JC. Progressive loss of pancreatic function in chronic pancreatitis is delayed by main pancreatic duct decompression – a longitudinal prospective analysis of the modified Peustow procedure. Ann Surg 1993; 217: 458-468

[60] Novis BH, Bornman PC, Girdwood AH et al. Endoscopic manometry of the pancreatic duct and sphincter zone in patients with chronic pancreatitis. Dig Dis Sc 1985; 30:225-228

[61] Okazaki K, Yamamoto Y, Ito K et al. Endoscopic measurement of papillary sphincter zone and pancreatic main ductal pressure in patients with chronic pancreatitis. Gastroenterology 1986; 91: 409-418

[62] Pandol SJ, Raraty M. Pathobiology of alcoholic pancreatitis. Pancreatology 2007; 7:105-114

[63] Partington PF, Rochelle REL. Modified Puestow procedure for retrograde drainage of the pancreatic duct. Ann Surg1960; 152: 1037-43

[64] Patel AG, Toyoma MT, Alvarez C et al. Pancreatic interstitial pH in human and feline chronic pancreatitis. Gastroenterology 1995; 109: 1639-1645

[65] Pessaux P, Kianmanesh R, Regimbeau JM et al. Frey procedure in the treatment of chronic pancreatitis: short term results. Pancreas 2006; 33: 354-358

[66] Salim AS. Perspectives in pancreatic pain. HPB Surg 1997; 10: 269-277

[67] Sanfey H, Bulkley B, Cameron JL. The role of oxygen derived free radicals in the pathogenesis of acute pancreatitis. Ann Surg 1984; 200:405-413

[68] Sarles H. Etiopathogenesis and definition of chronic pancreatitis. Dig Dis Sci 1986; 11(suppl): s91-107

[69] Shrikhande SV, Martignoni ME, Shrikhande M et al. Comparison of histological features and inflammatory cell reaction in alcoholic, idiopathic and tropical chronic pancreatitis. Br J Surg 2003; 90: 1565-1572

[70] Singh SM, Reber HA. The pathology of chronic pancreatitis. W J Surg 1990; 14: 2-10

[71] Stevens T, Conwell DL, Zuccaro G. Pathogenesis of chronic pancreatitis: an evidence-based review of past theories and recent developments. Am J Gastroenterol 2004; 99: 2256-2270

[72] Strate T, Bachman K, Busch P et al. Resection vs drainage in treatment of chronic pancreatitis: long term results of a randomized trial. Gastroenterology 2008; 134: 1406-1411

[73] Strate T, Knoefel WT, Yekebas E et al. Chronic pancreatitis: etiology, pathogenesis, diagnosis and treatment. Int J Colorectal Dis 2003; 18: 97-106

[74] Strate T, Taherpour Z, Bloechle C et al. Long-term follow-up of a randomized trial comparing the Beger and Frey procedures for patients suffering from chronic pancreatitis. Ann Surg 2005; 241: 591-598

[75] Ugljesic M, Bulajic M, Milosavljevic T et al. Endoscopic manometry of the sphincter of Oddi and pancreatic duct in patients with chronic pancreatitis. Int J Pancreatol. 1996; 19: 191-195

[76] Wells RG, Crawford JM. Pancreatic stellate cells. The new stars of chronic pancreatitis? Gastroenterol 1998; 115: 491-493

[77] Whitcomb DC, Schneider A. Hereditary pancreatitis: a model for inflammatory disease of the pancreas. Best Pract Res Clin Gastroenterol 2002; 16: 347-363

[78] Zhu ZW, Friess H, Wang L et al. Brain derived neurotrophic factor (BDNF) is upregulated and associated with pain in chronic pancreatitis. Dig Dis Sci 2001; 46: 1633-1639

[79] Warshaw AL. Pain in chronic pancreatitis: patients, patience and the impatient surgeon. Gastroenterol 1984; 86: 987-989

[80] Warshaw AL, Popp JL, Schapiro RH. Long-term patency, pancreatic function, and pain relief after lateral pancreaticojejunostomy for chronic pancreatitis. Gastroenterol 1980; 79: 289-293

[81] Yekebas EF, Bogoevski D, Honarpisheh H et al. Long-term follow-up in small duct chronic pancreatitis: a plea for extended drainage by "V-shaped excision" of the anterior aspect of the pancreas. Ann Surg 2006; 244:940-946

8

Appendiceal MALT Lymphoma in Childhood – Presentation and Evolution

Antonio Marte[1,*], Gianpaolo Marte[2], Lucia Pintozzi[1] and Pio Parmeggiani[1]
[1]Pediatric Surgery, 2nd University of Naples, Naples
[2]General Surgery, 2nd University of Naples, Naples
Italy

1. Introduction

Lymphoma of mucosa-associated lymphoid tissue (MALT lymphoma) was first described by Isaacson et al. in 1983 (Isaacson & Wright, 1984). According to the WHO lymphoma classification, the indolent B cell lymphoma of MALT type is classified as a marginal zone lymphoma, thus called because it originates from the B lymphocytes normally present in a distinct anatomical location (marginal zone) of the secondary lymphoid follicles (Harris et al., 2001). MALT lymphomas comprise up to 40% of adult non-Hodgkin lymphomas (NHL); the median age at occurrence is 60 years, with a female predominance (Anonymous, 1997). In paediatric age MALT lymphomas are very rare. We report on a case of MALT lymphoma involving the appendix in a 6-year-old immunocompetent girl and its evolution toward an inflammatory bowel disease (IBD) at a middle-term follow-up.

2. Case report

P.A., a 6-year-old girl, was referred to our institution in May 2005 with a diagnosis of appendicitis. The girl had been complaining of right lower abdominal pain for 6 months. More recently, the pain was exacerbated by walking and coughing. Abdominal ultrasound showed a slight effusion of the pelvic fossa. Her postnatal history showed some period of constipation spaced by regular daily evacuations. Blood examinations showed neutrophil leucocytosis. The patient underwent laparoscopic appendectomy using the three-trocar technique, three endo-loops and the Liga-Sure for the hemostasis. During the laparoscopic exploration no hyperplastic mesenteric lymphnode was found. The appendix appeared moderately hyperemic with a slight enlargement of two-thirds of its distal portion (Fig. 1).

The postoperative course was uneventful and the girl was discharged on day 1, without any complications. The appendix underwent a routine histological examination. The morphological appearance showed thickened lamina propria and submucosa, which were occupied by pseudonodules of immunocompetent cells (Fig. 2), characterized by lymphocytes with small nuclei with a narrow cytoplasmic rim and plasma cell (Fig. 3). Immunohistochemical studies revealed positivity for CD20 (CD20, pan B cell), and

---

* Corresponding Author

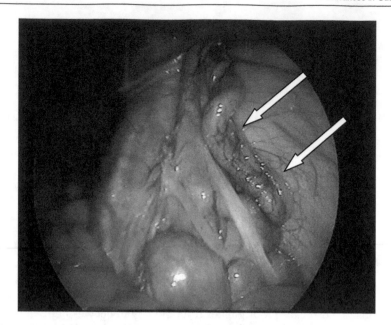

Fig. 1.

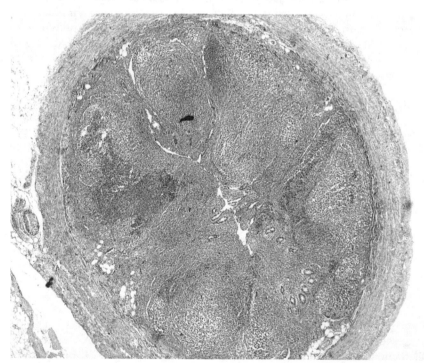

Fig. 2. Hematoxylin–eosin staining. The wall of appendix is thickened, and occupied by a compact nodular formation. The serous and muscular tunic appear thin.

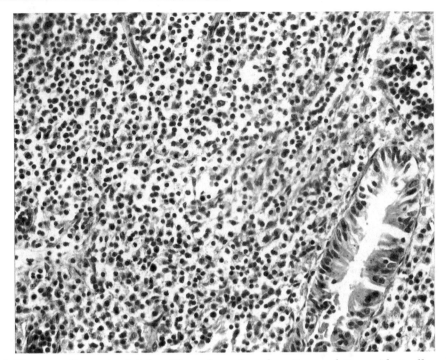

Fig. 3. Hematoxylin–eosin staining. Hyperdense lymphocytic population with small nuclei and narrow cytoplasmic rim and some plasmacytoid and monocytoid elements with great and hyperchromatic nuclei.

negativity for CD5 (CD5, Pan T cell, and B cell subsets) and CD10 using monoclonal antibodies, and positivity for anti-k (immunoglobulin light chain) using polyclonal antibodies, in addition to a low positivity to Ki-67 (proliferation-associated marker). Extensive further examination revealed that the lymphoma was restricted to the distal portion of the appendix (stage IA) and was not associated with any specific infection.

Abdominal MRI, OGDS, and capsule endoscopy of the ileum were all negative; the search for *H. pylori* was also negative. No chemotherapy was performed. After a 15-months follow-up, the patient was doing well (Marte et al., 2008). Calprotectin and clinical evaluation were repeated yearly showing no problem and the patient was asymptomatic. 3 year after, the yearly follow-up showed a slight increase of fecal calprotectin values (40μg/g) with recurrent abdominal pain and occasional episodes of diarrhea. The girl underwent a new clinical evaluation, small bowel radiological contrast study, videocapsule, OGDS, and colonoscopic examination. No fever or weight loss was present; erythrocyte sedimentation rate, C-reactive protein level were slightly higher. Perinuclear antineutrophil cytoplasmatic antibodies (pANCA) and Anti-Saccharomyces cerevisiae (ASCA) antibodies are not increased too.

The small bowel x-ray contrast, OGDS and videocapsule study demonstrated no abnormalities. Colon biopsies revealed a mild nonspecific IBD extending till 90 cm from the anal verge. (Fig.4,5,6,7)

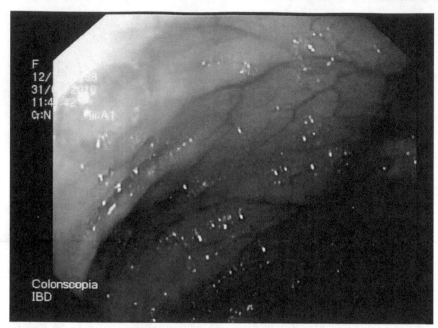

Fig. 4. Colonoscopy. Rectum and sigmoid colon: mucosal redness, nonspecific inflammatory pattern.

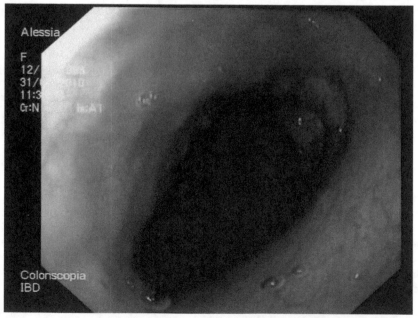

Fig. 5. Colonoscopy. Rectum and sigmoid colon: mucosal redness, nonspecific inflammatory pattern.

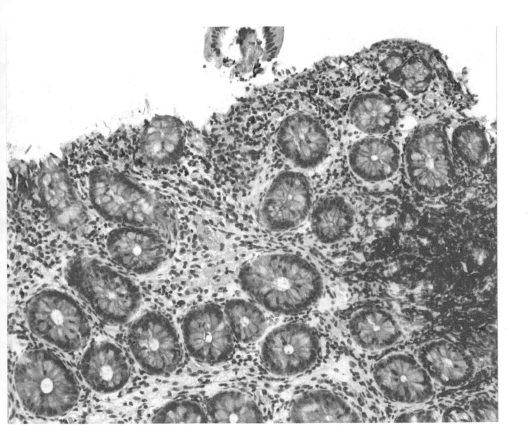

Fig. 6. Absent mucosal surface epithelium with focal reduction of the glands. The lamina propria is edematous, site of microbleeds and is infiltrated by elements of immunocompetent and heaps of eosinophils. (20 X). 90 cm from the anal verge.

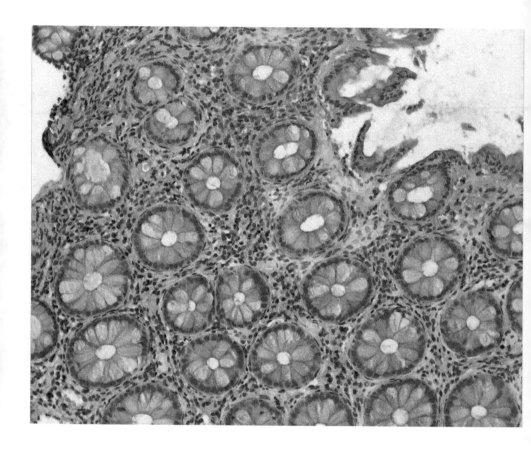

Fig. 7. Rectum (20X): 2 small erosions of the mucosa, glandular patrimony preserved, but low in mucus cells. The lamina propria is diffusely infiltrated by immunocompetent cells (lymphocytes and plasma cells).

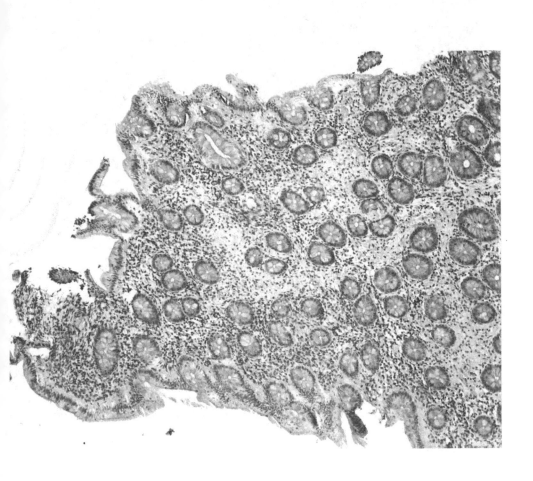

Fig. 8. Recto-sigmoid junction (10X). Mucosal home-based micro-inflammatory polyps. The glandular portion is moderately reduced. The lamina propria is edematous and infiltrated by immunocompetent elements.

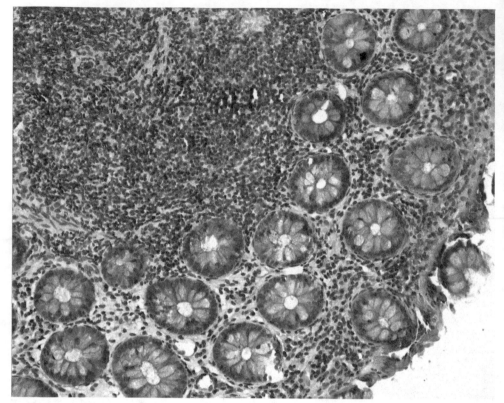

Fig. 9. Mucosal lymphocytes nodule. Glands, well structured, present a reduction of mucus cells. The lamina propria is infiltrated by immunocompetent elements. (20x). 15 cm from the anal verge.

A 6 weeks cycle of Mesalazine (5ASA), 2gr/day was administered to the patient obtaining the induction of remission and then repeated every 2 months for the prevention of recurrences. At present the patient is doing well and a strict clinical serologic follow-up with calprotectin, P-Anca and ASCA is scheduled every 6 months and, yearly, colonoscopy.

3. Discussion

Current knowledge of MALT lymphoma is largely based upon studies in adults. MALT lymphoma is rare in children; the available evidence consists mostly of isolated case reports, except for one series of ten cases (Corr et al., 1997), and another including a total of 48 cases (children and young adults) (Taddesse-Heath et al., 1997) and a pediatric NHL trial recruiting children and adolescents from Germany, Austria and Switzerland (Kaatsch et al., 2004). MALT often develops within the context of a pre-existing inflammatory response due to infection or to autoimmune disorder. Many studies show the relationship between *H. pylori* infection and gastric MALT lymphoma (Isaacson & Whright, 1984; Kurugoglu et al., 2002); some authors have reported a regression of MALT lymphoma in parotid gland (Alkan et al., 1996), lip gland (Berrebi et al., 1998), small intestine (Fischbach et al., 1997) and rectum (Matsudo et al., 1997) following *H. pylori* eradication. Other risk factors for MALT lymphoma include autoimmune diseases like Hashimoto thyroiditis or Sjogren syndrome, and Borrelia burgdorferi for skin lymphoma. A further prerequisite for the development of MALT lymphoma in children may be the presence of HIV infection (Teruya-Feldestein et al., 1995; Mo et al., 2004). In some patients no risk factors can be identified. The most common sites are the stomach and salivary glands. Others sites are: ocular adnexa, the lungs, thyroid and the skin (Zucca et al., 2000). Some retrospective analyses of histopathological results of appendectomy specimens performed for acute appendicitis in a large sample of patients, including children, report a prevalence of appendiceal malignant tumors ranging from 0.4 (Tchana et al., 2006) to 1.5% (Ravi et al., 2006). Among the malignant tumors, carcinoids have the highest incidence (Tchana et al., 2006; Ravi et al., 2006) and 70–90% of these tumors are discovered incidentally because they are usually restricted to the distal appendix (Akerstrom, 1989; Aranha & Greenle, 1980). From a review of the literature we found only one case of appendix lymphoma in paediatric age presenting with intussusception symptoms (Karabulut et al., 2005). Our report probably represents the first case of MALT lymphoma of the appendix found accidentally in a child during an appendectomy. MALT lymphomas manifest with aspecific symptoms. In our case, the clinical presentation was characterized by recurrent abdominal pain, and the only element of suspicion was the enlargement of the distal portion of the appendix. The subsequent evolution to a mild form of IBD could be considered as an evolution of the appendiceal malt-limphoma for which the phenomenon should be considered a prodromal presentation of a more extensive bowel disease which require a close follow-up and specific therapy (Aomatsu et al., 2011). Otherwise we can't exclude that the subsequent IBD could be an autonomous, subsequent disease considered that, also in this case, there are no data in the Literature. Furthermore, given the previous appendiceal malt-lymphoma, the efficacy of mesalazine alone, without the use of immunosuppressive drugs, can be considered a very favorable factor in our case. In conclusion, even if the occurrence of malignant appendiceal pathology in children is rare (Setty & Termuhlen, 2010), the probability that it is asymptomatic is very high. According to our experience, our case suggests that histological examination should always be performed following appendectomy in children and that if a MALT lymphoma were discovered, a close follow-up is strongly recommended, not only for the MALT lymphoma recurrence but also for its possible evolution towards an inflammatory bowel disease.

4. References

Akerstrom G (1989). Surgical treatment of patients with the carcinoid syndrome, *Acta Oncol* 28(3):409–414.

Alkan S, Karcher DS, Newman MA, Cohen P (1996). Regression of salivary gland MALT lymphoma after treatment for *H. pylori*, *Lancet* 348:268–269.

Anonymous (1997). A clinical evaluation of the international lymphoma study group classification of non Hodgkin's lymphoma. The non Hodgkin's lymphoma classification project, *Blood* 89:3909–3918.

Aomatsu T, Yoden A, Matsumoto K, Kimura E, Inoue K, Andoh A, Tamai H (2011). Fecal calprotectin is a useful marker for disease activity in pediatric patients with inflammatory bowel disease, *Dig Dis Sci.* Aug;56(8):2372-7.

Aranha GV, Greenle HB (1980). Surgical management of carcinoid tumors of the gastrointestinal tract, *Am Surg* 46(8):429–435.

Berrebi D, Lescoeue B, Faye A et al (1998). MALT lymphoma of labial minor salivary gland in an immunocompetent child with a gastric Helicobacter pylori infection, *J Pediatr* 133:290–292.

Corr P, Vaithilingum M, Thejpal R, Jeena P (1997). Paroid MALT lymphoma in HIV infected children, *J Ultrasound Med* 16:615–617.

Fischbach W, Tacke W, Greiner A et al (1997). Regression of immunoproliferative small intestinal disease after eradication of *H. pylori*, *Lancet* 349:31–32.

Harris NL, Jaffe ES, Stein H, Vardiman JW (2001). Pathology and genetics of tumors of the haemopoeitic and lymphoid tissues, WHO classification of tumors, *International Agency For Research On Cancer Press*, Lyon, pp 157–160.

Isaacson P, Wright DH (1984). Extranodal malignant lymphoma arising from mucosa associated lymphoid tissue, *Cancer* 53:2515–2524.

Kaatsch P, Spix C (2004). *Annual report 2004 (1980–2003)*. German childhood Cancer Registry.

Karabulut R, Sonmez K, Turkyilmaz Z, Yilmaz Y, Akyurek N, Basaklar AC, Kale N (2005). Mucosa associated lymphoma tissue lymphoma in the appendix, a lead point for intussusceptions, *J Pediatr Surg* 40(5):872–874.

Kurugoglu S, Mihmanli I, Celkan T, AkiH, Aksoy H, Korman U (2002). Radiological features in paediatric primary gastric MALT lymphoma and association with *H pylori*, *Pediatr Radiol* 32:82–87.

Marte A, Sabatino MD, Cautiero P, Accardo M, Romano M, Parmeggiani P (2008). Unexpected finding of laparoscopic appendectomy: appendix MALT lymphoma in children, *Pediatr Surg Int*. Apr;24(4):471-3.

Matsumoto T, Lida M, Shimizu M (1997). Regression of mucosa associated lymphoid tissue lymphoma of rectum after eradication of *H. pylori*, *Lancet* 350:115–116.

Mo JQ, Dimashkieh H, Mallery SR et al (2004) MALT lymphoma in children: case report and review of the literature, *Pediatr Dev Pathol* 7:407–413.

Ravi Marudanayagam, Geraint T Williams, Brian I Rees (2006). Review of the pathologiacal results of 2660 appendicectomy specimens, *J Gastroenterol* 41:745–749.

Setty BA, Termuhlen AM (2010). Rare pediatric non-Hodgkin lymphoma, *Curr Hematol Malig Rep*. Jul;5(3):163-8.

Taddesse-Heath L, Pittalunga S, Sorbara L et al (2003). Marginal zone B-cell lymphoma in children and young adults, *Am J Surg Pathol* 27:522–531.

Tchana SV, Detry O, Polus M, Thiry A, Detroz B, Maweja S, Hamoir E, Defechereux T, Cimbra C, De Roover A, Meurisse M, Honore P (2006). Carcinoid tumor of the appendix: a consecutive serie from 1237 appendectomies, *World J Gastroenterol* 7;12(41):6699–701.

Teruya-Feldstein J, Temeck BK, Sloas MM et al (1995). Pulmonary malignant lymphoma of mucosa associated lymphoid tissue (MALT) arising in a pediatric HIV-positive patient, *Am J Surg Pathol* 19:357–363.

Zucca E, Conconi A, Roggero E et al (2000). Non gastric MALT lymphomas: a survey of 369 european patients. The international extranodal lymphoma study group, *Ann Oncol* 11:99.

9

The Influence of Colonic Irrigation on Human Intestinal Microbiota

Yoko Uchiyama-Tanaka
Yoko Clinic
Japan

1. Introduction

It has been documented that the intestinal tract is inhabited by more than 10^{12} bacterial cells per gram of dry matter (Hayashi et al., 2002a; Langendijk et al., 1995; Suau et al., 1999), which is comprised of an estimated 400 to 500 bacterial species (Moor & Holdeman, 1974). The composition and activities of the indigenous intestinal microbiota are of paramount importance in human immunity, nutrition, and pathological processes, and therefore, the health of the individual (Van der Waaij et al., 1971). It is well established that the intestine is an important site of local immunity, and recent reports have suggested that it is a major site of extrathymic T cell differentiation (Cerf-Bensussan et al., 1985; Guy-Grand et al., 1991; Iiai eta al., 2002; Uchiyama-Tanaka, 2009). Numerous activated and quiescent lymphocytes are produced within gut-associated lymphatic tissues (GALT), such as Peyer's patches (Takahashi et al., 2005). Thus, it has been speculated that people who suffer from constipation and who harbor fecal residues in the intestine may have decreased local immune system function.

Colonic irrigations referred to as a colonics are a type of colonic hydrotherapy performed using an instrument in combination with abdominal massage, but without drugs or mechanical pressure. I previously reported that colonic irrigation may induce lymphocyte transmigration from GALT into the circulation, which may improve the functions of both the colon and immune system (Uchiyama-Tanaka, 2009). Colonic irrigation was developed about 40 years ago and no serious complications associated with its use have been reported. However, the impact of this method, which use a large amount of water, on the intestinal microbiota and serum electrolytes remains unknown. In this study, colonic irrigations were performed 3 times for each of the 10 subjects with no history of malignant or inflammatory disease.

2. Materials and methods

2.1 Study design and subjects

The procedures used in this study were in accordance with the guidelines of the Declaration of Helsinki for Human Experimentation, 2000 and all subjects provided informed consent. Ten outpatients from the Yoko Clinic (4 men and 6 women; mean age=38 ± 6 years; age range: 27–47 years) admitted to the hospital between April and May 2009 were enrolled in this study. None of the subjects had cancer or any active inflammatory disease.

2.2 Analysis of fecal microbiotauction

Fecal samples were collected before the first colonic irrigation and at 1 week after the third irrigation. These samples were analyzed using a kit from TechnoSuruga Laboratory Co., Ltd. (Shizuoka Japan). Fecal microbiota analysis targeted bacterial 16S rRNA genes with a terminal restriction fragment length polymorphism (T-RFLP) analysis program (Nagashima's method) (Ando et al., 2007; Nagashima et al. 2002, 2006). T-RFLP was performed as previously described by Nagashima et al. (2002, 2006). The 16S rRNA genes were amplified using a forward primaer, 516f [5'-TGCCAGCAGCCGCGGTA-3'] and a reverse primer, 1510r [5'-GGTTACCTTGTTACGACTT-3']. The 5' ends of the forward primer, 516f were labeled with 6'-carboxyfluorescein, which was synthesized by Applied Biosystems Japan (Tokyo, Japan). The purified PCR products (2 µL) were digested with 10 U of either BslI (New England BioLabs, Inc., Ipswich, MA, USA) at 55°C for 3 h. The lengths of terminal restriction fragments were determined with the ABI PRISM 3130xl Genetic Analyzer (Applied Biosystems, Tokyo, japan).

2.3 Laboratory determinations

Blood samples were collected from the subjects in a sitting position before the start and at 10 min after the third irrigation. Serum samples were analyzed using a commercial kit.

2.4 Colonic irrigations

Each patient underwent 3 colonic irrigations over a period 2 weeks. Same trained physician performed colonic irrigations for all subjects. Irrigations using an intestinal irrigation devide (Colon Hydromat Comfort: Herrmann Apparatebau GmbH, Kleinwallstadt, Germany) that circulated approximately 30–50 L of purified warm water (38°C) through a filter (Uchiyama-Tanaka, 2009). During an irrigation process, which lasts for approximately 1 hour, a subject is laid supine on a bed and given abdominal massage. Because colonic irrigations utilize a large amount of water introduced using a tube and abdominal massage, there are some contraindications, such as renal failure, heart failure, liver cirrhosis, severe hemorrhoids, after post-intestinal polypectomy, post-abdominal surgery and pregnacy. The principle of the Colon Hydromat Comfort's function is shown in Figure1.

Filtered hot water and ordinary water are mixed and passed into a patient's colon through the speculum. The sewage water flows out due to the pressure in the water-filled colon. Some pictures of fecal residues and intestinal epithelium during colon irrigations are shown below.

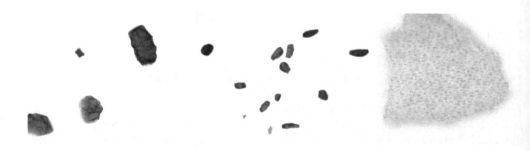

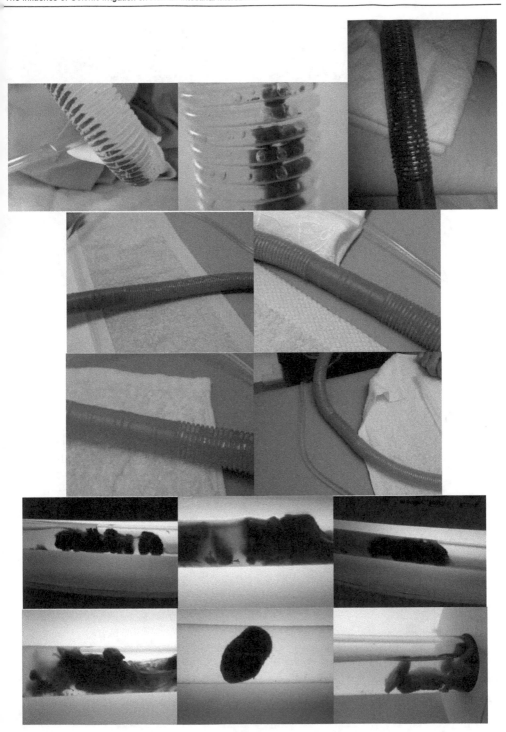

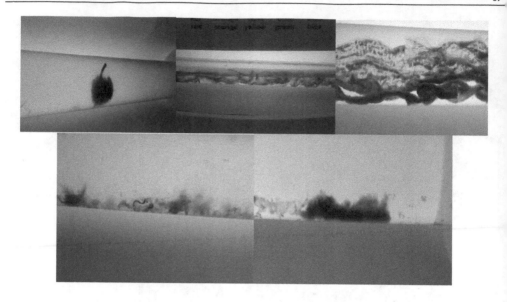

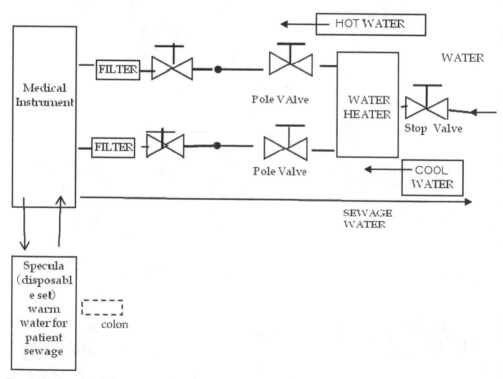

Fig. 1. Principle of the Colon Hydromat Comfort

2.5 Statistics

Results are given as means ± standard deviations (SD). Student's paired t-test was used to compare results before and after irrigations. P < 0.05 was considered statistically significant.

3. Results

Patient clinical characteristics are summarized in Table 1.

Patient	Age	Gender	Underlying disease	Symptom change
No. 1	44	Male	Pollen allergy	Symptom-free (after 7 times)
No. 2	47	Female	Constipation	Better
No. 3	45	Female	Ovarian cysts	Size Smaller (8 cm to 6 cm, after 3 times)
No. 4	47	Male	Atopic dermatitis	Decreased itching
No. 5	28	Male	Psoriasis	Better (still undergoing irrigation)
No. 6	38	Female	Constipation	Better
No. 7	38	Female	Constipation	Better
No. 8	32	Female	Face eruption	Better
No. 9	39	Female	Constipation	Better
No. 10	29	Male	Allergic Rhinitis	Decreased blowing of nose

Table 1. Subject's clinical characteristics and symptom changes after irrigations

Each patient underwent 3 colonic irrigations over a period of 2 weeks. Fecal samples were collected before the first colon irrigation and at 1 week after the third irrigation. The relative proportions of bacteria found in the fecal samples of each patient before and after colonic irrigation are shown in Table 2.

	1		2		3		4	
Presumed bacterium	b	a	b	a	b	a	b	a
Bifidobacterium	18.6	16.5	22.9	17.1	8.7	14.9	1.8	14.5
Lactobacillales	2.2	4.5	4.1	0	6.1	4	0	0
Bacteroides	23	17	21.3	20.9	31.7	31.6	44.4	38.3
Prevotella	9.1	2.8	7.8	8.9	0	0	0	0
Clostridium cluster IV	11.6	15.4	14.5	19.1	25.5	23	22.7	13.9
Clostridium subcluster XIVa	13	16.3	17.7	24.7	21.3	19.4	14.6	22.4
Clostridium cluster XI	2.6	4.2	0	0	0	0	2.4	2.3
Clostridium cluster XVIII	7	4.4	2	1.4	0	0	5.1	0
others	13	18.8	9.6	8	6.7	7.1	9.1	8.6

Table 2. Continued

5		6		7		8		9		10	
b	a	b	a	b	a	b	a	b	a	b	a
1.9	2	17.9	2.6	22.6	28.2	9.9	1	0	28.5	5.6	26.7
0	0	1.5	0	2.7	2.5	0	0	3.3	3.2	1.6	1.5
28.3	14.7	13.5	14.4	15.6	25.4	29.8	12.3	59.8	30.3	32.9	33
38.3	31.6	23.9	30.3	0	0	0	40.3	0	0	0	0
2.8	8.1	3.8	1.5	12.6	11.7	0	19.7	0	19.1	0	4.8
3.9	15.8	19	11.2	22.8	17.4	26.5	11.6	7.7	13	24.4	15.1
1.7	0	1	3.4	11.1	3	13.8	2.5	3.3	3.3	0	0
1.1	0	1.1	0.6	0	1.5	0	1.2	1.7	0	0	0
22	27.8	18.3	35.9	12.6	10.3	20	11.3	24.3	2.4	35.5	18.9

No 1-10: Patients in Table 1. b: Before colonic irrigations. a: After 3 times colonic irrigations

Table 2. The changes in the fecal microbiota between prior to and after 3 clonic irrigations

There were no significant differences in the overall quantities of fecal bacteria in samples collected before and after irrigations. There was also no tendency for changes int the proportions of Lactobacillales and *Bifidobacterium* and *Clostridium* subclusters. The proportions of these bacterial orders are shown in Table 3.

Presumed microbiota %	prior to (mean ± SD)	after	p
Bifidobacterium	10.99±8.85	15.29±10.74	p>0.05
Lactobacillales	2.15±1.99	1.57±1.84	p>0.05
Bacteroids	30.08±13.86	23.8±9.2	p>0.05
Prevotella	7.88±13.07	11.39±16.09	p>0.05
Clostridium IV	9.4±9.62	13.62±7.04	p>0.05
Clostridum XIVa	17.07±7.33	16.64±4.42	p>0.05
Clostridum XI	3.61±4.9	1.87±1.69	p>0.05
Clostridum XVIII	1.8±2.4	0.91±1.38	p>0.05
Others	17.13±8.85	14.92±10.42	p>0.05

Table 3. The mean changes in the microbiota between prior to and after 3 colonic irrigations

According to Collins et al. (1994), *Clostridium* clusters and subclusters cannot revide the unknown pole in intestine. For example, *Faecalibacterium prausnitzil* is an important bacteria as butyrate-producing bacterium in *Clostridium* cluster IV. In contrast, *Clostridium perfringens* is a well known as harmful bacterium in *Clostridium* cluster I. Lactobacillales and *Bifidobacterium* are considered to be healthy, beneficial fecal bacteria. In this study, beneficial bacteria decreased in some patients. Serum electrolytes after irrigations (sodium, potassium, and chlorine) exhibited no significant changes from their values before irrigation (data not shown). Patient symptoms were improved after irrigations (Table 1), and they did not experience any difficulties.

4. Discussion

This study showed that colonic irrigations are safe in terms of serum electrolytes for subjects with normal renal function and had a positive impact on these subjects' symptoms. However, these irrigations showed no tendency for any effects on the intestinal microbiota. Colonic irrigation was developed at the National Aeronautics and Space Administration and has been used worldwide in the care of allergic and pollen diseases, skin disorders, and constipation. I previously reported that colonic irrigation may induce lymphocyte transmigration from GALT into the circulation, which may improve the function of both the colon and the immune system functions (Uchiyama-Tanaka, 2009). The increase in the lymphocytes was suspected to be the result of lymphocytes transmigrating as intraepithelial lymphocytes from Peyer's patched and lymph nodes around the intestine as a result of irrigation and abdominal massage.

Based on my personal experience, patient symptoms can improve after colonic irrigations. However, it has been proposed that colon irrigations with large volumes of water may obliterate the microbiota and induce electrolyte abnormalities, but no studies support these claims. The results of this study suggests that after 3s colonic irrigations, the composition of the microbiota changes, but there is no tendency for the changes in the bacterial components.

Colonic irrigations are different from enemas for the following reasons: (a) they are not self-administered, but are administered by a professionally trained person; and (b) they are administered using a device that controls water flow and infuses the entire colon with water, in contrast to the more limited infusion of warm filtered water into the rectum. The water circulates throughout the colon and removes its contents while the patient lies on a bed. The temperature and pressure of water are closely monitored and regulated during a series of fills and releases to aid colonic peristalsis. Because this method involves a closed system, the waste materials are removed without any unpleasant odor or discomfort, which are usually associated with enemas.

The intestine is an important site of local immunity and nutrition (Iiai et al., 2002). It is a major site of extrathymic T cell differentiation, and numerous activated and quiescent lymphocytes are produced within GALT. The very important role of the intestine, as a part of the immune system is due to the intestinal microbiota. Thus, it has been speculated in peoplewho suffer from constipation and who harbor fecal residues, the intestine may have a diminished function in the immune system (Alveres, 2001, 1924).

The intestinal epithelium is the first line of defense system to encounter intestinal pathogens and dietary antigens. It has been speculated that when the intestine is filled with feces, there may be a reduced function of this immune system caused by toxins leaking from the gut, in addition to bacterial translocation from the gut to the systemic circulation caused by a breakdown of the intestinal wall. This breakdown can be caused by a variety of injuries to the body at further locations far from the gut.

It has been reported that increased gut permeability and bacterial translocation play a role in multiple organ failure (MOF: Swank & Deitch, 1996). Failure of the gut barrier is central to the hypothesis that toxins escaping from the gut lumen contribute to the activation of a host's immune inflammatory defense mechanisms, which subsequently leads to autointoxication and tissue destruction that are seen in the septic response characteristics of MOF (Swank & Deitch,1996; Garcia-Tsao et al., 1995; Purohit et al., 2008). Thus, colonic irrigation is useful for removing fecal residues.

Although irrigation is useful for establishing a "good" status in the intestine in terms of removing fecal residues, we should not expect too much from these irrigations. Factors like proper nutrition and food intake and a stress-free life style are also important in improving the microbiota, rather than colonic irrigations alone. One report showed that the microbiota of people on a strict vegetarian diet was very different from those on normal diets (Hayashi et al. 2002b). The removal of residual fecal matter in the colon may provide a break from a bad dietary cycle and highlight the importance of intestinal care in everyday life.

Colonic irrigation is relatively safe and is a good method for impressing upon patients the importance of intestinal care. But according to the results of this study, some patients' microbiota deteriorated. Although safe in terms of serum electrolytes, it should be noted that colonic irrigations should not be performed for patients with renal failure, heart disease, liver cirrhosis with ascites, recent abdominal surgery, pregnancy, and other conditions. In addition, excessive therapy such as everyday irrigations should be avoided. This may result in the loss of massive amount of digestive fluid. Except for the first 3 times of colonic irrigation, subsequent irrigations should be performed within a minimum 1 month interval.

This study was limited by its small study population. Some subjects showed reduced proportions in beneficial fecal bacteria, although their symptoms including allergic rhinorrhea, constipation, skin itching, and eczema, were improved. We should be careful with regard to the duration and number of irrigations administered and preferably take probiotics after colonic irrigation. If the patient is in a "good" status in terms of stool analysis, a single trial with an adequate duration would be sufficient.

Another limitation of this study was that the actual numbers of bacteria were not determined using these methods. T-RFLP is only useful for estimating the proportions of bacteria. Hence, we need a more efficient quantitative method for bacterial analysis in addition to the existing one with an advantageous cost versus performance.

In conclusion, colonic irrigation has no influence on serum electrolytes and may induce improvements in symptoms without any effects on the intestinal microbiota.

5. References

Alveres, WC. (2001). Origin of so-called autointoxication symptoms. *JAMA*.72: pp. 8-13.

Alverez, WC.; Freedlander. BL.(1924). The rate of progress of food residues through the bowel. *JAMA*. 83: pp. 576-580.

Ando, A.; Sakata, S., Koizumi, Y., Mitsuyama, K., Fujiyama, Y., Benno, Y.(2007). Terminal restriction fragment length polymorphism analysis of the diversity of fecal microbiota in patients with ulcerative colitis. *Inflamm Bowel Dis.* 13: pp. 955-962.

Cerf-Bensussan, N.; Guy-Grand, D., Griscelli, C. (1985). Intraepithelial lymphocytes of human gut: isolation, characterization and study of natural killer activity. *Gut.* 26: pp.81-88

Collins, MD.; Lawson, PA., Willems ,A., Cordoba, JJ., Fernandez-Garayzabal, J., Garcia, P., Cai, J., Hippe, H., Farrow, JAE.(1994). The Phylogeny of the Genus Clostridium: Proposal of Five New Genera and Eleven New Species Combinations. *Int J Syst Bacteriol*. 44: pp. 812-826.

Garcia-Tsao, G.; Lee, FY., Bardeb, GE., Cartun, R., West, AB. (1995) Bacterial translocation to mesenteric lymph nodes is increased in cirrhotic rats with ascites. *Gastroenterology* 108: pp. 1835-1841

Guy-Grand, D.; Cerf-Bensussan, N., Malissen, B., Malassis-Seris ,M., Briottet, C., Vassalli, P. (1991). Two gut intraepithelial CD8+ lymphocyte population with different T cell receptors. A role for the gut epithelium in T cell differentiation. *J Exp Med*. 173: pp. 471-481.

Hayashi, H.; Sakamoto, M. & Benno, Y. (2002). Phylogenetic analysis of human gut microbiota using 16S rDNA clone libraries and strictly anaerobic culture-based methods. *Microbiol Immunol*, 46: pp. 535-548

Hayashi, H.; Sakamoto, M., Bennno, Y. (2002). Fecal microbial diversity in a strict vegetarian as determined by molecular analysis and cultivation. *Microbiol Immunol* 46: pp.819-831.

Iiai, T.; Watanabe, H., Suda, T., Okamoto, H., Abo, T., Hatakeyama, K. (2002). CD161+T (NT) cells exist predominantly in human intestinal epithelium as well as in liver. *Clin Exp Immunol* 129: pp. 92-98.

Langendijk, PS.; Schut, F., Jansen, GJ., Raangs, GC., Kamphuius, GR., Wilkison ,MH., Welling, GW. (1995). Quantitative fluorescence in situ hybridization of Bifidobacterium spp. With genus-specific 16S rRNA-targeted probes and its application in fecal samples. *Appl Environ Microbiol* 61: pp. 3069-3075

Moor, WE.; Holdeman, LV.(1974). Human fecal flora: the normal flora of 20 Japanese-Hawaiians. *Appl Environ Microbiol*. 27: pp. 961-979

Nagashima, K.; Hisada ,T., Sato, M., Mochizuki, J. (2002). Application of new primer-enzyme combinations to terminal restriction fragment length polymorphism profiling of bacterial populations in human feces. *Appl Environ Microbiol* 69: pp. 1251-1262

Nagashima, K.; Mochizuki, J., Hisada, T., Suzuki, S., Shimomura, K. (2006). Phylogenetic analysis of 16S ribosomal RNA gene sequences from human fecal microbiota and improved utility of terminal restriction fragment length polymorphism profiling. *Bioscience Microflora*. 25: pp. 99-107.

Purohit, V.; Bode, JC., Bode, C., Brenner, DA., Choudhry, MA., Hamilton, F., Kang, YJ., Keshavarzin, A., Rao, R., Sartor, RB., Swanson, C., Turner, JR. (2008) Alcohol, intestinal bacterial growth, intestinal permeability to endotoxin, and medical consequences: Summary of a symposium. *Alcohol* 42: pp. 349-361

Suau, A.; Bonnet, R., Sutren, M., Godon, JJ., Gibson, G.R., Collins, MD., Dore, J. (1999). Direct analysis of genes encoding 16S rRNA from complex communities reveals many novel molecular species within the human gut. *Appl Environ Microbiol* 65: pp. 4799-4807

Swank, GM.; Deitch, EA. (1996) Role of the gut in multiple organ failure. Bacterial translocation and permeability changes. *World J Surg* 20: pp. 411-417

Takahashi, S.; Kawamura ,T., Kanda, Y., Taniguchi, T., Nishizawa, T., Iiai, T., Hatakeyama, K., Abo, T.(2005). Multipotential acceptance of Peyer's patches in the intestine for both thymus-derived T cells and extrathymic T cells in mice. *Immunol Cell Biol.* 83: pp.504-510.

Uchiyama-Tanaka, Y.; (2009). Colon irrigation and lymphocyte movement to peripheral blood. *Biochemical Research.* 30:pp. 311-314.

Van der Waaij, D.; Berghuis-de Vries, JM., Lekkerkerk van der ,Wees. (1971). Colonization resistance of digestive tract in conventional and antibiotic treated mice. *J Hyg.* 67: pp. 405-411.

Section 2

Diseases of the Liver and Biliary Tract

10

Pancreato-Biliary Cancers – Diagnosis and Management

Nam Q. Nguyen
Department of Gastroenterology, Royal Adelaide Hospital,
North Terrace, Adelaide, SA
Australia

1. Introduction

Pancreato-biliary cancers are relatively uncommon and in general, including cancers arise from the pancreas, bile duct and major ampullae. These tumours are uniformly carried a poor prognosis due to late presentation and surgical resection is only possible in less than 20% patients (David et al., 2009; Luke et al., 2009). Despites many medical advances in the imaging diagnosis, chemo-radio-therapy, surgical technique and post-operative care over the last 2 decades, the overall survival of patients with pancreato-biliary neoplasm has not improved significantly (Luke et al., 2009). The aim of the current chapter is to review and discuss current techniques and approaches to the diagnosis and management of pancreato-biliary neoplasm.

2. Clinico-pathology of pancreato-biliary tumours

2.1 Pancreatic carcinoma

In the Western world, pancreatic cancer is the fourth leading cause of cancer related mortality with the approximate incidence of 11 per 100 000, and ranks second after colorectal cancer among all gastrointestinal malignancies (Shaib et al., 2006). Men are more frequently affected than women and over 80% patients are diagnosed at the age older than 60 years. Almost 50% patients have distant metastases at the time of presentation with poor 5-year survival of 5% (Shaib et al., 2006). Recent data suggest that although the mortality rate for males has decreased by 0.4% from 1990 to 2005, the mortality rate for females has increased by 4.4% (Shaib et al., 2006; Jemal et al., 2009). The reason for this gender difference in mortality is unknown. Risk factors for pancreatic cancer include smoking, alcohol, diabetes mellitus, chronic pancreatitis, family history of pancreatic cancer. Patients with hereditary pancreatitis, Puetz-Jeghers syndrome, familial atypical multiple mole melanoma, familial breast and ovarian cancer, Li-Fraumeni syndrome, Fanconi anaemia, ataxia-telangiectasia, familial adenomatous polyposis, cystic fibrosis and possible hereditary non-polyposis colon cancer syndrome are also at higher risk of having pancreatic cancer (Shaib et al., 2006; Klapman and Malafa, 2008).

Ductal infiltrating adenocarcinoma is the most common type of pancreatic cancer with 78% located in the head, 11% in the body and 11% in the tail (Lillemoe et al., 2000; Ghaneh et al.,

2008). Less than 15% of pancreatic cancers are intraductal mucinous papillary neoplasm (IPMN), solid pseudopapillary neoplasm, pancreatoblastoma, mucinous cystadenocarcinoma, adenosquamous carcinoma and acinar cell carcinoma (Ghaneh et al., 2008). Given the preponderance pancreatic head location of the tumours, painless cholestatic symptoms are the most common presentation (Ghaneh et al., 2008). Anorexia, abdominal pain or mass and weight loss often indicate the presence of advanced disease.

2.2 Cholangiocarcinoma

This is rare malignant disease of the epithelial cells in the intra- and extrahepatic bile ducts and the incidence is increasing, especially the intra-hepatic subtype (Patel, 2001). In addition to liver flukes infestation, hepatitis B and C infections have recently been associated with rise of cholangiocarcinoma in the developing countries, and are thought to be responsible for the increasing incidence of intra-hepatic cholangiocarcinomas. In the western countries, primary sclerosing cholangitis and congenital anomalies such as Caroli's syndrome and choledochal cysts are the main predisposing risk factors for cholangiocarcinoma (Patel, 2006).

As with pancreatic cancer, most of the cholangiocarcinomas are unresectable at presentation and the prognosis for these patients is dismal. Clinical presentations of cholangiocarcinoma are dependent on tumour location (Patel, 2006). Extrahepatic tumours, including those involving the bifurcation usually show signs of biliary obstruction with jaundice and pale stools. In contrast, intra-hepatic cholangiocarcinomas more often present with late symptoms of malignancy such as weight loss, loss of appetite, and abdominal pain or mass.

2.3 Ampullary tumours

Compared to pancreatic carcinoma and cholangiocarcinoma, ampullary neoplasm is the least common and aggressive tumour. In general, ampullary tumour has better clinical outcomes even when the tumour is not resectable (Heinrich and Clavien 2010). Whilst ampullary tumours can occur sporadically, they are often seen in the context of genetic syndromes such as familial adenomatous polyposis and hereditary non-polyposis colorectal cancer, in whom the risk is 100 times more than the general population (Offerhaus et al., 1992). As endoscopic screening and surveillance program is adopted for these at-risk individuals, most tumours are adenomas at detection, though the potential of malignant transformation to carcinomas is high (Jean and Dua, 2003; Fischer and Zhou, 2004). Currently, there is no consensus on the management of ampullary tumors. Factors that impact treatment strategy include the patient's general health, tumor characteristics, and available expertise. Ampullary adenomas, especially those with high-grade dysplasia, warrant therapy because they are "time bombs" for malignancy and may already harbor malignancy missed on biopsy (Heinrich and Clavien 2010). Although endoscopic resection is widely embraced as first-line therapy in patients with benign ampullary tumors (Binmoeller et al., 1993; Beger et al., 1999; Cheng et al., 2004), the final treatment decision is based on the histological findings of the ampullectomized specimen. The presence of invasive carcinoma in the specimen indicates the need for definitive surgical resection. In patients who are poor candidates for surgery or who refuse surgery, endoscopic resection with ablative therapy can be considered despite unfavorable tumor characteristics (Nguyen et al. 2010). Endoscopic ampullectomy has also been reported to successfully eradicate large ampullary adenomas (Zadorova et al., 2001), early T1 ampullary adenocarcinoma

(Katsinelos et al., 2007), and even lesions with intraductal growth (Bohnacker et al., 2005). Given its tumour behaviour, clinical presentation and treatment modality are very different to that of pancreatic cancer and cholangiocarcinoma, ampullary tumours will not be discussed further in this chapter.

3. Investigations of pancreato-biliary cancers

The imaging modalities involve in the detection, staging and management of pancreatic cancer are computer tomography (CT), magnetic resonance imaging (MRI), endoscopic retrograde cholangiopancreatography (ERCP), endoscopic ultrasound (EUS) and positron emission tomography (PET) (Clarke et al., 2003; Chang et al., 2009; Peddu et al., 2009). The diagnosis can potentially be made by any, or a combination of the above modalities. The roles and relative importance of these imaging modalities have changed over the last few decades and continue to change with rapid technological advancement in medical imaging.

Base on current best available evidence, CT should be used as first line for diagnosis, staging and the assessment of resectability in pancreato-biliary cancer. MRI should be reserved for patients with iodine contrast allergy or who cannot be exposed to radiation or to be used as an adjunct to CT in patients with suspicious liver lesions that need to be to better characterized (Clarke et al., 2003; Peddu et al., 2009). MR cholangio-pancreatography (MRPC) is an essential part of the evaluation for cholangiocarcinoma as it can identify the luminal involvement of the cancer as well as the road map of the biliary tree (Patel, 2006). Such information is not only important in local staging but also critical in determining respectability, type of surgery and/or identifying the dominant obstructive ductal system for biliary drainage. In selected cases, cholangioscopy is helpful by providing direct endoscopic visualization of the intra-ductal lesion that responsible for the biliary stricture (Patel, 2006). The recent development of SpyGlass cholangioscopy system has also allowed tissue sample under direct vision.

EUS should be used for local staging and assessment of resectability if it remains inconclusive on non-invasive imaging modalities (Chang et al., 2009; Iglesias Garcia et al., 2009). It should also be used in patients with a high clinical suspicion of a lesion that has not been clearly demonstrated using other modalities. EUS-FNA should also be the biopsy route of choice in patients where a tissue diagnosis or tissue from regional lymph nodes may alter the course of treatment, or if neo-adjuvant treatment is contemplated. If there is disagreement between CT and EUS images, then laparotomy and trial of dissection should be considered (Chang et al., 2009). PET/CT should be used selectively such as when metastatic disease is suspected but has not been demonstrated with other imaging modalities (Nguyen and Bartholomeusz, 2011; Serrano et al. 2010). The availability and local expertise of each imaging modality will also influence their use. A suggested management algorithm for patients with suspected pancreato-biliary cancer is shown in Figure 1.

3.1 Tumour markers

The role of tumour marker in the diagnosis and management of pancreato-biliary cancers remains controversial (Balzano and Di Carlo, 2008). Carbohydrate antigen 19-9 (CA19-9), which is caused by the up-regulation of glycosyl transferase genes, is the most commonly used marker and can provide useful diagnostic and prognostic information (Duffy et al.

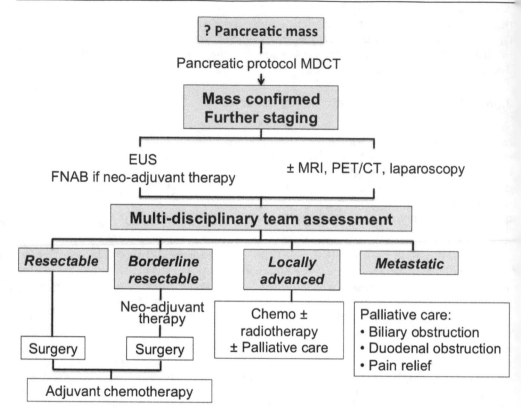

Fig. 1. Suggested algorithm for the evaluation and management of patients with suspected pancreatic.

2010). Its sensitivity (70%-90%) and specificity (43%-91%) for diagnosing pancreatic cancer are only modest and can be falsely increased by high serum bilirubin (Duffy et al. 2010). However, for those with confirmed pancreatic cancer, high serum CA19-9 is associated with a worse survival (Park et al., 2008). Similarly, in patients who undergo curative resection for pancreatic cancer, a normalizing post-operative CA19-9 level is associated with a longer median and disease-free survival compared to those with persistently high level (Duffy et al., 2008; Balzano and Di Carlo, 2008).

3.2 Tissue sampling

A distinct advantage of EUS is its ability to obtain tissue via fine needle aspiration (FNA). This approach is superior to percutaneous biopsy (via US or CT guided) in the investigation of pancreato-biliary malignancies with higher diagnostic yield (84% vs. 62%) and significantly lower risk of tumour seeding from the needle tract (<2% vs. 16%) (Paquin et al., 2005). Apart from biopsy of the primary tumour, it also has the ability to biopsy lymph nodes, liver lesions and ascitic fluid, which is critical in accurate staging and avoiding unnecessary resection (Figure 2). For pancreatic head lesions, the possibility of seeding is eliminated, as the needle track is included in the resection specimen (Yamao et al., 2005). In

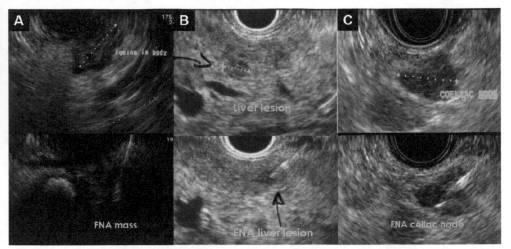

Fig. 2. Examples of EUS-guide FNA of a pancreatic mass in the body (panel A), a liver lesion (panel B) and pathological celiac node (panel C).

contrast, for lesions in the pancreatic body and tail, where the needle track is not resected, the risks and benefits of pre-operative biopsy should be carefully assessed on an individual basis. Due to its anatomical position, tissue acquisition from biliary lesion via EUS guided FNA is more difficult and in general, the diagnostic yield is lower than that for pancreatic cancer and is dependent on the location of the lesion. As it is easier to visualize and access the distal biliary lesions, the diagnostic yield is significantly higher in distal compared with proximal lesions (81% vs 59%) (Mohamadnejad et al. 2011).

3.3 Cholangioscopy

In cases where the diagnosis of the biliary stricture remains unclear after conventional MDCT, MRI and EUS evaluation, directly visualization of the appearance of the ductal strictures and biopsy can be helpful in differentiating benign from malignant disorders (Figure 3). Although video "mother-baby" cholangioscope provides high quality images, it is fragile and often lack of accessory channel for tissue sampling (Nguyen, 2009; Nguyen et al., 2009). The diagnostic yield of malignancy based on cholangioscopic appearance of the intra-ductal lesion varied from 70% to 88% (Nguyen, 2009; Nguyen et al., 2009). Currently, tissue sampling is only possible with the single-operator disposable SpyGlass system, which has a 1.2mm accessory channel. Although SpyGlass guided tissue sample is successful in up to 96% of cases, its overall accuracy in confirming a malignant stricture is only modest (49% of cases) (Nguyen, 2009; Nguyen et al., 2009). This is mainly due to the poor sensitivity of SpyGlass guided biopsy in the diagnosis of malignancy from extrinsic cancers (8%) as compared to that of intrinsic cancers (66%) (Nguyen, 2009; Nguyen et al., 2009).

4. Therapeutic approaches for pancreato-biliary cancers

Patients with suspected or confirmed diagnosis of pancreato-biliary malignancy should be assessed by a multidisciplinary team and stratified as resectable, borderline resectable,

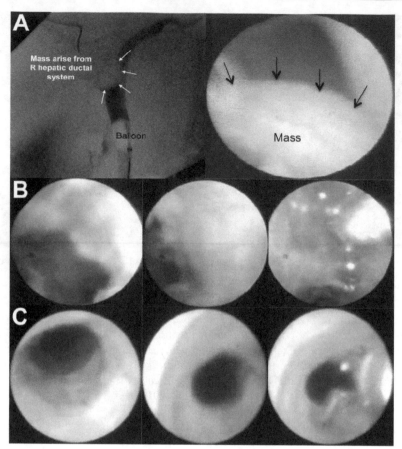

Fig. 3. Cholangioscopic images from SpyScope for investigation of suspected biliary strictures. A case of a hepatoma causing a polypoid protrusion into the right hepatic duct at the hilum, mimicking a cholangiocarcinoma on cholangiography (panel A). A case of cholangiocarcinoma in the upper common bile duct (CBD) stricture, confirmed on SpyGlass guided biopsy (panel B). A case of mid-CBD stricture in a patient with primary sclerosing cholangitis, which appeared benign on SpyScope and was confirmed on biopsy (panel C).

locally advanced unresectable or metastatic disease. Treatment should be planned according to local expertise and established guidelines, as resectable and borderline patients should be referred to surgeons, unresectable and metastatic patients should be referred to medical and radiation oncologists and palliative care teams. Endoscopic interventions to alleviate biliary or duodenal obstruction are also important in improving the performance status and quality of life in these patients. A multidisciplinary approach to pancreato-biliary malignancy is necessary to improve the overall outcome of these patients, especially for borderline resectable or unresectable disease as neo-adjuvant chemo-radiation therapy may play a role in down-staging and the conversion to potentially resectable, and in some case "curable", disease (Verslype et al., 2007; Chang et al., 2008). The therapeutic approach for pancreatic cancers is summarized in Figure 1.

4.1 Surgery

Surgical resection remains the only possibility of cure for pancreato-biliary cancers as chemotherapy and radiotherapy offering only a modest survival benefit. Patients who undergo complete surgical resection for localized, non-metastatic adenocarcinoma of the pancreas have a 5-year survival rate of approximately 20 to 25%, and a median survival of 22 months (Cameron et al., 2006). Unfortunately less than 20% of patients with pancreatic cancer have disease amendable to surgical resection at the time of presentation (Yeo et al., 1997) because patients often present at an advanced stage with widespread metastatic or locally advanced disease. The type of resection depends on the location of the tumours with Whipple's procedures are most commonly performed as most cancers locate in the head of pancreas.

Similarly, the type and extend of resection for cholangiocarcinoma depends on the location of the tumour. The indication and type of resection of intra-hepatic cholangiocarcinoma is similar to those of liver cancers. In contrast, curative surgery for extra-hepatic cholangiocarcinoma is rare and is only possible for distal ductal tumours (Witzigmann et al., 2008; Lang et al., 2009). Hilar tumours involving the bifurcation are usually contraindicated for surgery and have very poor prognosis. Even in patients whose resection is considered successful, the overall five-year survival rate in the range of 25–30% (Lang et al., 2009).

4.2 Chemo-radiotherapy

Given the high loco-regional recurrence rate and a tendency towards early liver metastasis after pancreatic resection, adjuvant chemotherapy has been employed though its benefits remain controversial with mixed results until recently (Brennan, 2004; Zuckerman and Ryan, 2008). Of the six randomized controlled trials that examined the effects of adjuvant chemotherapy after pancreatic resection (Kalser and Ellenberg, 1985; Moertel et al., 1994; Neoptolemos et al., 2001; Neoptolemos et al., 2004; Oettle et al., 2007; Regine et al., 2008), only two trials were able to demonstrate a survival benefit of adjuvant chemotherapy (Neoptolemos et al., 2001; Neoptolemos et al., 2004). In the ESPAC-1 study, the survival of patients treated with adjuvant 5-Fluorouracil (5-FU) was significantly longer than that without adjuvant chemotherapy (20.1 months vs 15.5 months) (Neoptolemos et al., 2001; Neoptolemos et al., 2004). Subsequent meta-analysis supports the results of ESPAC-1 trial and indicated that 5-FU reduced the risk of death by 25% (Stocken et al., 2005). More recently, German investigators (Oettle et al., 2007) have demonstrated a disease-free survival advantage of patients who received gemcitabine adjuvant chemotherapy (13.4 months vs 6.9 months), but not the overall survival (22.1 months vs 20.2 months). Given the encouraging data from these trials (Neoptolemos et al., 2001; Neoptolemos et al., 2004; Oettle et al., 2007), adjuvant chemotherapy with either 5-FU or gemcitabine or both is increasingly used in patients with resected pancreatic cancer (Fogelman et al., 2004; Goldstein et al., 2004). Compared with 5-FU, gemcitabine is better tolerated with lesser incidence of grade 3 and 4 haematological toxicity (Oettle et al., 2007; Palmer et al., 2007).

Similarly, in order to convert borderline resectable to resectable tumors or to increase the probability of complete microscopic tumor resection, neo-adjuvant chemo-radiotherapy has also been evaluated (Gillen et al., 2010; Heinrich et al., 2010; van Tienhoven et al., 2011;

Vinciguerra 2011). A recent systematic review evaluating retrospective and prospective studies on neo-adjuvant chemo-radiotherapy from 1966 to 2009 included a total of 111 studies and 4,394 patients suggests that up to one third of patients with previously borderline resectable cancers are eligible for resection after neoadjuvant treatment (Gillen et al. 2010). More importantly, these patients were found to have comparable median survival as those who undergoing resection followed by adjuvant therapy (20.1 vs. 23.6 months, respectively). In contrast, neoadjuvant therapy did not seem to improve overall outcome for patients with resectable cancer at presentation (Gillen et al. 2010).

In contrast to pancreatic cancer, cholangiocarcinoma has been shown to be resistant to common chemotherapy (Anderson and Kim, 2009). Numerous drugs have been tested alone and in combination, and thus far, the response rate has been unacceptably low. Although gemcitabine chemotherapy is often given to patients with unresectable cholangiocarcinoma, the survival benefit has not been proven in a randomised controlled trial (Gruenberger et al. 2010).

5. Palliative endoscopic interventions

Given that up to 80-85% of pancreato-biliary cancers are unresectable and the survival benefit of chemo-radiation therapy is very modest, palliative treatment plays a very important role in the care of these patients. Relief of symptoms secondary to gastro-duodenal obstruction, jaundice and pain are essential to improve their quality of life and overall survival. In the past, surgical palliative approaches, such as gastric bypass and hepatico-enteric decompression, are more common used as the diagnosis of unresectable disease is frequently made in the operating room. With the recent improvement in pre-operative staging, diagnostic laparotomy is rarely performed and biliary or gastro-duodenal obstruction is mostly managed by minimally invasive endoscopic interventions.

5.1 Alleviation of biliary obstruction

Currently, endoscopic biliary stenting is the treatment of choice for unresectable pancreato-biliary cancers with obstructive jaundice (Figure 4). Endoscopic placement of plastic stent(s) was equally effective as surgical technique in palliating obstructive jaundice, but endoscopic stent was associated with fewer procedural complications and death (Taylor et al., 2000). More recently, the invention of larger diameter self-expandable metallic (SEM) biliary stents provides longer stent patency for drainage. Compared to plastic stents, SEM stents are significantly less likely to be occluded and thus, minimized the number of repeated ERCP. As with plastic stents, endoscopic placement of SEM stents has been shown to provide similar overall survival to surgical decompression but is more cost-effective and better quality of life (Knyrim et al., 1993; Prat et al., 1998). The concurrent use of chemotherapeutic agents in patients palliated with SEM stents does not increase the risk for ascending cholangitis (Nakai et al., 2005).

Percutaneous trans-hepatic stenting (PTHS) is often reserved for patients in whom ERCP has failed due to a higher complication rate as well as poorer quality of life (Pinol et al., 2002). More recently, the advent of EUS assisted ductal drainage and stenting has significantly improved the success rate of endoscopic approach and thus, reduced the need for PTHS. This approach involves puncturing a dilated intra-hepatic duct, under direct EUS

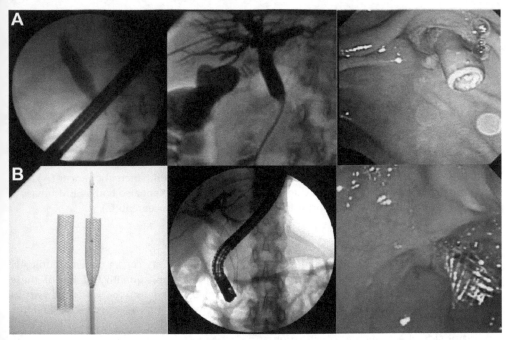

Fig. 4. Examples of biliary obstruction from pancreatic cancer requiring biliary drainage using plastic biliary stent (panel A) and SEM biliary stent (panel B).

guidance, to pass a guide wire into the duodenum, which then allows successful canulation of the biliar tree via ERCP and stenting (Shami and Kahaleh, 2007). In cases of duodenal obstruction, direct biliary drainage from a dilated intrahepatic duct into the stomach or duodenum via a SEM is an effective alternative for palliation with reasonable safety profile (Iwamuro et al., 2010; Nguyen-Tang et al. 2010). Surgical biliary bypass is only considered for patients who have relatively preserved functional status with obstructive jaundice and have failed on endoscopic stent placement.

5.2 Alleviation of gastro-duodenal obstruction

Although gastric bypass is commonly performed for unresectable patients with gastro-duodenal obstruction, the introduction of self-expanding metallic duodenal stents has changed the options for palliation (Figure 5). Current data suggest that placement of self-expandable metallic duodenal stents for malignant gastric outlet obstruction is successful in 98% of cases with a median duration of patency of 10 months (van Hooft et al., 2009). Serious complications from duodenal stenting, such as gastrointestinal bleeding or perforation, are rare with long-term stent dysfunction occurs in 14% of patients and migration in only 2% (van Hooft et al., 2009). Compared with palliative surgery, stent placement provides a shorter hospital stay, earlier resumption of oral intake, fewer complications and lower hospital costs (Maetani et al., 2004; Maetani et al., 2005). Currently, surgical palliation is often reserved for patients who are expected have a long life-expectancy and need both biliary and gastric bypass.

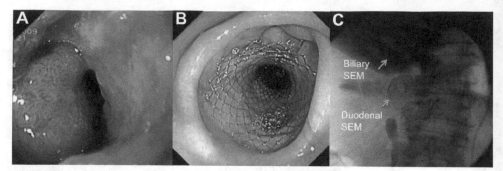

Fig. 5. A case of duodenal obstruction caused by locally advanced pancreatic cancer (A) and was successfully treated with a SEM duodenal stent (B).This patient also had a SEM biliary stent inserted for biliary drainage prior to the duodenal stent placement (C).

5.3 Alleviation of pain

Approximately 70% of patients with unresectable pancreato-biliary cancer develop clinically important pain, which can significantly reduce the quality and quantity of life of these patients (Andren-Sandberg et al., 1999). Good pain relief is, therefore, an essential part of effective palliative care. Although opioid analgesics are most commonly used as the first line pain relieved medication, one third of patients experience inadequate control of pain with significant side effects such as constipation and drowsiness (Andren-Sandberg et al., 1999). In these patients, neurolytic celiac plexus block under radiological or surgical guidance with absolute alcohol can be performed with up to 90% success rate (Mercadante et al., 2003; Wong et al., 2004; Noble and Gress, 2006). Recent studies have shown that EUS-guided neurolysis is equally effective but has significantly fewer serious complications associated with surgical or percutaneous approaches (O'Toole and Schmulewitz, 2009; Puli et al., 2009)

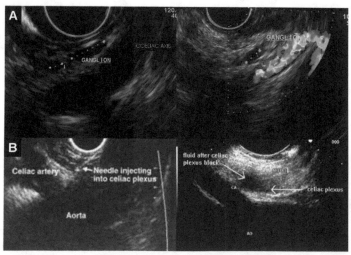

Fig. 6. Celiac ganglia can be visualized clearly on EUS imaging (panel A). Examples of EUS guided celiac ganglion blockage with alcohol injection (panel B).

(Figure 6). A recent double-blind randomized controlled study has also found that celiac plexus block is superior than systemic analgesic therapy in providing pain relief and improving quality of life (Wong et al., 2004). Thus, EUS-guided celiac neurolysis should be considered in all patients who have abdominal pain related to the pancreato-biliary cancer.

6. Conclusions

Despite the recent advances in diagnostic modalities, chemo-radiotherapy, surgical and post-operative care, the overall prognosis of pancreato-biliary malignancies has barely changed over the last few decades. The management of these patients is often complex and requires expertise in many fields. Thus, multidisciplinary teams are necessary to optimize the overall care. As the majority of these patients are diagnosed in advanced stages, good palliative care measures are essential to the management. Fortunately, a number of advances in endoscopic techniques have been made to improve the quality of life of these patients and avoid unnecessary surgery.

7. References

Anderson, C. and R. Kim (2009). "Adjuvant therapy for resected extrahepatic cholangiocarcinoma: a review of the literature and future directions." *Cancer Treat Rev* 35(4): 322-7.

Andren-Sandberg, A., A. Viste, A. Horn, D. Hoem and H. Gislason (1999). "Pain management of pancreatic cancer." *Ann Oncol* 10 Suppl 4: 265-8.

Balzano, G. and V. Di Carlo (2008). "Is CA 19-9 useful in the management of pancreatic cancer?" *Lancet Oncol* 9(2): 89-91.

Beger, H. G., F. Treitschke, F. Gansauge, N. Harada, N. Hiki and T. Mattfeldt (1999). "Tumor of the ampulla of Vater: experience with local or radical resection in 171 consecutively treated patients." *Arch Surg* 134(5): 526-32.

Binmoeller, K. F., S. Boaventura, K. Ramsperger and N. Soehendra (1993). "Endoscopic snare excision of benign adenomas of the papilla of Vater." *Gastrointest Endosc* 39(2): 127-31.

Bohnacker, S., U. Seitz, D. Nguyen, F. Thonke, S. Seewald, A. deWeerth, R. Ponnudurai, S. Omar and N. Soehendra (2005). "Endoscopic resection of benign tumors of the duodenal papilla without and with intraductal growth." *Gastrointest Endosc* 62(4): 551-60.

Brennan, M. F. (2004). "Adjuvant therapy following resection for pancreatic adenocarcinoma." *Surg Oncol Clin N Am* 13(4): 555-66, vii.

Cameron, J. L., T. S. Riall, J. Coleman and K. A. Belcher (2006). "One thousand consecutive pancreaticoduodenectomies." *Ann Surg* 244(1): 10-15.

Chang, D. K., N. D. Merrett and A. V. Biankin (2008). "Improving outcomes for operable pancreatic cancer: is access to safer surgery the problem?" *J Gastroenterol Hepatol* 23(7 Pt 1): 1036-45.

Chang, D. K., N. Q. Nguyen, N. D. Merrett, H. Dixson, R. W. Leong and A. V. Biankin (2009). "Role of endoscopic ultrasound in pancreatic cancer." *Expert Rev Gastroenterol Hepatol* 3(3): 293-303.

Cheng, C. L., S. Sherman, E. L. Fogel, L. McHenry, J. L. Watkins, T. Fukushima, T. J. Howard, L. Lazzell-Pannell and G. A. Lehman (2004). "Endoscopic snare papillectomy for tumors of the duodenal papillae." *Gastrointest Endosc* 60(5): 757-64.

Clarke, D. L., S. R. Thomson, T. E. Madiba and C. Sanyika (2003). "Preoperative imaging of pancreatic cancer: a management-oriented approach." *J Am Coll Surg* 196(1): 119-29.

David, M., C. Lepage, J. L. Jouve, V. Jooste, M. Chauvenet, J. Faivre and A. M. Bouvier (2009). "Management and prognosis of pancreatic cancer over a 30-year period." *Br J Cancer* 101(2): 215-8.

Duffy, M. J., C. Sturgeon, R. Lamerz, C. Haglund, V. L. Holubec, R. Klapdor, A. Nicolini, O. Topolcan and V. Heinemann (2010). "Tumor markers in pancreatic cancer: a European Group on Tumor Markers (EGTM) status report." *Ann Oncol* 21(3): 441-7.

Fischer, H. P. and H. Zhou (2004). "Pathogenesis of carcinoma of the papilla of Vater." *J Hepatobiliary Pancreat Surg* 11(5): 301-9.

Fogelman, D. R., J. Chen, J. A. Chabot, J. D. Allendorf, B. A. Schrope, R. D. Ennis, S. M. Schreibman and R. L. Fine (2004). "The evolution of adjuvant and neoadjuvant chemotherapy and radiation for advanced pancreatic cancer: from 5-fluorouracil to GTX." *Surg Oncol Clin N Am* 13(4): 711-35, x.

Ghaneh, P., E. Costello and J. P. Neoptolemos (2008). "Biology and management of pancreatic cancer." *Postgrad Med J* 84(995): 478-97.

Gillen, S., T. Schuster, C. Meyer Zum Buschenfelde, H. Friess and J. Kleeff (2010). "Preoperative/neoadjuvant therapy in pancreatic cancer: a systematic review and meta-analysis of response and resection percentages." *PLoS Med* 7(4): e1000267.

Goldstein, D., S. Carroll, M. Apte and G. Keogh (2004). "Modern management of pancreatic carcinoma." *Intern Med J* 34(8): 475-81.

Gruenberger, B., J. Schueller, U. Heubrandtner, F. Wrba, D. Tamandl, K. Kaczirek, R. Roka, S. Freimann-Pircher and T. Gruenberger (2010). "Cetuximab, gemcitabine, and oxaliplatin in patients with unresectable advanced or metastatic biliary tract cancer: a phase 2 study." *Lancet Oncol* 11(12): 1142-8.

Heinrich, S. and P. A. Clavien (2010). "Ampullary cancer." *Curr Opin Gastroenterol* 26(3): 280-5.

Heinrich, S., B. Pestalozzi, M. Lesurtel, F. Berrevoet, S. Laurent, J. R. Delpero, J. L. Raoul, P. Bachellier, P. Dufour, M. Moehler, A. Weber, H. Lang, X. Rogiers and P. A. Clavien (2010). "Adjuvant gemcitabine versus NEOadjuvant gemcitabine/oxaliplatin plus adjuvant gemcitabine in resectable pancreatic cancer: a randomized multicenter phase III study (NEOPAC study)." *BMC Cancer* 11: 346.

Iglesias Garcia, J., J. Larino Noia and J. E. Dominguez Munoz (2009). "Endoscopic ultrasound in the diagnosis and staging of pancreatic cancer." *Rev Esp Enferm Dig* 101(9): 631-8.

Iwamuro, M., H. Kawamoto, R. Harada, H. Kato, K. Hirao, O. Mizuno, E. Ishida, T. Ogawa, H. Okada and K. Yamamoto "Combined duodenal stent placement and endoscopic ultrasonography-guided biliary drainage for malignant duodenal obstruction with biliary stricture." *Dig Endosc* 22(3): 236-40.

Jean, M. and K. Dua (2003). "Tumors of the ampulla of Vater." *Curr Gastroenterol Rep* 5(2): 171-5.

Jemal, A., R. Siegel, E. Ward, Y. Hao, J. Xu and M. J. Thun (2009). "Cancer statistics, 2009." *CA Cancer J Clin* 59(4): 225-49.

Kalser, M. H. and S. S. Ellenberg (1985). "Pancreatic cancer. Adjuvant combined radiation and chemotherapy following curative resection." *Arch Surg* 120(8): 899-903.

Katsinelos, P., J. Kountouras, G. Chatzimavroudis, C. Zavos, G. Paroutoglou, R. Kotakidou, K. Panagiotopoulou and B. Papaziogas (2007). "A case of early depressed-type ampullary carcinoma treated by wire-guided endoscopic resection." *Surg Laparosc Endosc Percutan Tech* 17(6): 533-7.

Klapman, J. and M. P. Malafa (2008). "Early detection of pancreatic cancer: why, who, and how to screen." *Cancer Control* 15(4): 280-7.

Knyrim, K., H. J. Wagner, J. Pausch and N. Vakil (1993). "A prospective, randomized, controlled trial of metal stents for malignant obstruction of the common bile duct." *Endoscopy* 25(3): 207-12.

Lang, H., G. C. Sotiropoulos, G. Sgourakis, K. J. Schmitz, A. Paul, P. Hilgard, T. Zopf, T. Trarbach, M. Malago, H. A. Baba and C. E. Broelsch (2009). "Operations for intrahepatic cholangiocarcinoma: single-institution experience of 158 patients." *J Am Coll Surg* 208(2): 218-28.

Lillemoe, K. D., C. J. Yeo and J. L. Cameron (2000). "Pancreatic cancer: state-of-the-art care." *CA Cancer J Clin* 50(4): 241-68.

Luke, C., T. Price, C. Karapetis, N. Singhal and D. Roder (2009). "Pancreatic cancer epidemiology and survival in an Australian population." *Asian Pac J Cancer Prev* 10(3): 369-74.

Maetani, I., S. Akatsuka, M. Ikeda, T. Tada, T. Ukita, Y. Nakamura, J. Nagao and Y. Sakai (2005). "Self-expandable metallic stent placement for palliation in gastric outlet obstructions caused by gastric cancer: a comparison with surgical gastrojejunostomy." *J Gastroenterol* 40(10): 932-7.

Maetani, I., T. Tada, T. Ukita, H. Inoue, Y. Sakai and J. Nagao (2004). "Comparison of duodenal stent placement with surgical gastrojejunostomy for palliation in patients with duodenal obstructions caused by pancreaticobiliary malignancies." *Endoscopy* 36(1): 73-8.

Mercadante, S., E. Catala, E. Arcuri and A. Casuccio (2003). "Celiac plexus block for pancreatic cancer pain: factors influencing pain, symptoms and quality of life." *J Pain Symptom Manage* 26(6): 1140-7.

Moertel, C. G., L. L. Gunderson, J. A. Mailliard, P. J. McKenna, J. A. Martenson, Jr., P. A. Burch and S. S. Cha (1994). "Early evaluation of combined fluorouracil and leucovorin as a radiation enhancer for locally unresectable, residual, or recurrent gastrointestinal carcinoma. The North Central Cancer Treatment Group." *J Clin Oncol* 12(1): 21-7.

Mohamadnejad, M., J. M. DeWitt, S. Sherman, J. K. LeBlanc, H. A. Pitt, M. G. House, K. J. Jones, E. L. Fogel, L. McHenry, J. L. Watkins, G. A. Cote, G. A. Lehman and M. A. Al-Haddad "Role of EUS for preoperative evaluation of cholangiocarcinoma: a large single-center experience." *Gastrointest Endosc* 73(1): 71-8.

Nakai, Y., H. Isayama, Y. Komatsu, T. Tsujino, N. Toda, N. Sasahira, N. Yamamoto, K. Hirano, M. Tada, H. Yoshida, T. Kawabe and M. Omata (2005). "Efficacy and safety of the covered Wallstent in patients with distal malignant biliary obstruction." *Gastrointest Endosc* 62(5): 742-8.

Neoptolemos, J. P., J. A. Dunn, D. D. Stocken, J. Almond, K. Link, H. Beger, C. Bassi, M. Falconi, P. Pederzoli, C. Dervenis, L. Fernandez-Cruz, F. Lacaine, A. Pap, D.

Spooner, D. J. Kerr, H. Friess and M. W. Buchler (2001). "Adjuvant chemoradiotherapy and chemotherapy in resectable pancreatic cancer: a randomised controlled trial." *Lancet* 358(9293): 1576-85.

Neoptolemos, J. P., D. D. Stocken, H. Friess, C. Bassi, J. A. Dunn, H. Hickey, H. Beger, L. Fernandez-Cruz, C. Dervenis, F. Lacaine, M. Falconi, P. Pederzoli, A. Pap, D. Spooner, D. J. Kerr and M. W. Buchler (2004). "A randomized trial of chemoradiotherapy and chemotherapy after resection of pancreatic cancer." *N Engl J Med* 350(12): 1200-10.

Nguyen-Tang, T., K. F. Binmoeller, A. Sanchez-Yague and J. N. Shah (2010). "Endoscopic ultrasound (EUS)-guided transhepatic anterograde self-expandable metal stent (SEMS) placement across malignant biliary obstruction." *Endoscopy* 42(3): 232-6.

Nguyen, N. Q. (2009). "Application of per oral cholangiopancreatoscopy in pancreatobiliary diseases." *J Gastroenterol Hepatol* 24(6): 962-9.

Nguyen, N. Q. and D. F. Bartholomeusz "18F-FDG-PET/CT in the assessment of pancreatic cancer: is the contrast or a better-designed trial needed?" *J Gastroenterol Hepatol* 26(4): 613-5.

Nguyen, N. Q., K. F. Binmoeller and J. N. Shah (2009). "Cholangioscopy and pancreatoscopy (with videos)." *Gastrointest Endosc* 70(6): 1200-10.

Nguyen, N. Q., J. N. Shah and K. F. Binmoeller "Outcomes of endoscopic papillectomy in elderly patients with ampullary adenoma or early carcinoma." *Endoscopy* 42(11): 975-7.

Noble, M. and F. G. Gress (2006). "Techniques and results of neurolysis for chronic pancreatitis and pancreatic cancer pain." *Curr Gastroenterol Rep* 8(2): 99-103.

O'Toole, T. M. and N. Schmulewitz (2009). "Complication rates of EUS-guided celiac plexus blockade and neurolysis: results of a large case series." *Endoscopy* 41(7): 593-7.

Oettle, H., S. Post, P. Neuhaus, K. Gellert, J. Langrehr, K. Ridwelski, H. Schramm, J. Fahlke, C. Zuelke, C. Burkart, K. Gutberlet, E. Kettner, H. Schmalenberg, K. Weigang-Koehler, W. O. Bechstein, M. Niedergethmann, I. Schmidt-Wolf, L. Roll, B. Doerken and H. Riess (2007). "Adjuvant chemotherapy with gemcitabine vs observation in patients undergoing curative-intent resection of pancreatic cancer: a randomized controlled trial." *Jama* 297(3): 267-77.

Offerhaus, G. J., F. M. Giardiello, A. J. Krush, S. V. Booker, A. C. Tersmette, N. C. Kelley and S. R. Hamilton (1992). "The risk of upper gastrointestinal cancer in familial adenomatous polyposis." *Gastroenterology* 102(6): 1980-2.

Palmer, D. H., D. D. Stocken, H. Hewitt, C. E. Markham, A. B. Hassan, P. J. Johnson, J. A. Buckels and S. R. Bramhall (2007). "A randomized phase 2 trial of neoadjuvant chemotherapy in resectable pancreatic cancer: gemcitabine alone versus gemcitabine combined with cisplatin." *Ann Surg Oncol* 14(7): 2088-96.

Paquin, S. C., G. Gariepy, L. Lepanto, R. Bourdages, G. Raymond and A. V. Sahai (2005). "A first report of tumor seeding because of EUS-guided FNA of a pancreatic adenocarcinoma." *Gastrointest Endosc* 61(4): 610-1.

Park, J. K., Y. B. Yoon, Y. T. Kim, J. K. Ryu, W. J. Yoon and S. H. Lee (2008). "Survival and prognostic factors of unresectable pancreatic cancer." *J Clin Gastroenterol* 42(1): 86-91.

Patel, T. (2001). "Increasing incidence and mortality of primary intrahepatic cholangiocarcinoma in the United States." *Hepatology* 33(6): 1353-7.

Patel, T. (2006). "Cholangiocarcinoma." *Nat Clin Pract Gastroenterol Hepatol* 3(1): 33-42.

Peddu, P., A. Quaglia, P. A. Kane and J. B. Karani (2009). "Role of imaging in the management of pancreatic mass." *Crit Rev Oncol Hematol* 70(1): 12-23.

Pinol, V., A. Castells, J. M. Bordas, M. I. Real, J. Llach, X. Montana, F. Feu and S. Navarro (2002). "Percutaneous self-expanding metal stents versus endoscopic polyethylene endoprostheses for treating malignant biliary obstruction: randomized clinical trial." *Radiology* 225(1): 27-34.

Prat, F., O. Chapat, B. Ducot, T. Ponchon, G. Pelletier, J. Fritsch, A. D. Choury and C. Buffet (1998). "A randomized trial of endoscopic drainage methods for inoperable malignant strictures of the common bile duct." *Gastrointest Endosc* 47(1): 1-7.

Puli, S. R., J. B. Reddy, M. L. Bechtold, M. R. Antillon and W. R. Brugge (2009). "EUS-guided celiac plexus neurolysis for pain due to chronic pancreatitis or pancreatic cancer pain: a meta-analysis and systematic review." *Dig Dis Sci* 54(11): 2330-7.

Regine, W. F., K. A. Winter, R. A. Abrams, H. Safran, J. P. Hoffman, A. Konski, A. B. Benson, J. S. Macdonald, M. R. Kudrimoti, M. L. Fromm, M. G. Haddock, P. Schaefer, C. G. Willett and T. A. Rich (2008). "Fluorouracil vs gemcitabine chemotherapy before and after fluorouracil-based chemoradiation following resection of pancreatic adenocarcinoma: a randomized controlled trial." *Jama* 299(9): 1019-26.

Serrano, O. K., M. A. Chaudhry and S. D. Leach "The role of PET scanning in pancreatic cancer." *Adv Surg* 44: 313-25.

Shaib, Y. H., J. A. Davila and H. B. El-Serag (2006). "The epidemiology of pancreatic cancer in the United States: changes below the surface." *Aliment Pharmacol Ther* 24(1): 87-94.

Shami, V. M. and M. Kahaleh (2007). "Endoscopic ultrasonography (EUS)-guided access and therapy of pancreatico-biliary disorders: EUS-guided cholangio and pancreatic drainage." *Gastrointest Endosc Clin N Am* 17(3): 581-93, vii-viii.

Stocken, D. D., M. W. Buchler, C. Dervenis, C. Bassi, H. Jeekel, J. H. Klinkenbijl, K. E. Bakkevold, T. Takada, H. Amano and J. P. Neoptolemos (2005). "Meta-analysis of randomised adjuvant therapy trials for pancreatic cancer." *Br J Cancer* 92(8): 1372-81.

Taylor, M. C., R. S. McLeod and B. Langer (2000). "Biliary stenting versus bypass surgery for the palliation of malignant distal bile duct obstruction: a meta-analysis." *Liver Transpl* 6(3): 302-8.

van Hooft, J. E., M. J. Uitdehaag, M. J. Bruno, R. Timmer, P. D. Siersema, M. G. Dijkgraaf and P. Fockens (2009). "Efficacy and safety of the new WallFlex enteral stent in palliative treatment of malignant gastric outlet obstruction (DUOFLEX study): a prospective multicenter study." *Gastrointest Endosc* 69(6): 1059-66.

van Tienhoven, G., D. J. Gouma and D. J. Richel (2011). "Neoadjuvant chemoradiotherapy has a potential role in pancreatic carcinoma." *Ther Adv Med Oncol* 3(1): 27-33.

Verslype, C., E. Van Cutsem, M. Dicato, S. Cascinu, D. Cunningham, E. Diaz-Rubio, B. Glimelius, D. Haller, K. Haustermans, V. Heinemann, P. Hoff, P. G. Johnston, D. Kerr, R. Labianca, C. Louvet, B. Minsky, M. Moore, B. Nordlinger, S. Pedrazzoli, A. Roth, M. Rothenberg, P. Rougier, H. J. Schmoll, J. Tabernero, M. Tempero, C. van de Velde, J. L. Van Laethem and J. Zalcberg (2007). "The management of pancreatic cancer. Current expert opinion and recommendations derived from the 8th World

Congress on Gastrointestinal Cancer, Barcelona, 2006." *Ann Oncol* 18 Suppl 7: vii1-vii10.

Vinciguerra, V. (2011). "Adjuvant and neoadjuvant therapy for pancreatic cancer." *Oncology (Williston Park)* 25(2): 192-3.

Witzigmann, H., H. Lang and H. Lauer (2008). "Guidelines for palliative surgery of cholangiocarcinoma." *HPB (Oxford)* 10(3): 154-60.

Wong, G. Y., D. R. Schroeder, P. E. Carns, J. L. Wilson, D. P. Martin, M. O. Kinney, C. B. Mantilla and D. O. Warner (2004). "Effect of neurolytic celiac plexus block on pain relief, quality of life, and survival in patients with unresectable pancreatic cancer: a randomized controlled trial." *Jama* 291(9): 1092-9.

Yamao, K., A. Sawaki, N. Mizuno, Y. Shimizu, Y. Yatabe and T. Koshikawa (2005). "Endoscopic ultrasound-guided fine-needle aspiration biopsy (EUS-FNAB): past, present, and future." *Journal of Gastroenterology* 40(11): 1013-1023.

Yeo, C. J., J. L. Cameron, T. A. Sohn, K. D. Lillemoe, H. A. Pitt, M. A. Talamini, R. H. Hruban, S. E. Ord, P. K. Sauter and J. Coleman (1997). "Six hundred fifty consecutive pancreaticoduodenectomies in the 1990s: pathology, complications, and outcomes." *Ann Surg* 226(3): 248-257.

Zadorova, Z., M. Dvofak and J. Hajer (2001). "Endoscopic therapy of benign tumors of the papilla of Vater." *Endoscopy* 33(4): 345-7.

Zuckerman, D. S. and D. P. Ryan (2008). "Adjuvant therapy for pancreatic cancer: a review." *Cancer* 112(2): 243-9.

11

Hepatic Encephalopathy

Om Parkash, Adil Aub and Saeed Hamid
Aga Khan University, Karachi
Pakistan

1. Introduction

The liver is the most important organ for the well-functioning of other organs because of its vital role in nutrition, metabolism and secretion. Any disturbance in normal homeostasis of liver as it happens in acute liver failure (ALF) and chronic liver disease (cirrhosis) will lead to extra hepatic manifestations of liver disease, among them one is encephalopathy. And this encephalopathy caused by liver abnormality is known as Hepatic encephalopathy (HE).(1) HE occurs in 50-70% of patients with chronic liver disease and this is one of the sign of decompensated chronic liver disease. Occurrence of HE associated with poor prognosis with survival of approximately 42% at 1 year.(2)

1.1 Definition

Hepatic encephalopathy(HE) is defined as a reversible and metabolically induced neuropsychiatric complication, most commonly associated with cirrhosis, but may also be a complication of acute or chronic liver disease.(3) The affected patients exhibit alterations in psychomotor functions, personality changes, cognitive impairment and disturbed sleep pattern. Although, precise pathophysiologic mechanisms are not well understood, severe liver damage or the presence of Porto-systemic shunts are thought to be the major mechanisms involved.(4)

According to the classification proposed by the working party in 1998, HE can be graded into 3 types:

1. Type A HE (associated with acute liver failure);
2. Type B HE (observed in patients with Porto-systemic bypass and no intrinsic hepato-cellular disease);
3. Type C HE (associated with cirrhosis or portal-hypertension or Porto-systemic shunt).

    Type C HE can be further divided into three categories:

    i.   Episodic HE (Spontaneous; recurrent; precipitated)
    ii. Persistent HE (Mild; Severe; Treatment dependent)
    iii. Minimal or Overt HE(3)

Overt HE (OHE) is a syndrome of neuropsychiatric abnormalities that can be detected by bedside clinical tests in contrast to minimal HE (MHE) that requires specific psychometric tests for detection.(5) Defining type-C HE into minimal or overt, episodic or persistent and precipitated or spontaneous is clinically relevant since the management of each category is very different. Nowadays MHE has been recognized as the major factor in impairing the health related quality of life (HRQOL) in patients with cirrhosis.(6, 7) And MHE has prognostic significance because it predicts the occurrence of overt HE and is not useful predictor for mortality in cirrhosis.(8)

2. Pathophysiology

The pathophysiology of hepatic encephalopathy is intricate and exact mechanisms leading to HE are not clearly understood. Hepatic encephalopathy pathogenesis has many components which include ammonia, inflammatory cytokines, benzodiazepine like compounds and manganese like substances which impair neuronal function.(9) The role of ammonia has dominated explanations for the pathogenesis of HE but it cannot single handedly explain all the neurological changes seen in HE. Evidence regarding other concurrent factors has emerged over the years and it is thought that these factors either work alone or in synergy to cause astrocytes to swell and fluid to accumulate in brain which causes the symptoms of HE(10). Some factors and conditions also appear to precipitate HE (Box A).

2.1 The ammonia theory

Ammonia is produced predominantly from dietary nitrogenous components, bacterial metabolism of these nitrogenous products in the colon and in small intestine from glutamine by glutaminase enzyme.(11) Eventually this ammonia from gastrointestinal tract enters portal circulation for its final destination of urea cycle in the liver to be converted as urea which will subsequently be excreted by kidneys.(12) Under normal conditions, ammonia is eliminated through urea formation in the liver but in patients with acute liver failure, brain and muscle cells are also involved in the metabolism. Elevated levels of ammonia may cause severe toxicity so it must be removed from the body.(13) Because of liver disease and portosystemic collaterals in cirrhosis, ammonia concentration in blood rises hence crosses the blood brain barrier.(14) In Brain, astrocytes are the only cells capable of metabolizing ammonia and express the enzyme glutamine synthase for the conversion of ammonia into glutamine. So, ammonia detoxification in astrocytes leads to accumulation of glutamine which being an osmolyte, causes movement of water inside the astrocyte and causes cerebral edema i-e 'Trojan horse' hypothesis(14-16). Some of the studies had shown the ammonia induced expression of aquaporin water channel on astrocytes. (17)

This has been seen in autopsies of patients with cirrhosis in which brain tissue had shown swollen astrocytes with enlarged nuclei along with displacement of chromatin to the perimeter of the cell, this condition is known as Alzheimer type II astrocytosis.(18) Acute insult of ammonia leads to calcium dependent glutamate release from astrocytes, which causes increased neuronal activity (as seen in Type A HE). A prolonged exposure to ammonia leads to glutamine induced osmotic stress, which causes compensatory release of myoinositol and taurine from the astrocytes, which may lead to down regulation of glutamate receptors and neuroinhibitory state of HE (as seen in Type C HE). Elevated intracellular ammonia levels also results in altered neurotransmission by agonizing GABA tone.(19)

Hyper ammonia lead to abnormal cerebral blood flow and glucose metabolism and this had been seen in studies of single photon emission tomographic (SPECT) in which redistribution of blood flow form cerebral cortex to subcortical regions had been demonstrated. This abnormality lead to different HE features.(17, 20)

2.2 Inflammation

The partial credit also goes to the inflammation because majority of the cirrhotic patients in the presence of infection develop the HE. This association of markers of inflammatory response in state of systemic inflammatory response (SIRS) and HE, has been demonstrated in different studies.(21, 22) In one of the clinical study, it has been seen that HE or neuropsychological dysfunction improves after the resolution of SIRS.(23) Despite this exact mechanism of inflammation leading to HE is still not known as yet, but possibly it is hypothesized that cytokine mediated changes in blood brain barrier (BBB) permeability, altered glutamate uptake by astrocyte and altered expression of GABA receptors.(23)

TNF released in response to inflammation has been correlated to the symptoms of HE. It causes Astrocytes to release inflammatory cytokines (i-e IL-1, IL-6) which impairs the endothelial Blood-Brain barrier and increases ammonia diffusion into astrocytes. (24)

2.3 Neurosteroids and GABA/Benzodiazepine receptor complex theory

Neurosteroids are mainly produced by myelinating glial cells in response to increased expression of peripheral type benzodiazepine receptor (Trasnslocator proteins), which are activated by ammonia, inflammation and manganese. Neurosteroids increase chloride influx and thereby enhance GABAergic tone, causing symptoms in patients with Type C HE.(25, 26)

GABA mediates its action through GABA-receptor complex (GRC) and acts as an inhibitory neurotransmitter. Increased sensitivity of the trasnslocator proteins also enhances the activation of GABA-GRC complex, hence causing inhibition of neurotransmission.(14, 27) Increased GABAergic tone has been associated with the pathogenesis of HE and this was proved by the reports which had revealed the beneficial effects of benzodiazepine antagonist (Flumazenil).(28) There is an excess of benzodiazepine like compounds in HE that are derived from synthesis by intestinal flora, dietary vegetables and medications.(29, 30) Moreover natural benzodiazepines also accumulate in brain and furthermore cirrhotic patients have the poor capability of clearing the benzodiazepine like compounds.(31) These compounds bind to GABA receptor complex inducing GABA release and neuro-inhibition. A study by Stewart et al group had shown that ammonia itself bind to the GABA receptor complex.(32) It may also potentiate benzodiazepines by up regulating expression of peripheral type benzodiazepine receptor that trigger synthesis of neuro-steroids, which are strong GABA agonists.(33)

Hence GABAergic tone is more likely attributed to elevated levels of benzodiazepines like compounds in patients with cirrhosis.

BCCA and false neurotransmitter theory: Brain neurotransmission is regulated by CNS concentration of amino acids and their precursor. In cirrhotic patients, plasma concentrations of aromatic amino acids (tryptophan, tyrosine, and phenalanine) are elevated and branch chain amino acids (Leucine, isoleucine and valine) concentration are reduced. Aromatic as well as branch chain amino acids share a common transport mechanism into the CNS and as a consequence of increased of aromatic amino acids, neuronal levels may be increased leading to the production of false neurotransmitter subsequently leading to HE.(34)

Serotonin theory: Serotonin, a neurotransmitter which is widely distributed in CNS, has been implicated in the pathogenesis of HE. In cirrhotic patients it has been seen that serotonin metabolism is altered hence leading to serotonergic synaptic deficit. Serotonergic pathway in brain is important for regulation of sleep, locomotion and circadian rhythmicity.(35) Serotonin metabolism is intricately and selectively sensitive to the degree of portosystemic shunting and hyperammonaemia, therefore suggesting a role for serotonin in early neuropsychiatric symptoms of HE.(36)

Zinc theory: Zinc (Zn) element is a component/substrate of urea cycle enzymes. It is assumed that this element is reduced in patients with liver cirrhosis. Zn supplementation increases activities of ornithine transcarbamalyse increasing excretion of ammonia ions. Interestingly till now there is conflicting evidence for this hypothesis of Zn supplementation in He patients.(37, 38)

2.4 Oxidative and nitrosative stress

Exposure of astrocytes to ammonia, inflammatory cytokines, hyponatremia and benzodiazepines leads to enhanced production of RNS & ROS via the Calcium dependent N-methyl-D-aspartate (NMDA) pathway. RNS and ROS cause tyrosine nitration, leading to altered BBB permeability and astrocyte swelling. (39, 40)

2.5 Manganese theory

In normal healthy individuals, Maganese is cleared by liver and excreted into the bile. Manganese is known to stimulate the Translocator proteins located on astrocytes, leading to enhanced neurosteroid synthesis. In cirrhotic patients, it accumulates in the basal ganglia because of decreased excretion of Maganese due to portosystemic shunting and promotes formation of Alzheimer's type 2 astrocytes.(41) Brain magnetic resonance imaging (MRI) in cirrhotic patients has shown changes which are due to accumulation of Maganese in basal ganglia particularly in the palladium, putamen and caudate nucleus.(41)

3. Precipitating factors: (Box A)

The Most of HE episodes are precipitated by an event rather than spontaneous, with infection anywhere in body being the common, though its frequency is decreasing. Hence careful history and examination are necessary to identify the precipitating or contributing factors for HE, most of the time these factors are evident.(42)

Gastrointestinal bleeding commonly precipitates the HE even if it is controlled or stopped bleeding. Sometimes occult chronic gastrointestinal blood loss can also lead to HE, which needs to be evaluated and treated accordingly.(42)

Dehydration is again a very common precipitating factor in cirrhotic patients leading to HE because some of the patients ascites, are diuretics. And aggressive diuresis do induce dehydration leading to metabolic alkalosis and electrolyte imbalances.

• GI Bleeding	• Constipation
• Electrolyte imbalance	• Hypovolemia
• Trauma	• Dehydration
• Infection	• Medications (sedatives, diuretics, psychotropic,)
• Sepsis	• Uremia
• Dietary protein Overload	

Box A. Precipitating Factors for HE

It has also been seen that transjuglar intrahepatic portosystemic shunt (TIPS) in some of the cases can lead to HE. Few other precipitating factors which can sometimes lead to HE, need to be looked into by taking careful history and examination and shown in Box (A)

4. Clinical features

The clinical signs and symptoms of HE may range from mild cognitive impairment to profound coma. These include forgetfulness, alteration in sleep-wake cycle, changes in personality and emotions, hyperreflexia and drowsiness. In more severe cases disorientation, constructional apraxia , asterixis, seizures and eventually coma may develop.(43) It is very important to exclude other causes of altered mental status or encephalopathy (Box B) in suspected patients for appropriate management of HE.

• Subdural Hematoma
• Drug or alcohol intoxication
• Wilson's disease
• Hypoglycemia
• Wernicke's encephalopathy
• CNS Sepsis
• Postictal Confusion

Box B. Differential Diagnosis for HE

Clinically, the most commonly employed criteria used for grading is the West Haven criteria (Table 1) which defines HE semi quantitatively into four grades, based on the presence of specific clinical signs and symptoms and their severity. Further classification of comastose or unconscious patients can be done by using Glasgow Coma Scale which provides a more objective assessment of the conscious state of the patient.(4)

5. Diagnosis

Checking for Elevated Blood ammonia levels is the most commonly used parameter for assessment, but they may also be elevated due to other possible causes (i-e tourniquet use, delayed processing and cooling of sample, disorders related to ammonia and proline metabolism). In acute liver failure, arterial ammonia levels >150 mg/dl may be predictive of brain edema and herniation. However, measurement of arterial ammonia over venous ammonia offers no advantage in Chronic liver disease.(3, 44)

Grade	Intellectual function	Neuromuscular function
0	Normal	Minor abnormalities
1	Personality changes, attention deficits, irritability, depressed state	Tremor and incoordination
2	Changes in sleep-wake cycle, cognitive dysfunction, lethargy, behavioral changes	Asterixis, Speech abnormalities, Ataxic gait
3	Disorientation, unconsciousness, amnesia	Nystagmus, Clonus, Muscular rigidity
4	Stupor and Coma	Unresponsiveness to noxious stimuli, Oculocephalic reflex

Table 1. West Haven classification for grading of HE(1)

Neuropsychometric evaluation usually is done via 'paper and pencil tests' and 'computerized tests'. The routinely used paper and pencil tests include psychometric HE scores (PHES) and The Repeatable Battery for the Assessment of neurological status (RBANS). PHES has been endorsed as a 'gold standard' for diagnosis of MHE and is used to diagnose the cognitive changes that characterize MHE. RBANS in addition to diagnosing the cognitive issues, also scores patient's memory.(45) Some computerized psychometric tests like 'The inhibitory control test' and 'CDR computerized assessment system' are gaining popularity as promising diagnostic tests due to their effectiveness and convenience(46). However, the value of these psychometric tests is limited by methodological problems, training and education, demographic dependence and lack of standardization.(43)

Neurophysiological assessment is done via Electroencephalography (EEG) and the Critical flicker frequency test (CFF). EEG is associated with decreased electrical activity and shows diffuse slowing of alpha waves with eventual development of delta waves.(47) CCF, a light based test, is used for a rapid and reliable quantification of HE. Based on the principle of hepatic retinopathy, it represents the frequency at which discrete light pulses are first perceived by the patient. A CCF of below 39 Hz is diagnostic for MHE and the test results are not dependent on sex, occupation and education level.(48)

Imaging Modalities include different Magnetic resonance techniques(T1-weighted imaging, proton spectroscopy, magnetic transfer ratio, T2- weighted FLAIR sequence and diffusion weighted imaging) to measure cerebral edema, changes in brain activity and concentration of different substances(i-e glutamine, choline). A CT scan can be used to exclude subdural hematoma or other cerebrovascular events that may mimic HE.(48)

6. Treatment

HE treatment has evolved over the last 5 decades and medical science had seen many breakthroughs during this tenure. Treatment can be tailored around multiple key management principles which parallel the pathophysiology of the disease and these principles are:(42)

Management of precipitating factors,

Reduction of ammonia

Modulation intestinal flora

Modulation of neurotransmission

Correction of nutritional deficiencies

Reduction of inflammation/infection

Many treatment options are available for the treatment of HE with the mainstay to eliminate the underlying factors that precipitate HE. It is recommended that all patients should receive the empiric therapy (Box C) for HE, based on the principle of reducing the production and absorption of ammonia. Some strategies that are commonly applied to stop precipitating events are the following:

1. in patients with HE induced by gastrointestinal hemorrhage, stop the bleeding with vasoactive drugs, an endoscopic therapy or an angiographic shunt (TIPS), correct the anemia with a blood transfusion and use a nasogastric tube to facilitate upper gastrointestinal cleansing;
2. Promptly start Antibiotics therapy for infections;
3. Resolve constipation by cathartic and/or bowel enema, electrolyte abnormalities by discontinuing diuretics and correct hypo- or hyperkalemia;
4. Correct deterioration of renal function by stopping diuretics, treating dehydration and discontinuing nephrotoxic drugs
5. if HE is precipitated by the administration of exogenous sedatives, discontinue benzodiazepines and start flumazenil.(49)

- Lactulose (15-30ml orally, twice daily)
- Rifaximin (550mg orally, twice daily)
- Neomycin (500mg orally, four times daily)
- Metronidazole (250mg orally, four times daily)
- Vancomycin (250mg orally, four times daily)
- Sodium Benzoate(5 mg orally, twice daily)
- Flumazenil (1-3 mg IV)

Box C. Empiric Treatment for Hepatic encephalopathy(48)

7. Reduction of ammonia and modulation of neurotransmission

7.1 Nonadsorable disaccharides

Nonadsorable disaccharides (Lacutlose and Lactitol) especially Lactulose are considered the first line therapy for HE despite lack of well-designed randomized controlled trial. They are metabolized by the colonic bacteria and form by products that reduce the colonic PH, hence interfering with mucosal uptake of glutamine and reducing the synthesis and absorption of ammonia. There are other proposed mechanism of lactulose in HE such as lactulose modifies the colonic flora which in turn results in shift of urease containing bacteria with lactobacillus, fourfold increased fecal nitrogen excretion due to increase stool volume and it also helps in reduction of formation potentially toxic short chain fatty acids e.g propionate or butyrate.(50-53)

Lactulose can also be administered orally through a nasogastric tube to unresponsive patients as well as rectally through enemas.

The most common side effects associated with over use include dehydration, electrolyte imbalance and abdominal cramping. Previously it is known to cause no improvement in psychometric test performance and mortality(54). Few years back a study conducted in India had shown significant improvement and health related quality of life and psychometric improvement in patients with HE especially with minimal HE.(7)

The lactulose has got some role in preventing recurrent episodes of HE. It was proved by an open label RCT study from India by Sarin group, which suggested that lactulose is also effective in preventing recurrent episodes of HE.(55)

The recommended dose of lactulose is about 15-30ml given twice a day. Lactitol, an alternative to lactulose is considered equally effective and is used in patients intolerant of lactulose, but it is not available in some countries.(56, 57)

7.2 Antibiotics

Patients intolerant to nonabsorable disaccharides are generally treated with antibiotics, to suppress the bacteria involved in ammonia genesis. There are few antibiotics which have been used for the treatment of HE which had shown limited benefit, which include neomycin, metronidazole, oral vancomycin and very recently Rifaximin.(54)

In fact neomycin was used for treatment of HE for many years based on earlier studies then in early 1990's a double blind randomized controlled trial had no improvement in HE. And also because of its limited systemic absorption which would lead to ototoxicity and nephrotoxicity has lost its use in HE in liver cirrhosis. (58)

Rifaximin, a minimally absorbed oral antibiotic has been approved by FDA for the treatment of chronic HE, on the basis of results of a multicenter, randomized, controlled trials and met analysis.(59) Recently a RCT had shown benefit in prevention of recurrent hepatic encephalopathy over period of 6 months follow up. Subsequently further studies had also shown role of Rifaximin in improving the health related quality of life in patients with HE similarly improvement in Psychometric tests and simulated driving tests.(60-62) The use of this antibiotic is increasing due to few adverse effects and no known drug interactions. The recommended adult daily dose is 1200 mg/day, usually in three divided doses.

Some small studies have also reported the effectiveness of vancomycin and metronidazole, but the data to support their use is not enough.(54)

7.3 Other agents

Acarbose; a hypoglycemic agent and an intestinal a-glucosidase inhibitor which causes decrease in blood ammonia levels and improves mild HE in patients with cirrhosis.(63) It has also been hypothesized that Acarbose promotes the proliferation of intestinal saccharolytic bacterial flora while reducing proteolytic flora that produce mercaptans, benzodiazepine like substances and ammonia as well. This theory was answered in a randomized cross over trial by Gentile S et al group in Italy.(63)

Probiotics and synbiotics modify the gut bacterial flora and reduce ammonia levels. Their use however is still being investigated.(64)

7.4 Agents causing alteration in ammonia metabolism (L-Ornithine L-Aspartate and benzyl benzoate)

Urea cycle plays a key role in ammonia metabolism and its excretion by forming urea in periportal hepatocytes or synthesis of glutamine in perivenous hepatocytes. But in cirrhosis, the activities of carbamyl phosphate synthetase enzyme (Urea synthesis) and of glutamine synthesis (glutamine synthesis) are impaired hence as compensation glutamine increased which in turn lead to increased level of ammonia. Therefore ornithine aspartate and benzoate has been used for reducing the ammonia levels by increasing the metabolism to glutamine and hippurate respectively.

L-ornithine-L-aspartate (LOLA) activates urea cycle and enhances ammonia clearance. LOLA induces an increase of liver and muscle ammonia metabolism, leading to decreased blood levels, and is able to cross the blood-brain barrier, increasing the cerebral ammonia disposal.(65) One or two sachets of LOLA should be administered three times daily.(4)

Other ammonia excretors like sodium benzoate, sodium phenyl acetate and sodium phenyl butyrate are also reported to show improvement but clear efficacy has not been established yet. Sodium phenyl acetate and Ammonal are the only drugs approved by the Food and Drug Administration for the treatment of acute hyperammonemia and associated encephalopathy in patients with urea cycle disorders.(66)

7.5 Agents used in neurotransmission hypothesis

Branch chain amino acids (BCCA): As it has been hypothesized that in liver cirrhosis, there has been reversal of aromatic amino acids (AAA) to BCCA which could lead to encephalopathy in patients with cirrhosis. Encephalopathy is presumably caused by increase in levels of AAA for monoamine neurotransmission which lead to transformed neuronal excitability and causing HE. Hence numbers of studies have been done to evaluate the effects of BCCA on HE. BCCA can be given orally as well as in infusion form.(67, 68)

Agents used for GABA hypothesis pathway: GABA receptor complex is the principal inhibitory network in nervous system and seems to be a contributor to neuronal inhibition in HE. This GABA receptor complex contains barbiturates and benzodiazepine receptor sites, chloride channels and a GABA binding site. In cirrhosis, there is an evidence for increase in benzodiazepine receptor ligands in subjects with HE, therefore effects of benzodiazepine receptor antagonist have been evaluated.(69, 70)

Flumazenil, a $GABA_A$ receptor antagonist also improves the symptoms in patients with grade 3 or 4 HE but its use is limited due to adverse effects(71). It has been seen that response to treatment with flumazenil is rapid onset with few minutes and then with few hours, more than half of these patients deteriorated with 2-3 hours.(72, 73) Because of its short duration effect and variable results of different studies, flumazenil cannot be recommended as routine therapy.

7.6 Other treatment options

7.6.1 Nutritional intervention

In the past, dietary protein restriction was considered an important component of the treatment of HE. Recent evidence however suggests that excessive restriction can raise serum ammonia levels, as a result of reduced muscular ammonia metabolism.(74) It has also been seen that majority of the patients with advanced liver disease had severe protein calorie malnutrition due to multifactorial reasons including the decreased oral intake, catabolic state etc.(75)

A high-protein diet is therefore recommended for improving the symptoms of HE. The European society for Parenteral and Enteral nutrition recommended an energy intake of 35/40 kcal/kg body weight per day and that patients must eat at least 1.2g/kg of protein daily along with Branched-chain amino acids (BCAA's) and vegetable-based protein.(76) Vegetable and dairy based proteins are preferred to animal proteins because of a high calorie-to-nitrogen ratio. Vegetable based proteins increase colonic motility and enhances intestinal nitrogen clearance. They also reduce colonic PH, which prevents ammonia absorption into gut.(77)

Zinc increases the activity of ornithine transcarbamylase (an enzyme in urea cycle) so zinc supplementation is also recommended for HE especially in patients who don't show any response to lactulose or neomycin.(38)

7.6.2 Prognosis once recovered from HE

Patients who recovered from HE can have persistent and cumulative neurologic deficits despite achieving normal mental status after receiving medical therapy. Study for North America had shown that patients with overt HE had persistent deficits in working memory, response inhibition and learning when assessed by psychometric tests. Recurrent episodes are associated with severity of underlying disease.(78, 79)

Conclusion: HE includes variety of neuropsychiatric symptoms and signs among patients with CLD leading to liver failure. Occurrence of HE indicates worse prognosis and should be kept on liver transplant list wherever it is available. Initial treatment includes the identification and correction of precipitating factors such as electrolyte imbalances, GI bleeding, medications, and sepsis. The main treatment modalities include the nonabsorbable disaccharide, principally lactulose and antibiotics like metronidazole or Rifaximin nowadays.

8. References

[1] Nevah   MI,   Fallon   MB.   Hepatic   encephalopathy,   Hepatorenal   syndrome,
       Hepatopulmonary syndrome and Systemic complications of Liver disease.
       Feldman: Sleisenger and Fordtran's Gastrointestinal and Liver Disease,

Pathophysiology/Diagnosis/Management 9th ed: Saunders, An Imprint of Elsevier 2010. p. 1543-46.

[2] Bustamante J, Rimola A, Ventura PJ, Navasa M, Cirera I, Reggiardo V, et al. Prognostic significance of hepatic encephalopathy in patients with cirrhosis. J Hepatol. 1999 May;30(5):890-5.

[3] Ferenci P, Lockwood A, Mullen K, Tarter R, Weissenborn K, Blei AT. Hepatic encephalopathy--definition, nomenclature, diagnosis, and quantification: final report of the working party at the 11th World Congresses of Gastroenterology, Vienna, 1998. Hepatology. 2002 Mar;35(3):716-21.

[4] Cash WJ, McConville P, McDermott E, McCormick PA, Callender ME, McDougall NI. Current concepts in the assessment and treatment of hepatic encephalopathy. QJM. Jan;103(1):9-16.

[5] Bajaj JS, Wade JB, Sanyal AJ. Spectrum of neurocognitive impairment in cirrhosis: Implications for the assessment of hepatic encephalopathy. Hepatology. 2009 Dec;50(6):2014-21.

[6] Groeneweg M, Quero JC, De Bruijn I, Hartmann IJ, Essink-bot ML, Hop WC, et al. Subclinical hepatic encephalopathy impairs daily functioning. Hepatology. 1998 Jul;28(1):45-9.

[7] Prasad S, Dhiman RK, Duseja A, Chawla YK, Sharma A, Agarwal R. Lactulose improves cognitive functions and health-related quality of life in patients with cirrhosis who have minimal hepatic encephalopathy. Hepatology. 2007 Mar;45(3):549-59.

[8] Romero-Gomez M, Boza F, Garcia-Valdecasas MS, Garcia E, Aguilar-Reina J. Subclinical hepatic encephalopathy predicts the development of overt hepatic encephalopathy. Am J Gastroenterol. 2001 Sep;96(9):2718-23.

[9] Munoz SJ. Hepatic encephalopathy. Med Clin North Am. 2008 Jul;92(4):795-812, viii.

[10] Norenberg MD, Jayakumar AR, Rama Rao KV, Panickar KS. New concepts in the mechanism of ammonia-induced astrocyte swelling. Metab Brain Dis. 2007 Dec;22(3-4):219-34.

[11] Gerber T, Schomerus H. Hepatic encephalopathy in liver cirrhosis: pathogenesis, diagnosis and management. Drugs. 2000 Dec;60(6):1353-70.

[12] Butterworth RF. Complications of cirrhosis III. Hepatic encephalopathy. J Hepatol. 2000;32(1 Suppl):171-80.

[13] Cooper AJ, Plum F. Biochemistry and physiology of brain ammonia. Physiol Rev. 1987 Apr;67(2):440-519.

[14] Sundaram V, Shaikh OS. Hepatic encephalopathy: pathophysiology and emerging therapies. Med Clin North Am. 2009 Jul;93(4):819-36, vii.

[15] Haussinger D, Kircheis G, Fischer R, Schliess F, vom Dahl S. Hepatic encephalopathy in chronic liver disease: a clinical manifestation of astrocyte swelling and low-grade cerebral edema? J Hepatol. 2000 Jun;32(6):1035-8.

[16] Olde Damink SW, Jalan R, Dejong CH. Interorgan ammonia trafficking in liver disease. Metab Brain Dis. 2009 Mar;24(1):169-81.

[17] Rama Rao KV, Norenberg MD. Aquaporin-4 in hepatic encephalopathy. Metab Brain Dis. 2007 Dec;22(3-4):265-75.

[18] Pilbeam CM, Anderson RM, Bhathal PS. The brain in experimental portal-systemic encephalopathy. I. Morphological changes in three animal models. J Pathol. 1983 Aug;140(4):331-45.

[19] Mas A. Hepatic encephalopathy: from pathophysiology to treatment. Digestion. 2006;73 Suppl 1:86-93.

[20] Jalan R, Olde Damink SW, Lui HF, Glabus M, Deutz NE, Hayes PC, et al. Oral amino acid load mimicking hemoglobin results in reduced regional cerebral perfusion and deterioration in memory tests in patients with cirrhosis of the liver. Metab Brain Dis. 2003 Mar;18(1):37-49.

[21] Blei AT. Infection, inflammation and hepatic encephalopathy, synergism redefined. J Hepatol. 2004 Feb;40(2):327-30.

[22] Rolando N, Wade J, Davalos M, Wendon J, Philpott-Howard J, Williams R. The systemic inflammatory response syndrome in acute liver failure. Hepatology. 2000 Oct;32(4 Pt 1):734-9.

[23] Shawcross DL, Davies NA, Williams R, Jalan R. Systemic inflammatory response exacerbates the neuropsychological effects of induced hyperammonemia in cirrhosis. J Hepatol. 2004 Feb;40(2):247-54.

[24] Moldawer LL, Marano MA, Wei H, Fong Y, Silen ML, Kuo G, et al. Cachectin/tumor necrosis factor-alpha alters red blood cell kinetics and induces anemia in vivo. FASEB J. 1989 Mar;3(5):1637-43.

[25] Ahboucha S, Butterworth RF. The neurosteroid system: an emerging therapeutic target for hepatic encephalopathy. Metab Brain Dis. 2007 Dec;22(3-4):291-308.

[26] Baulieu EE. Neurosteroids: a novel function of the brain. Psychoneuroendocrinology. 1998 Nov;23(8):963-87.

[27] Ahboucha S, Butterworth RF. Pathophysiology of hepatic encephalopathy: a new look at GABA from the molecular standpoint. Metab Brain Dis. 2004 Dec;19(3-4):331-43.

[28] Reversal of hepatic coma by benzodiazepine antagonist (Ro 15-1788). Lancet. 1985 Jun 8;1(8441):1324-5.

[29] Lighthouse J, Naito Y, Helmy A, Hotten P, Fuji H, Min CH, et al. Endotoxinemia and benzodiazepine-like substances in compensated cirrhotic patients: a randomized study comparing the effect of rifaximine alone and in association with a symbiotic preparation. Hepatol Res. 2004 Mar;28(3):155-60.

[30] Zeneroli ML, Venturini I, Corsi L, Avallone R, Farina F, Ardizzone G, et al. Benzodiazepine-like compounds in the plasma of patients with fulminant hepatic failure. Scand J Gastroenterol. 1998 Mar;33(3):310-3.

[31] Zeneroli ML, Venturini I, Stefanelli S, Farina F, Miglioli RC, Minelli E, et al. Antibacterial activity of rifaximin reduces the levels of benzodiazepine-like compounds in patients with liver cirrhosis. Pharmacol Res. 1997 Jun;35(6):557-60.

[32] Stewart CA, Reivich M, Lucey MR, Gores GJ. Neuroimaging in hepatic encephalopathy. Clin Gastroenterol Hepatol. 2005 Mar;3(3):197-207.

[33] Ahboucha S, Layrargues GP, Mamer O, Butterworth RF. Increased brain concentrations of a neuroinhibitory steroid in human hepatic encephalopathy. Ann Neurol. 2005 Jul;58(1):169-70.

[34] Fischer JE, Rosen HM, Ebeid AM, James JH, Keane JM, Soeters PB. The effect of normalization of plasma amino acids on hepatic encephalopathy in man. Surgery. 1976 Jul;80(1):77-91.

[35] Lozeva V, Montgomery JA, Tuomisto L, Rocheleau B, Pannunzio M, Huet PM, et al. Increased brain serotonin turnover correlates with the degree of shunting and hyperammonemia in rats following variable portal vein stenosis. J Hepatol. 2004 May;40(5):742-8.

[36] Lozeva-Thomas V. Serotonin brain circuits with a focus on hepatic encephalopathy. Metab Brain Dis. 2004 Dec;19(3-4):413-20.

[37] Yoshida Y, Higashi T, Nouso K, Nakatsukasa H, Nakamura SI, Watanabe A, et al. Effects of zinc deficiency/zinc supplementation on ammonia metabolism in patients with decompensated liver cirrhosis. Acta Med Okayama. 2001 Dec;55(6):349-55.

[38] Marchesini G, Fabbri A, Bianchi G, Brizi M, Zoli M. Zinc supplementation and amino acid-nitrogen metabolism in patients with advanced cirrhosis. Hepatology. 1996 May;23(5):1084-92.

[39] Hermenegildo C, Monfort P, Felipo V. Activation of N-methyl-D-aspartate receptors in rat brain in vivo following acute ammonia intoxication: characterization by in vivo brain microdialysis. Hepatology. 2000 Mar;31(3):709-15.

[40] Schliess F, Gorg B, Haussinger D. Pathogenetic interplay between osmotic and oxidative stress: the hepatic encephalopathy paradigm. Biol Chem. 2006 Oct-Nov;387(10-11):1363-70.

[41] Rose C, Butterworth RF, Zayed J, Normandin L, Todd K, Michalak A, et al. Manganese deposition in basal ganglia structures results from both portal-systemic shunting and liver dysfunction. Gastroenterology. 1999 Sep;117(3):640-4.

[42] Frederick RT. Current concepts in the pathophysiology and management of hepatic encephalopathy. Gastroenterol Hepatol (N Y). 2011 Apr;7(4):222-33.

[43] Haussinger D. [Hepatic encephalopathy: clinical aspects and pathogenesis]. Dtsch Med Wochenschr. 2004 Sep 3;129 Suppl 2:S66-7.

[44] Bernal W, Hall C, Karvellas CJ, Auzinger G, Sizer E, Wendon J. Arterial ammonia and clinical risk factors for encephalopathy and intracranial hypertension in acute liver failure. Hepatology. 2007 Dec;46(6):1844-52.

[45] Weissenborn K, Ennen JC, Schomerus H, Ruckert N, Hecker H. Neuropsychological characterization of hepatic encephalopathy. J Hepatol. 2001 May;34(5):768-73.

[46] Mardini H, Saxby BK, Record CO. Computerized psychometric testing in minimal encephalopathy and modulation by nitrogen challenge and liver transplant. Gastroenterology. 2008 Nov;135(5):1582-90.

[47] Montagnese S, Amodio P, Morgan MY. Methods for diagnosing hepatic encephalopathy in patients with cirrhosis: a multidimensional approach. Metab Brain Dis. 2004 Dec;19(3-4):281-312.

[48] Prakash R, Mullen KD. Mechanisms, diagnosis and management of hepatic encephalopathy. Nat Rev Gastroenterol Hepatol. Sep;7(9):515-25.

[49] Riggio O, Ridola L, Pasquale C. Hepatic encephalopathy therapy: An overview. World J Gastrointest Pharmacol Ther. Apr 6;1(2):54-63.

[50] Ferenci P, Herneth A, Steindl P. Newer approaches to therapy of hepatic encephalopathy. Semin Liver Dis. 1996 Aug;16(3):329-38.

[51] Riggio O, Varriale M, Testore GP, Di Rosa R, Di Rosa E, Merli M, et al. Effect of lactitol and lactulose administration on the fecal flora in cirrhotic patients. J Clin Gastroenterol. 1990 Aug;12(4):433-6.

[52] Mortensen PB. The effect of oral-administered lactulose on colonic nitrogen metabolism and excretion. Hepatology. 1992 Dec;16(6):1350-6.

[53] Mortensen PB, Holtug K, Bonnen H, Clausen MR. The degradation of amino acids, proteins, and blood to short-chain fatty acids in colon is prevented by lactulose. Gastroenterology. 1990 Feb;98(2):353-60.

[54] Bajaj JS. Management options for minimal hepatic encephalopathy. Expert Rev Gastroenterol Hepatol. 2008 Dec;2(6):785-90.

[55] Sharma BC, Sharma P, Agrawal A, Sarin SK. Secondary prophylaxis of hepatic encephalopathy: an open-label randomized controlled trial of lactulose versus placebo. Gastroenterology. 2009 Sep;137(3):885-91, 91 e1.

[56] Blanc P, Daures JP, Rouillon JM, Peray P, Pierrugues R, Larrey D, et al. Lactitol or lactulose in the treatment of chronic hepatic encephalopathy: results of a meta-analysis. Hepatology. 1992 Feb;15(2):222-8.

[57] Camma C, Fiorello F, Tine F, Marchesini G, Fabbri A, Pagliaro L. Lactitol in treatment of chronic hepatic encephalopathy. A meta-analysis. Dig Dis Sci. 1993 May;38(5):916-22.

[58] Strauss E, Tramote R, Silva EP, Caly WR, Honain NZ, Maffei RA, et al. Double-blind randomized clinical trial comparing neomycin and placebo in the treatment of exogenous hepatic encephalopathy. Hepatogastroenterology. 1992 Dec;39(6):542-5.

[59] Jiang Q, Jiang XH, Zheng MH, Jiang LM, Chen YP, Wang L. Rifaximin versus nonabsorbable disaccharides in the management of hepatic encephalopathy: a meta-analysis. Eur J Gastroenterol Hepatol. 2008 Nov;20(11):1064-70.

[60] Bass NM, Mullen KD, Sanyal A, Poordad F, Neff G, Leevy CB, et al. Rifaximin treatment in hepatic encephalopathy. N Engl J Med. 2010 Mar 25;362(12):1071-81.

[61] Sidhu SS, Goyal O, Mishra BP, Sood A, Chhina RS, Soni RK. Rifaximin improves psychometric performance and health-related quality of life in patients with minimal hepatic encephalopathy (the RIME Trial). Am J Gastroenterol. 2011 Feb;106(2):307-16.

[62] Bajaj JS, Heuman DM, Wade JB, Gibson DP, Saeian K, Wegelin JA, et al. Rifaximin improves driving simulator performance in a randomized trial of patients with minimal hepatic encephalopathy. Gastroenterology. 2011 Feb;140(2):478-87 e1.

[63] Gentile S, Guarino G, Romano M, Alagia IA, Fierro M, Annunziata S, et al. A randomized controlled trial of acarbose in hepatic encephalopathy. Clin Gastroenterol Hepatol. 2005 Feb;3(2):184-91.

[64] Liu Q, Duan ZP, Ha DK, Bengmark S, Kurtovic J, Riordan SM. Synbiotic modulation of gut flora: effect on minimal hepatic encephalopathy in patients with cirrhosis. Hepatology. 2004 May;39(5):1441-9.

[65] Poo JL, Gongora J, Sanchez-Avila F, Aguilar-Castillo S, Garcia-Ramos G, Fernandez-Zertuche M, et al. Efficacy of oral L-ornithine-L-aspartate in cirrhotic patients with hyperammonemic hepatic encephalopathy. Results of a randomized, lactulose-controlled study. Ann Hepatol. 2006 Oct-Dec;5(4):281-8.

[66] Jalan R, Wright G, Davies NA, Hodges SJ. L-Ornithine phenylacetate (OP): a novel treatment for hyperammonemia and hepatic encephalopathy. Med Hypotheses. 2007;69(5):1064-9.

[67] Naylor CD, O'Rourke K, Detsky AS, Baker JP. Parenteral nutrition with branched-chain amino acids in hepatic encephalopathy. A meta-analysis. Gastroenterology. 1989 Oct;97(4):1033-42.

[68] Marchesini G, Dioguardi FS, Bianchi GP, Zoli M, Bellati G, Roffi L, et al. Long-term oral branched-chain amino acid treatment in chronic hepatic encephalopathy. A randomized double-blind casein-controlled trial. The Italian Multicenter Study Group. J Hepatol. 1990 Jul;11(1):92-101.

[69] Basile AS, Harrison PM, Hughes RD, Gu ZQ, Pannell L, McKinney A, et al. Relationship between plasma benzodiazepine receptor ligand concentrations and severity of hepatic encephalopathy. Hepatology. 1994 Jan;19(1):112-21.

[70] Basile AS, Hughes RD, Harrison PM, Murata Y, Pannell L, Jones EA, et al. Elevated brain concentrations of 1,4-benzodiazepines in fulminant hepatic failure. N Engl J Med. 1991 Aug 15;325(7):473-8.

[71] Goulenok C, Bernard B, Cadranel JF, Thabut D, Di Martino V, Opolon P, et al. Flumazenil vs. placebo in hepatic encephalopathy in patients with cirrhosis: a meta-analysis. Aliment Pharmacol Ther. 2002 Mar;16(3):361-72.

[72] Barbaro G, Di Lorenzo G, Soldini M, Giancaspro G, Bellomo G, Belloni G, et al. Flumazenil for hepatic encephalopathy grade III and IVa in patients with cirrhosis: an Italian multicenter double-blind, placebo-controlled, cross-over study. Hepatology. 1998 Aug;28(2):374-8.

[73] Gyr K, Meier R, Haussler J, Bouletreau P, Fleig WE, Gatta A, et al. Evaluation of the efficacy and safety of flumazenil in the treatment of portal systemic encephalopathy: a double blind, randomised, placebo controlled multicentre study. Gut. 1996 Aug;39(2):319-24.

[74] Vaquero J, Chung C, Cahill ME, Blei AT. Pathogenesis of hepatic encephalopathy in acute liver failure. Semin Liver Dis. 2003 Aug;23(3):259-69.

[75] Charlton M. Branched-chain amino acid enriched supplements as therapy for liver disease. J Nutr. 2006 Jan;136(1 Suppl):295S-8S.

[76] Plauth M, Cabre E, Riggio O, Assis-Camilo M, Pirlich M, Kondrup J, et al. ESPEN Guidelines on Enteral Nutrition: Liver disease. Clin Nutr. 2006 Apr;25(2):285-94.

[77] Amodio P, Caregaro L, Patteno E, Marcon M, Del Piccolo F, Gatta A. Vegetarian diets in hepatic encephalopathy: facts or fantasies? Dig Liver Dis. 2001 Aug-Sep;33(6):492-500.

[78] Bajaj JS, Schubert CM, Heuman DM, Wade JB, Gibson DP, Topaz A, et al. Persistence of cognitive impairment after resolution of overt hepatic encephalopathy. Gastroenterology. 2010 Jun;138(7):2332-40.

[79] Riggio O, Ridola L, Pasquale C, Nardelli S, Pentassuglio I, Moscucci F, et al. Evidence of persistent cognitive impairment after resolution of overt hepatic encephalopathy. Clin Gastroenterol Hepatol. 2011 Feb;9(2):181-3.

12

Adverse Reactions and Gastrointestinal Tract

A. Lorenzo Hernández[1], E. Ramirez[1]
and Jf. Sánchez Muñoz-Torrero[2]
[1]University Autonoma of Madrid
[2]University of Extremadura
Spain

1. Introduction

Adverse drug reactions are common and there is an increasing interest in recognizing them. There are several studies that try to identify epidemiology, true incidence in hospitalized and not hospitalized patients and the main concerns about their causes and possible solutions. Gastrointestinal tract, mainly haemorrhages and peptic disease are the most common site of adverse drug reactions; that´s the reason why we should recognize this problem and how to manage. Also we try to review the most common drugs affecting gastrointestinal tract. Less common and, usually less severe, liver disease and pancreatitis can be produced by adverse drug reactions. In this chapter we review theses aspects of adverse drug events, particularly, those related to drugs affecting gastrointestinal tract.

2. Definition of adverse drug reactions

An adverse drug event is an unwanted and unintended medical event related to the use of medications. An adverse drug event is considered an adverse drug reaction (ADR) when there is a causal link between the event and use of the drug. An adverse drug reaction is considered serious when the patients outcome is one of the following: death, life-threatening, hospitalization (initial or prolonged), disability –significant, persistent or permanent change, impairment, damage or disruption in the patient's body function/structure or physical activities or quality of life, congenital anomaly or require intervention to prevent permanent impairment or damage [Supplementary information in Appendix 1].

Causality assessment is necessary to determine the likehood that a drug caused a suspected ADR. There are a number of different methods used to judge causation, the first attempts were proposed by Karch and Lasagna (1977), Lecenthal et al. (1979) and Naranjo et a.l (1981). Most of these approaches to assigning causality are based on the following clinical features: temporal relationship between drug exposure and the onset of adverse drug event, characteristic symptoms and laboratory abnormalities and/or histology, and challenge-dechallenge-rechallenge (improvement after stopping the suspected drug and reappearance after starting the agent in question).

ADRs can be considered "on-target" effects, if they are result of exaggerated pharmacology that may be managed by dose reduction or other therapeutic modifications, i.e. hypoglycemia associated with antidiabetic agents. "Off-target" toxicities are frequently more problematic because they may not be predicted from pharmacology and toxicology studies, and they may occur only after prolonged exposure, i.e. hypersensibility reactions associated to antiepileptics. Unexpected ADRs that first appear after marketing authorization of the medication continue trouble clinicians, regulators, and drug sponsors. The most notably cause is the use by large number of patients, providing sufficient statistical power to detect rare events. Other factors include use in special populations, drug inte ractions, renal and hepatic insufficiency, long duration of use and drug withdrawal.

3. Epidemiology of adverse drug reactions

Adverse drug reactions (ADRs) are considered to be among the leading causes of morbidity and mortality. Around 5-25% of hospitals admissions are estimated to be due to ADRs and about 6-15% of hospitalized patients experience serious ADRs (SADRs) causing significant prolongation of hospital stay and projected that adverse drug events are the fourth to sixth leading cause of death in the United States. Most studies are focused on rates of serious and fatal events in hospitalized patients, probably because tracking of ADRs is more established in the inpatients setting. An English study (Kane-Gill, 2010) found an increase in hospitalizations caused by ADR in about 76.8% in ten years. A recent study of administrative health-care data found an annual ADR prevalence rate of 0.5% among ambulatory-care patients; however, the authors acknowledge this is probably an underestimate of true ADR rates. Ambulatory-care patients experiencing an ADR were younger on average than hospitalized patients.

Risk factors of suffering adverse drug events are: women, elderly and polipharmacy mainly. Women were more likely than men to have ADRs in both outpatients and inpatients settings. In the study from Zopf (2008), the OR of women from suffering ADR was 1.562; (95% CI 0.785, 2.013). Other risk factors implicated in adverse drug reactions are elderly, drug-drug interactions, polipharmacy and renal insufficiency. In the study of Sanchez Muñoz (2011), also drug-drug interactions were as important as age and renal insufficiency in producing adverse drug reactions.

Patients affected by adverse dug events are admitted in internal medicine department and geriatrics quite often, but patients hospitalized in Intensive care units and pediatrics also suffer from these problems.

4. Severity of adverse drug reactions – Fatal adverse drug reaction

It has been estimated than fatal ADRs are expected in approximately 0.32% of hospitalized patients, and complications from drug therapy are the most common adverse event in hospitalized patients. If true, then ADRs are the 4th leading cause of death—ahead of pulmonary disease, diabetes, AIDS, pneumonia, accidents, and automobile deaths. However, some studies show greater severity prevalence and fatality rate. In the hospital setting the study from Kaurr, (Kaurr,2011) observed grade severe of adverse reaction in 13.4% patients. In the study from Sánchez Muñoz-Torrero (2010) the reactions were severe in 17% and fatal in 1.6% of hospitalized patients.

These statistics do not include the number of ADRs that occur in ambulatory settings. The exact number of ADRs is not certain and is limited by methodological considerations. However, whatever the true number is, ADRs represent a significant public health problem. In a Sweden study there were reviewed the death reports in one year in relation with adverse drugs reactions. They found 3.1% of deaths associated with fatal adverse drug events, mostly haemorraghes. 89% of patients died at hospital meanwhile only 35% of patients dead at hospital with no relation with drug events.

So most of studies trying to establish epidemiology and cost of adverse drug reactions demonstrate that these events are harmful and we have to make great efforts to diminish the incidence and morbidity.

5. Cost of adverse drug reactions

In western countries, drug-related illnesses account 5% to 10% of inhospital costs, and being associated with a substantial increase in morbidity and mortality. In addition to their impact on human health, ADRs also have significant impact on healthcare costs. These costs are essentially hospital costs, in particular arising from an increase in length of stay caused by an ADR. Although has been estimated that the occurrence of an ADR during hospitalization or leading to hospitalization is responsible in U.S.A. (data from 1997) for a cost of approximately 2800 Euros in an additional length of stay of 2.2 days, several studies have also pointed out that the structure of ADR cost is heterogeneous, a factor which must be taken into account when developing preventive strategies. Although data of costs were not calculated, Sanchez Muñoz-Torrero et al (2010) study found an increase in hospital staying in almost 9 days (18±17 days vs 9.6±5.8, $p<0.001$), which accounts for more direct and indirect costs of the hospitalization. Also another Spanish (Carrasco Garrido et al, 2010) study found an increase in 19% of hospital costs associated with the appearance of adverse drug events.

6. Potential causes implicated in adverse drug reactions

Older patients are particularly vulnerable to drug-related illness because they are usually on multiple drug regimens, which expose them to the risk of drug interactions (Mallet et al, 2007), and because age is associated with changes in pharmacokinetics and pharmacodinamics (Aronson, 2007).

Onder et al. (2010) developed and validated a risk stratification model (The GerontoNet ADR Risk Score) to identify patients 65 years or older who are at risk for an ADR during hospitalization. They used data from the Italian Group of Pharmacoepidemiology in the Elderly to develop an ADR risk score. The ADR risk score was then validated in a sample of older adults who were admitted to 4 university hospitals in Europe. The number of drugs and history of an ADR were the strongest predictors of ADRs, followed by heart failure, liver disease, presence of 4 or more conditions, and renal failure (Table 1).

Recently Sánchez Muñoz-Torrero et al found that renal function and drug–drug interactions were statistically significant associated with the appearance of ADR. Also duration of hospitalization was associated but it wasn't possible to establish that if duration of hospitalization was the cause or the consequence of ADR. Recently Hamilton et al (2011) reviewed the adverse drug reactions in older people with potentially inappropriate prescriptions.

Variable	OR (95% CI)	Points
≥4 Comorbid conditions	1.31 (1.04-1.64)	1
Heart failure	1.79 (1.39-2.30)	1
Liver disease	1.36 (10.6-1.74)	1
No. of drugs		
≤5	1 [Reference]	0
5-7	1.90 (1.35-2.68)	1
≥8	4.07 (2.93-5.65)	4
Previous ADR	2.41 (1.79-3.23)	2
Renal failure	1.21 (0.96-1.51=	1

Abbreviations: ADR, adverse drug reactions; CI, confidence interval; OR, odd ratio.

Table 1. Variables included in the Score (adapted from Onder *et al*)

7. Main drugs implicated in reactions

Drug classes most frequently associated with ADRs in both inpatients and outpatient populations are non steroidal anti-inflamatory drugs (NSAIDs), diuretic, anticoagulants, antiobiotics and antineoplastic agents.

Antibiotic and vaccination reactions are more frequent in the 0 –to-9 year age group.

In adults and elderly people, there a great variety of drugs causing adverse drug reactions. However, it depends the type of hospitalization, the deparment, etc, the type of adverse reactions and drugs implicated are quite different. Pimohamed et al. (2004) found that aspirin was the casual agent in 18% of cases of all admission for ADRs, while other NSAIDs and diuretics were implicates in 12% and 27% respectively. The most common ADRs of NSAIDs were GI bleeding, peptic ulcerations, haemorrhagic cerebrovascular accident, renal impairment, wheezing and rash. Grenouillet-Delacre et al. (2007) found that psychotropic drugs, immunosuppressive drugs, anticoagulants and antibiotics were more than 50% of life-threatening adverse drug reactions at admission to medical intensive care. In Spain, antibiotic and anticoagulants are the drugs more frequently implicated in ADRs appeared during hospitalization but in another epidemiologic study (Carrasco Garrido, 2010) found that main drugs implicated in admission into the hospital were antineoplastics and immunosuppressive therapy. However there are very few studies that show antineoplastics and immunosuppressive therapies as the cause of adverse drug reactions although they are being increasingly used and promote the appearance of infections, medullar aplasia, etc. Also cardiovascular drugs, mainly diuretics and hypotensors drugs account for some common ADRs.

8. Drugs reactions affecting gastrointestinal tract

ADR that cause damage in gastrointestinal tract usually produce GI bleeding/peptic ulcerations, diarrhea (mainly associated to antibiotics), pancreatitis and liver toxicity. About 40% of ADR affect gastrointestinal and liver in hospitalized patients. As said before, gastrointestinal bleeding is the most frequent ADRs causing hospitalization or produced during hospitalization. In this issue, we try to review the ADRs affecting gastrointestinal tract.

8.1 GI bleeding

Mainly non steroidal anti-inflammatory drugs and antiplatelet/anticoagulants are implicated in gastrointestinal bleeding. The most frequent lesion is gastric erosions (about 40.2%), combination of gastric ulcer and gastric erosions (16.1%), gastric ulcer (15.0%), duodenal ulcer (13.8%), normal (13.8%) and duodenal erosions (1.1%). In a recent study 26% of patients admitted because of gastrointestinal bleeding had antiplatelet or anticoagulants as the cause of bleeding. The distribution of lesions was quite similar to the study from Devy, being gastric ulcer the most common lesion involved in the bleeding. Inhibition of cyclooxygenase, leading to inhibition of gastric prostaglandin synthesis, and impaired GI defense mechanisms represent additional mechanisms of drug-induced GI bleeding. In the particular setting of Intensive Care Units (ICUs) the most frequent lesion found in patients is the stress-related mucosal bleeding, in which another causes apart from drugs are implicated. In the study from Wikman-Jorgensen (2011) mortality of upper gastrointestinal bleeding was 3,5%, all in patients with great comorbidity which limited treatment of bleeding.

Drugs most frequently causing bleeding were aspirin in 36%, acenocumarol in 27%, clopidogrel in 18%. Combination of aspirin and clopidogrel are responsible of 6% of upper gastrointestinal bleeding. Aspirin is the drug more frequently implicated but it may chance in the future because of the increasing use of doble antiplatelet treatments and new anticoagulants (Rivaroxaban, Apixaban and Dabigatran). It is possible than in the near future we begin to see hemorrhages with dabigatran because of the recent approval in USA for the use of treatment in atrial fibrillation, including patients with low risk of thromboembolism. The risk of bleeding is bigger with Rivaroxaban as shown in the prophylaxis studies, but the approval for AF is pending.

Also lower gastrointestinal bleeding is increasing because of use of AINES mainly. New techniques for diagnosing lesions in small and large intestine are proving this increase in lower gastrointestinal bleeding. AINES can cause diverticulum perforation, mucosal inflammation, ulceration, causing bleeding in the intestine. Use of aspirin, clopidogrel or anticoagulants and the lower intestinal bleeding is an issue that has to be studied because of its frequency, use and potential harmful in small and large intestine. There's little information about its presentation and management.

8.2 Diarrhea

Diarrhoea may be defined by frequency or grams of loose grames per day: 3–5 times per day and/or loose stools 200–300 grams/day (250 mL/day).

It's estimated that diarrhoea accounts for the 7% of ADRs. There are lot of drugs producing diarrhea as a secondary effect: metformin, some chemotherapies, antibiotics, mainly clavulanic, clindamicin, immunosuppressant… Most of them cause diarrhea only while taking, or only at the beginning of prescription, but some are associated with chronic diarrhoea as metformin. However, the possibility of a drug causing a severe diarrhea is less common except in the case of antibiotics, hipomotility drugs, steroids, proton pump inhibitors because of the possibility of Clostridium difficile diarrhea.

Mechanisms of drugs producing diarrhoea are multiple: osmotic, secretory, motor, exudative, malabsorptive, infectious/inflammatory, and others. Examples of osmotic diarrhoea are enteral nutrition feeding, magnesium salts, etc. Examples of secretory diarrhoea (increase in intestinal ion secretion or diminution in intestinal ion absorption) are digoxin, quinidine, propafenone and theophiline. Examples or rapid intestinal transit are procinetic and macrolids. Exudative diarrhoea (changes in permeability and integrity of intestinal mucosa) are NSAIDs and antineoplastic. Drug-related malabsorption of fats, carbohydrates, and/or bile can also lead to diarrhea. Examples include octreotide (at high doses), highly active antiretroviral therapy, tetracycline, NSAIDs, and antineoplastic agents. Drug-induced infectious/inflammatory diarrhea includes microbial proliferation, pseudomembranous colitis, and histologic colitis. The risk of antibiotic associated diarrhea is higher with broad-spectrum agents (particularly those with antianaerobic activity and activity against Enterobacteriaceae), agents with high luminal concentrations (although oral/enteral administration is not necessarily a risk), longer duration of therapy, and use of multiple antibiotics.

8.3 Constipation and hypomotility

Anticholinergic drugs are responsible of constipation as well as other adverse reactions in patients, particularly elderly patients. Also opioids prescribed for cancer patients, chronic pain, etc are responsible of constipation which can produce paralitic ileum. In the setting of ICU patients hipomotility and constipation appears in 50-80 % of patients, particularly those with mechanically ventilated.

8.3.1 Hypomotility

Hypomotility is produced mainly abnormalities in propulsive motility, disturbances in esophageal and gastric motility, reduction in lower esophageal sphincter pressure. Exogenous cathecolamines can reduce antral contractions and small bowel peristalsis and alter motility patterns. Opioids inhibit neurotransmitters release and altering water and electrolyte absorption.

8.3.2 Constipation

Constipation is produced by changes in neuronal or motor function in the intestine. The most common cause is opioids. They inhibit the release of acetylcholine from the myenteric plexus and promote in the opioid receptors in the intestine a decreased motility and increase in intestinal fluid absorption. Other drugs implicated in constipation are antihistamines, calcium channel blockers, diuretics, tricyclic antidepressants.

8.4 Pancreatitis

Drug induced pancreatitis accounts for 0.1-2% of pancreatitis. Between 1968 and 1993 a total of 525 different drugs from many different substance classes have been reported to the WHO because they were suspected to induce pancreatitis as an unwanted side effect, The three drugs that are responsible of more cases of pancreatitis are mesalazine, azathioprine and simvastatine. Previously recognized patients with more risk of pancreatitis are pediatric and elderly patients, women, advanced HIV disease and inflammatory bowel disease. The interesant review from Balani (2008) showed a table with drugs commonly implicated in pancreatitis: ACE inhibitors, ARA-2, loop diuretics and thiazides, statins, bezafibrate, some antibiotics, pentamidine, azathioprine, mercaptopurine, aminosalicylates, anticonvulsivants and antipsychotics, estrogens, carbimazole, some antineoplastics, codeine, sulindac.

In critically ill patients there's also a review of drugs implicated in pancreatitis (Lat, 2010):

8.4.1 Drugs with a likely association

Drugs with a likely association: Asparaginase, azathioprine, cimetidine, corticosteriopids, corticotrophin, cytarabin, dapsone, didanosine, enalapril, estrogens, furosemide, isonizid, mercaptopurine, mesalamine, methyldope, metronidazole, omeprazol, opiates, pentamidine, pravastatin, salycilates, simvastatin, sulfasalizine, sulfamethoxazole/trimethoprim, sulindac, tetracycline, valproic acid.

8.4.2 Drugs with a potential or questionable association

Drugs with a potential or questionable association: acetaminophen, amiodarone, ampicilin, benzapril, carbamazepine, captopril, ceftriaxone, clarithromycin, cyclosporine, diphenoxylate, cisplatinerythromycin, fluvastatin, gemfibrozil, interferon, ribavirin, ketoprofen, lisinopril, ketoprofen, lisinopril, lovastatin, metformin, naproxen, thiazides, octerotide, penicillin, procainamide, propofol, propoxyphene, ramipril, ranitidine, rifampin.

8.5 Drug-Induced Liver Injury (DILI)

Hepatotoxicity and drug-induced liver injury (DILI) are terms used interchangeably. DILI can be defined as a liver injury induced by a drug or herbal medicines leading to liver test abnormalities or liver dysfunction with reasonable exclusion of other competing etiologies. Most cases of DILI are due to idiosyncratic or unexpected reactions. In contrast to paracetamol-induced hepatotoxicity, which occurs with dose-dependent overdose of the drug. Idiosyncratic drug reactions have been traditionally considered dose independent. However, drugs with well-documented idiosyncratic DILI have been shown to have a dose-dependent component. Idiosyncratic DILI, excluding injury caused by acetaminophen overdose, accounts for 7–15% of the cases of acute liver failure in Europe and the United States and is the most frequent reason for the withdrawal of an approved drug from the market. Estimates of the rate of incidence of DILI leading to hospital referral vary from 2.4 per 100,000 person-years (in a retrospective population-based study of 1.64 million UK subjects) to 13.9 per 100,000 inhabitants (in a prospective analysis in France). Complementary or alternative medicines are used by at least 20% of individuals in Western, Eastern, and African cultures, and reports of DILI have increased. Given its rarity, DILI may not be identified during clinical trials and may come to light only after the culprit drug has obtained market approval and large numbers of patients have been exposed. In addition, in preregistration clinical trials, mild asymptomatic liver injuries, often characterized by asymptomatic elevations in liver enzymes, are commonly seen. However, drugs capable of inducing severe DILI as well as drugs that have a low potential for causing severe injury (e.g., aspirin and heparin) can generate similar patterns of liver injury. It is therefore necessary to develop an approach that can distinguish drugs that are likely to cause severe DILI from drugs that are unlikely to do so.

RUCAM algorithm (Roussel Uclaf Causality Assessment Method) was the first algorithm developed specifically for DILI. After the meeting sponsored by the CIOMS (Paris, 1989), with the support of Russel Uclaf pharmaceutical company, the terminology and diagnosis criteria for causality assessment was proposed. The algorithm was validated using external cases with positive rechallenge (49 cases) and 28 controls (patients with acute liver damage not related to drugs) with available information before occurrence of re-exposure, with results of high sensitivity (86%), specificity (89%), positive predictive value (93%) and negative predictive value (78%) [Algorithm RUCAM are showed in Table 1 and 2 of Appendix 2].

International DILI Expert Working Group of clinicians and scientists reviewed current DILI terminology and diagnostic criteria so as to develop more uniform criteria that could be define and characterize the spectrum of clinician syndromes that constitute DILI. In Appendix 2 of supplementary information you will find threshold criteria for definition of a case as being DILI (Box 1), the pattern of liver injury (Box 2), severity (Box 3), causality assessment (Box 4), and chronicity (Box 5). Consensus was also reached on approaches to characterizing DILI in the setting of chronic liver diseases (Box 6), including autoimmune hepatitis (Box 7).

A very large number of different drugs have been associated with liver injury. There is a clear difference in the documentation or the evidence for hepatotoxicity associated with these drugs. Isoniazid, phenytoin, disulfiram, amoxicillin/clavulanate, halothane and chlopromazine are drugs with well characterized hepatotoxicity. More recently antibiotics (amoxicillin/clavunalate, erytromicin, flucloxacillin, trimethoprim-sulpha, nitrofurantoin, isoniazid and rifampicin), analgesics and NSAIDs (diclofenac, dextropropoxyphene, paracetamol, ibuprofen) probably the most common type of drugs associated with DILI. In hospitalized patients, antineoplasic agents seem to commonly lead to DILI and are probably underreported. In a Spanish pharmacovigilance prospective program based on laboratory signals at hospital all patients with liver test abnormalities (x 3 upper limits of normal) were evaluated being antibiotics (19.5%), hormonal contraceptives (14.6%) and anticancer agents (10%) were the most frequent drug-groups associated to liver injury. In out-patients, the single most common drug implicated in ine series was diclofenac. Among patients with acute liver failure resulting from drugs in the US who underwent liver transplantation, paracetamol (acetaminophen) was the most common causative drug, followed by isoniazid, propylthiouracil, phenytoin and valproate.. Herbal and dietary supplements are implicated in approximately 11% of patients who developed acute serious liver disease of unknown cause in Spain.

The expectrum of DILI is varied, acute liver injury with or without jaundice, chronic hepatitis, although rare, liver cirrhosis has been reported to occur with long-standing drug treatment suspected to have caused DILI, and approximately 25-30% of DILI present with symptom of immunoallergic drug reactions. Table 2 showed the most common types of liver injury that have been identified with drugs.

9. Drugs for gastrointestinal diseases and their implication in adverse reactions

Most of adverse reactions with drugs used for treating gastrointestinal diseases are proton pump inhibitors. New antiTNF drugs, steroids and immunosuppressant in general used for

Type	Drugs
Acute liver injury	Isoniazid, disulfiram, paracetamol
Chronic hepatitis	Phenytoin, isoniazid
Autoimmune hepatitis	Minocycline, nitrofurantoin
Granulomatous hepatitis	Carbamazepine, quinidine
Steatohepatitis	Amiodarone, valproate
Cholestatic hepatitis	Flucloxacillin, amoxicillin/clavulanate
Bland cholestasis	Estrogens, nimesulide
Ductopenia	Amoxicillin, Trimethoprim-sulpha
Fibrosis	Methotrexate
Nodular regenerative hyperplasia	Azathioprine, 6-thioguanine

Table 2. Types of DILI (adapted from Björnsson)

inflammatory bowel disease cause also adverse drug reactions but the extended use of IBP makes them responsible of most of the adverse reactions with gastrointestinal drugs: hypergastrinemia, hypomagnesemia, tumors and, recently, enteric infections, pneumonia and osteoporosis (Maffei, 2007). There is a controversy about the probability of some of theses adverse drug reactions with IBPs. In the recent review by Thomson (2010) they failed to found risk of carcinoid tumors, cancer or nosocomial pneumoniae. There still controversy about the risk of osteoporosis with the long term use of IBPs.

10. Strategies to diminish adverse drugs reactions

The main strategies for reducing adverse drug reactions are: drug interaction calculators, renal insufficiency calculators, prescribing programs and collaboration between pharmacists, pharmacologists and clinical physicians.

The world Health Organization defines pharmacovigilance as the science and activities related to the detection, assessment, understanding, and prevention of adverse affects or any other possible drug-related problem. The field has grown significantly in recent years as postapproval safety studies for new medication become increasingly required, encompassing retrospective analysis of heath-care claims databases, meta-analysis, patients registries, and prospective case-control studies.

Recognition, reporting and careful characterization of these troubling, often unexpected ADRs are vital to future prevention of these event because detection of patterns and common features of ADRs can enhance our understanding of new mechanism and risk factors. The expansion of electronic database capabilities in hospital and primare-care setting offers the promise of better safety-based detection and monitoring systems that can detect ADRs earlier and prevent ADRs in the future. Hospital informatics systems linking to electronic medical records and including patient genotype with medication ordering and dispensing will reduce medication errors and inappropriate prescribing while improving detection of ADRs. Also, the review of prescription by pharmacists can achieve a diminution in the appearance of adverse drug reactions.

It´s also important to recognize people specially susceptible to ADRs: elderly, women, polipharmacy, renal insufficiency and presence of drug-drug interactions. In this special population we have to be careful with prescription of new drugs and its dosing.

11. Conclusions

Adverse drug reactions is a very frequent problem that affects specially the gastrointestinal tract, being GI bleeding the most common adverse drug reaction causing hospital admission. Patients predisposed to suffer ADRs are elderly, women, renal insufficiency, polipharmacy and drug-drug interactions. Drugs used for treat gastrointestinal disease are quite sure but can b e implicated in ADRs as IBPs, imunosupre4ssants used for autoimmune hepatitis or inflammatory bowel disease. Recognition of this problem is increasing in frequency and new drugs can be responsible for new ADRs. Collaboration between clinician, pharmacists and pharmacology specialists is needed.

12. Appendix 1

ICH Guideline on E2D post-approval drug safety defined an adverse drug reaction (ADR) and a serious adverse drug reactions (SADR) as follows:

An adverse drug reaction, as established by regional regulations, guidance and practices, is concern noxious and unintended responses to a medicinal product. The phrase "responses to a medicinal product" means that a causal relationship between a medicinal product and an adverse event is at least a reasonable possibility (refer to the ICH E2A guideline). A reaction, in contrast to an event, is characterized by the fact that a causal relationship between the drug and the occurrence is suspected. For regulatory reporting purposes, if an event is spontaneously reported, even if the relationship is unknown or unstated, it meets the definition of an adverse drug reaction".

Serious adverse event /ADR. In accordance with ICH E2A guideline, a serious adverse event or reaction is any untoward medical occurrence that at any dose:

• Results in death
• is life-threatening (NOTE: The term "life-threatening" in the definition of "serious" refers to an event/reaction in which the patient was at risk of death at the time of the event/reaction; it does not refer to an event/reaction which hypothetically might have caused death if it were more severe),
• is a congenital anomaly/birth defect,
• is a medically important event or reaction.

Medical and scientific judgment should be exercised in deciding whether other situations should be considered serious, such as important medical events that might not be immediately life-threatening or result in death or hospitalization but might jeopardize the patient or might require intervention to prevent one of the other outcomes listed in the definition above. Examples of such events are intensive treatment in a emergency room or at home for allergic bronchospasm, blood dyscrasias or convulsions that do not result in hospitalization or development of drug dependency or drug abuse.

13. Appendix 2

Subject Information	
1. Temporal relationship of start of drug to ALT>2x ULN	Score
Initial treatment 5–90 days; subsequent treatment course: 1–15 days	2
Initial treatment <5 or >90 days; subsequent treatment course: >15 days	1
From cessation of drug: ≤15 days, or ≤15 days after subsequent treatment	1
Otherwise	0
2. After drug cessation- difference between peak ALT and upper limits normal	
Decreases >50% within 8 days	3
Decreases >50% within 30 days	2
No information or decrease >50% after >30 days, or inconclusive	0
Decrease <50% after 30 days or recurrent increase	-2
3. Risk factors	
No alcohol use	0
Alcohol use	1
Age ≤55 years	0
Age >55 years	1
4. Concomitant drug	
No concomitant drug administered	0
Concomitant drug with suggestive or compatible time of onset	-1
Concomitant known hepatotoxin with suggestive or compatible time of onset	-2
Concomitant drug with positive rechallenge or validated diagnostic test	-3
5. Nondrug causes: Six are primary: recent hepatitis A, B, or C, biliary obstruction, acute alcoholic hepatitis (AST > 2x ALT), recent hypotension	
Secondary group: Underlying other disease; possible CMV, EBV or HSV infection	
All primary and secondary causes reasonably ruled out:	2
All 6 primary causes ruled out	1
4 or 5 primary causes ruled out	0
< 4 primary causes ruled out (max. negative score for items 4 and 5: –4)	-2
Nondrug cause highly probable	-3
6. Previous information on hepatotoxicity of the drug in question	
Package insert or labelling mention	2
Published case reports but not in label	1
Reaction unknown	0
7. Rechallenge	
Positive (ALT doubles with drug in question alone)	3
Compatible (ALT doubles with same drugs as given before initial reaction) +1	1
Negative (Increase in ALT but <2x ULN, same conditions as when reaction occurred)	-2
Not done, or indeterminate result	0
Total (range of algebraic sum: –8 to +14)	
Score Interpretation: Highly probable >8; Probable 6–8; Possible 3–5; Unlikely 1–2; Excluded <0	

Table 1. RUCAM Hepatocellular Injury Scale

Subject Information	
1. Temporal relationship of start of drug to ALP>2x ULN	Score
Initial treatment 5–90 days; subsequent treatment course: 1–90 days	2
Initial treatment <5 or >90 days; subsequent treatment course: >90 days	1
From cessation of drug: ≤30 days, or ≤30 days after subsequent treatment	1
Otherwise	0
2. After drug cessation - difference between peak ALP or total bilirubin and ULN	
Decreases ≥50% within 180 days	2
Decreases <50% within 180 days	1
Persistence or increase or no information	0
If drug is continued – inconclusive	0
3. Risk factors	
No alcohol use	0
Alcohol use	1
Age ≤55 years	0
Age >55 years	1
4. Concomitant drug	
No concomitant drug administered	0
Concomitant drug with suggestive or compatible time of onset	-1
Concomitant known hepatotoxin with suggestive or compatible time of onset	-2
Concomitant drug with positive rechallenge or validated diagnostic test	-3
5. Nondrug causes: Six are primary: recent hepatitis A, B, or C, biliary obstruction, acute alcoholic hepatitis (AST > 2x ALT), recent hypotension	
Secondary group: Underlying other disease; possible CMV, EBV or HSV infection	
All primary and secondary causes reasonably ruled out:	2
All 6 primary causes ruled out	1
4 or 5 primary causes ruled out	0
< 4 primary causes ruled out (max. negative score for items 4 and 5: –4)	-2
Nondrug cause highly probable	-3
6. Previous information on hepatotoxicity of the drug in question	
Package insert or labelling mention	2
Published case reports but not in label	1
Reaction unknown	0
7. Rechallenge	
Positive (ALT doubles with drug in question alone)	3
Compatible (ALT doubles with same drugs as given before initial reaction) +1	1
Negative (Increase in ALT but <2x ULN, same conditions as when reaction occurred)	-2
Not done, or indeterminate result	0
Total (range of algebraic sum: –8 to +14)	
Score Interpretation: Highly probable >8; Probable 6–8; Possible 3–5; Unlikely 1–2; Excluded <0	

Table 2. RUCAM Cholestatic or Mixed Liver Injury Scale

Any one of the following:
• More than or equal to fivefold elevation above the upper limit of normal (ULN) for alanine aminotransferase (ALT)
• More than or equal to twofold elevation above the ULN for alkaline phosphatase (ALP) (particularly with accompanying elevations in concentrations of 5'-nucleotidase or γ-glutamyl transpeptidase in the absence of known bone pathology
driving the rise in ALP level)
• More than or equal to threefold elevation in ALT concentration and simultaneous elevation of bilirubin concentration exceeding 2× ULN
Level of evidence: 2b (exploratory/retrospective cohort studies)

Box 1. clinical chemistry criteria for drug-induced liver injury (DILI) (adapted from Aithal et al. 2011)

• Pattern of liver injury is based on earliest identified liver chemistry elevations that qualify as DILI (Box 1)
• Pattern of liver injury is defined using R value where R =(ALT/ULN)/(ALP/ULN). This will require estimation of alanine aminotransferase (ALT) (aspartate transaminase is used when ALT is unavailable) and alkaline phosphatase (ALP) from the same serum sample
• ALT activity = patient's ALT/upper limit of normal (ULN); ALP activity = patient's ALP/ULN; R = ALT activity/ALP activity
• Hepatocellular pattern of DILI = R ≥ 5
• Mixed pattern of DILI = R > 2 and < 5
• Cholestatic pattern of DILI = R ≤ 2
• Histological summary should be recorded separately (if liver biopsy has been performed). However, the liver biopsy interpretation will generally not replace the R value for purposes of classification
Level of evidence: 2b (retrospective cohort studies)

Box 2. criteria for classifying the clinical pattern of drug induced liver injury (DILI) (adapted from Aithal et al. 2011)

Category	Severity	Description
1	Mild	Elevated alanine aminotransferase/alkaline phosphatase (ALT/ALP) concentration reaching criteria for DILI* but bilirubin concentration <2× upper limit of normal (ULN)
2	Moderate	Elevated ALT/ALP concentration reaching criteria for DILI* and bilirubin concentration ≥2× ULN, or symptomatic hepatitis
3	Severe	Elevated ALT/ALP concentration reaching criteria for DILI*, bilirubin concentration ≥2× ULN, and one of the following: • International normalized ratio ≥1.5 • Ascites73 and/or encephalopathy, disease duration <26 weeks, and absence of underlying cirrhosis31 • Other organ failure considered to be due to DILI
4	Fatal or transplantation	Death or transplantation due to DILI

Box 3. DILI severity index (adapted from Aithal et al. 2011)

• The Roussel Uclaf Causality Assessment Method (RUCAM) scale should be used for causality assessment (Appendix 2)

• If more than one drug is suspected to be causing DILI, the RUCAM scale should be applied to each drug separately. If such assessments are not practical (e.g., antituberculosis medications), all the drugs involved may be implicated as a single entity.

• If more than one drug is rated "possible" or higher by RUCAM, evaluation should be sought by a specialist to rank the drugs by order of likelihood of causing DILI. This may be done on the basis of the signature pattern of DILI and a review of the literature.

Level of evidence: 1b (validating cohort studies)

Box 4. DILI causality assessment (adapted from Aithal et al. 2011)

• Initial clinical episode met the criteria to qualify as acute DILI (Box 1)

• Initial episode on causality assessment has been considered possible, probable, or highly probable DILI on the basis of Roussel Uclaf Causality Assessment Method scoring criteria (Appendix 2).

Persistent DILI is defined as evidence of continued liver injury after withdrawal of the causative agent, beyond 3 months of follow-up for hepatocellular and mixed DILI, and beyond 6 months for cholestatic DILI

• Chronic DILI is defined as evidence of continued liver injury after withdrawal of the causative agent beyond 12 months of follow-up, regardless of the classification of DILI

• There is no new risk factor other than exposure to the suspect drug that would explain the persistence of liver injury, and other causes of chronic liver diseases have been excluded

Level of evidence: 4 (prognostic cohort studies of modest quality)

Box 5. Characteristics of persistent and chronic druginduced liver injury (DILI) (adapted from Aithal et al. 2011)

• Evidence of chronic liver disease is established on the basis of validated methods such as clinical evidence of cirrhosis, histological evidence of chronic liver disease, and imaging in cases of vascular disorder and tumours, as appropriate

• Evidence of drug intake for an appropriate duration preceding the appearance of symptoms, signs, or test results suggestive of chronic liver disease

• Exclusion of other etiologies of chronic disease (outlined in Supplementary Appendix 2, table S3)

Level of evidence: 1b (prospective/validating cohort studies with good follow-up)

Box 6. characteristics of drug-associated chronic liver disease (adapted from Aithal et al. 2011)

• The score is ≥6 points on simplified diagnostic criteria for AIH (scores >6 points with the simplified criteria can be obtained if liver biopsy is performed. Hennes *et al.*()consider a probable diagnostic score to be ≥6)

• Injury resolves on withdrawal of medication that triggered the AIH, with or without immunosuppressive therapy to induce remission

• No relapse within a period of 1 year after withdrawal of all immunosuppressants. This criterion needs further confirmation and cannot be considered pathognomonic because it is quite variable depending on the cohorts analyzed

Level of evidence: 2b (exploratory cohort study)

Box 7. Characteristics of drug-induced autoimmune hepatitis (AIH) (adapted from Aithal et al. 2011)

14. References

Aithal GP, Day CP. Hepatic adverse drug reactions. En: Pharmacovigilance. Chichester: John Wiley & Sons Ltd; p. 429-43 (2006.).

Aithal, G.P., Watkins P.B., Andrade, R.J., Larrey, D., Molokhia, M., Takikawa, H., Hunt, C.M., Wilke, R.A:, Avigan, M., Kaplowitz, N., Bjornsson, E. and Daly, A.K. Case definition and phenotype Standardization in Drug-induced Liver Injury. Clin Pharmacol Ther.89(6): 806-815.

Aronson, J.K. Adverse drug reactions – no farewell to harms. Br J Clin Pharmacol. ;63(2):131-135 (2007).

Balani AR, Grendell JH.Drug Saf. 2008;31(10):823-37.Drug-induced pancreatitis : incidence, management and prevention.

Bates, D.W., Spell, N., Cullen, D.J., Birdick, E., Laird, N., Petersen, L.A., Small, S.D., Boddie, J., Sweitzer, B.J., Leape, L.L. The cost of adverse drug events in hospitalized patients. JAMA. 277(4): 307-311 (2007).

Benichou C, Danan G, Flahault A. Causality assessment of adverse reactions to drugs--II. An original model for validation of drug causality assessment methods: case reports with positive rechallenge. J Clin Epidemiol. 1993 Nov;46(11):1331-1336

Beppu K, Osada T, Shibuya T, Watanabe SPathogenic mechanism of NSAIDs-induced mucosal injury in lower gastrointestinal tract. Nihon Rinsho. 2011 Jun;69(6):1083-7

Björnsson, E., Jerlstad, P., Bergqvist, A. & Olsson, R. Fulminant drug-induced hepatic failure leading to death or liver transplantation in Sweden. Scand. J. Gastroenterol. 40, 1095-1101 (2005).

Björnsson E. Review article: drug-induced liver injury in clinical practice. Aliment Pharmacol ther; 32: 3-12 (2010)

Budnitz, D.S., Pollock, D.A., Weidenbach, K.N., Mendelsohn, A.B., Schoeder, T.J., Annest, J.L. National surveillance of emergency department visits for outpatient adverse drug events. JAMA. 296 (15), 1858-1866 (2006).

Carrasco-Garrido P*, López de Andrés A, Hernández Barrera V, Gil de Miguel A, Jiménez García R. Trends of adverse drug reactions related hospitalizations in Spain (2001-2006). BMC Health Services Research 2010, 10:287.
http://www.biomedcentral.com/1472-6963/10/287

Cecile M, Seux V, Pauly V, Tassy S, Reynaud-Levy O, Dalco O, Thirion X, Soubeyrand J, Retornaz F. Adverse drug events in hospitalized elderly patients in a geriatric medicine unit: study of prevalence and risk factors. Rev Med Interne. 2009 May;30(5):393-400.

Cheng, C.M. Hospital systems for detection and prevention of adverse drug events. Clin Pharmacol Ther. 89: 779-781 (2011)

Clark K, Byfieldt N, Dawe M, Currow DC. Treating Constipation in Palliative Care: The Impact of Other Factors Aside From Opioids. Am J Hosp Palliat Care. 2011 May 23.

Classen, D.C., Pestotnik, S.L., Evans, R.S., Loyds, J.F., Burke, J.P. Adverse drug events in hospitalized patients. Excess length of stay, extra cost, and attributable mortality. JAMA. 277 (4),301-6 (1997).

Classen, D.C., Pestonik, S.L., Evans, R.S., Burke, J.P. Computerized surveillance of adverse drug event in hospital patients. Qua.l Saf. Health Care. 14, 221-226 (2005).

Danan G, Benichou C. Causality assessment of adverse reactions to drugs--I. A novel method based on the conclusions of international consensus meetings: application to drug-induced liver injuries. J Clin Epidemiol. 1993 Nov;46(11):1323-1330.

de Abajo, F.j., Montero, D., Madurga, M. & García Rodríguez, L.A. Acute and clinically relevant drug-induced liver injury: a population based case-control study. Br. J. Clin. Pharmacol. 58, 71–80 (2004).

De Valle MB, Av Klinteberg V, Alem N, Olsson R, Björnsson E. Drug-induced liver injury in a Swedish University hospital out-patient hepatology clinic. Aliment Pharmacol Ther 2006; 24: 1187-95

Devi DP, Sushma M, Guido S. Drug-induced upper gastrointestinal disorders requiring hospitalization: a five-year study in a South Indian hospital. Pharmacoepidemiol Drug Saf. 2004 Dec;13(12):859-62

Devlin JW, Mallow-Corbett S, Riker RR. Adverse drug events associated with the use of analgesics, sedatives, and antipsychotics in the intensive care unit. Crit Care Med. 2010 Jun;38(6 Suppl):S231-43.

Fontana RJ, Watkins PB, Bonkowsky HL, Chalasani N, Davern T, Serrano J, Rochon J; DILIN Study Group Drug-induced Liver Injury Network (DILIN) prospective study: rationale, design and condunt. Drug Saf; 32: 55-68 (2009)

Frazier, T.H. & Krueger, K.j. Hepatotoxic herbs: will injury mechanisms guide treatment strategies? Curr. Gastroenterol. Rep. 11, 317–324 (2009).

Gautier, S., Bachelet, H., Bordet, R., Caron, J. The cost of adverse drug reactions. Expert Opinion on Pharmacotherapy. 4(3): 319-326 (2003)

Gurwitz, J.H., Field, T.S., Harold, L.R., Rothschild, J., Debellis, K., Seger, A.C., Cadoret, C., Fish, L.S., Garber, L., Kelleher, M., Bates, D.W. Incidence and preventability of adverse drug events among elder persons in the ambulatory setting. JAMA. 289 (9), 1107–1116 (2003).

Grenouillet-Delacre, M., Verdoux, H., Moore, N., Haramburu, F., Miremont-Salamé, G., Etienne, G., Robinson, P., Gruson, D., Hilbert, G., Gabinski, C., Bégaud, B., Molimard, M. Life-threatening adverse drug reactions at admission to medical intensive care: a prospective study in a teaching hospital. Intensive Care Med. Dec;33(12):2150-7 (2007).

Hamilton H, Gallagher P, Ryan C, Byrne S, O'Mahony D. Potentially inappropriate medications defined by STOPP criteria and the risk of adverse drug events in older hospitalized patients.Arch Intern Med. 2011 Jun 13;171(11):1013-9.

Ibanez L, Perez E, Vidal X, Laporte JR. Prospective surveillance of acute serious liver disease unrelated to infectious, obstructive, or metabolic diseases: epidemiological and clinical features, and exposure to drugs. J Hepatol ; 37: 592–600 (2002)

ICH Guideline on E2D Postapproval Safety Data Management: Definitions and Standards for Expedited Reporting. London, 20 November 2003 CPMP/ICH/3945/03.

ICH Guideline on E2A Clinical Safety data Management: definitions and Standards for expedited Reporting E2A. Current Step 4 version, dated 27 October 1994 (CPMP/ICH/377/95)

Johnson, J.A., Bootman, J.L. Drug-related morbidity and mortality; a cost of illness model. Arch. Intern. Med. 155, 1949-56 (1995).

Kane-Gill, S.L., Van Den Bos, J. & Handler, S.M. Adverse drug reactions in hospital and ambulatory are setting identified using a large administrative database. Ann. Pharmacother. 44, 983-993 (2010).

Karch, F.E., Lasagna, L. Toward the operational identification of adverse drug reactions. Clin. Pharmacol. Ther. Mar;21(3):247-254 (1977).

Kaur S, Vinod Kapoor,[1] Rajiv Mahajan,[1] Mohan Lal,[2] and Seema Gupta. Monitoring of incidence, severity, and causality of adverse drug reactions in hospitalized patients with cardiovascular disease. Indian J Pharmacol. 2011 February; 43(1): 22–26.

Kongkaew C, Noyce PR, Ashcroft DM. Hospital admissions associated with adverse drug reactions: a systematic rview of prospectgive observational studies. Ann Pharmacother. 2008 Jul;42(7):1017-25.[1]

Kunac DL, Kennedy J, Austin N, Reith D. Incidence, preventability, and impact of Adverse Drug Events (ADEs) and potential ADEs in hospitalized children in New Zealand: a prospective observational cohort study. Paediatr Drugs. 2009;11(2):153-60.

Kurahara K, Matsumoto T, Iida M.. Characteristics of nonsteroidal anti-inflammatory drugs-induced colopathy Nihon Rinsho. 2011 Jun;69(6):1098-103.

Kutty P, Woods CW, Arlene C. Sena, Stephen R. Benoit, Susanna Naggie,,Joyce Frederick, Sharon Evans, Jeffery Engel, and L. Clifford McDonald. Risk Factors for and Estimated Incidence of Community-associated Clostridium diffi cile Infection, North Carolina, USA1Emerging Infectious Diseases • www.cdc.gov/eid • Vol. 16, No. 2, February 2010

Lancashire RJ, Cheng K, Langman MJ. Discrepancies between population-based data and adverse reaction reports in assessing drugs as causes of acute pancreatitis. Aliment Pharmacol Ther 2003 Apr 1;17(7):887–93.

Lammert C, Einarsson S, Saha C, Niklasson A, Bjornsson E, Chalasani N. Relationship between daily dose of oral medications and idiosyncrativ drug-induced liver injury: sear for signals. Hepatology 2008; 47: 2003-9

Larrey D. Epidemiology and individual susceptibility to adverse drug reactions affecting the liver. Semin Liver Dis; 22: 145–55 (2002).

Lat I, Foster DR, Erstad B. Drug-induced acute liver failure and gastrointestinal complications.Crit Care Med. 2010 Jun;38(6 Suppl):S175-87

Lazarou, J., Pomeranz, B.H., Corey, P.N. Incidence of adverse drug reactions in hospitalized patients: a meta-analysis of prospective studies. JAMA. 279 (15), 1200-5 (1998).

Leape, L.L., Brennan, T.A., Laird, N., Lawthers, A.G., Localio, A.R., Barnes, B.A., Hebert, L., Newhouse, J.P., Weiler, P.C., Hiatt, H. The nature of adverse events in hospitalized patients: results of the Harvard Medical Practice Study II. NEJM. 324 (6), 377-84 (1991).

Leung FW, Rao SS. Approach to fecal incontinence and constipation in older hospitalized patients. Hosp Pract (Minneap). 2011 Feb;39(1):97-104.

Leventhal, J.M., Hutchinson, T.A., Kramer, M.S., Feinstein, A.R. An algorithm for the operational assessment of adverse drug reactions. III. Results of tests among clinicians. JAMA. Nov 2;242(18):1991-1994 (1979).

Maffei M, Desmeules J, Cereda JM, Hadengue A. Side effects of proton pump inhbitors (PPIs). Rev Med Suiss 2007; 5(3): 1934-36, 1938.

Mallet, L, Spinewine, A, Huang, A. The challenge of managing drug interactions in elderly people. Lancet. 370(9582):185-191 (2007).

Mannesse, C.K., Derkx, F.H., de Ridder, M.A., Man in 't Veld, A.J., van der Cammen, T.J. Contribution of adverse drug reactions to hospital admission of older patients. Age Ageing. 29(1):35-39 (2000).

Meier Y, Cavallaro M, Roos M, et al. Incidence of drug-induced liver injury in medical inpatients. Eur J Clin Pharmacol; 61: 135–43 (2005).

Mino-León D, Galván-Plata ME, Doubova SV, Flores-Hernandez S, Reyes-Morales H. A pharmacoepidemiological study of potential drug interactions and their determinant factors in hospitalized patients. Rev Invest Clin. 2011 Mar-Apr;63(2):170-8.

Naranjo, C.A., Busto, U., Sellers, E.M., Sandor, P., Ruiz, I., Roberts, E.A., et al. A method for estimating the probability of adverse drug reactions. Clin. Pharmacol. Ther. Ago;30(2):239-245 (1981).

Nitsche CJ, Jamieson N, Lerch MM, Mayerle JV. Drug induced pancreatitis. Best Practice & Research Clinical Gastroenterology 24 (2010) 143–155

O'Grady, j.G. Acute liver failure. Postgrad. Med. J. 81, 148–154 (2005).

Onder, G., Petrovic, M., Tangíísuram, B., Meinardi, M.C., Markito-Notenboom W.P., Somers, S., Rajkumar, C., Bernabei, R., van der Cammen T.J.M. Development and Validation of a Score to Assess Risk of Adverse Drug Reactions Among In-Hospital Patients 65 years or older. Arch. Intern. Med. 170(13): 1142-1148 (2010).

Ostapowicz, G. et al. Results of a prospective study of acute liver failure at 17 tertiary care centers in the United States. Ann. Intern. Med. 137, 947–954 (2002).

Ouwerkerk J, Boers-Doets COuwerkerk J, Boers-Doets C. Best practices in the management of toxicities related to anti-EGFR agents for metastatic colorectal cancer. Eur J Oncol Nurs. 2010 Sep;14(4):337-49

Pirmohamed M, James S, Meakin S, Green C, Scott AK, Walley TJ, Farrar K, Park BK & Breckenridge AM. Adverse drug reactions as a cause of admission to hospital: prospective analysis of 18 820 patients. BMJ. 329,15-9 (2004).

Ramachandran, R. & Kakar, S. Histological patterns in drug-induced liver disease. J. Clin. Pathol. 62, 481–492 (2009).

Ramirez E, Carcas AJ, Borobia AM, Lei SH, Piñana, E, Fudio S & Frias J A Pharmacovigilance Program From Laboratory Signals for the Detection and Reporting of Serious Adverse Drug Reactions in Hospitalizad Patients. Clin Pharmacol Ther. 87 (1): 74-86.

Russo MW, Galanko jA, Shrestha R, Fried MW & Watkins P. Liver transplantation for acute liver failure from drug induced liver injury in the United States. Liver Transpl. 10, 1018–1023 (2004).

Sánchez Muñoz-Torrero JF, Barquilla P, Velasco R, Fernández Capitán MC, Pacheco N, Vicente L, & all. Adverse drug reactions in internal medicine units and associated risk factors. Eur J Clin Pharmacol (2010) 66:1257–1264

Sgro, C. et al. Incidence of drug-induced hepatic injuries: a French populationbased study. Hepatology 36, 451–455 (2002).

Tai-Yin Wu, Min-Hua Jen, Alex Bottle, Mariam Molokhia, Paul Aylin, Derek Bell, Azeem Majeed. Ten-year trends in hospital admissions for adverse drug reactions in England 1999–2009 J R Soc Med 2010: 103: 239–250. DOI 10.1258/jrsm.2010.100113

Watkins, P.B., Seligman, P.j., Pears, j.S., Avigan, M.I. & Senior, j.R. Using controlled clinical trials to learn more about acute drug-induced liver injury. Hepatology 48, 1680–1689 (2008).

Wawruch M, Macugova A, Kostkova L, Luha J, Dukat A, Murin J, Drobna V, Wilton L, Kuzelova M The use of medications with anticholinergic properties and risk factors for their use in hospitalised elderly patients. Pharmacoepidemiol Drug Saf. 2011 Jun 13. doi: 10.1002/pds.2169.

Wester K, Jönsson A, Spigset O, Druid H, Hägg S. Incidence of fatal adverse drug reactions: a population based study. Br J Clin Pharmacology 2008 / 65:4 / 573–579

White, R.A., Xu, H., Denny, J.C., Roden , D.M., Krauss, R.M., McCarty, C.A., Davis, R.L., Skaar, T., Lamba, J., Savoga, G. The emerging role of electronic medical records in pharmacogenomics. Clin. Pharmmacol. Ther. 89, 379-386 (2011)

Wikman-Jorgensen, López-Calleja E, Safont-Gasó P, Matarranz-del-Amo M, Andrés Navarro R & Merino-Sánchez J. Antiagregation and anticoagulation, relationship with upper gastrointestinal bleeding. Rev Esp Enferm Dig 2011; 103: 360-365.

Zopf Y, Rabe C, Neubert A, Hahn EG, Dormann H. Risk factors associated with adverse drug reactions following hospital admission: a prospective analysis of 907 patients in two German university hospitals. Drug Saf. 2008;31(9):789-98.

13

Recontructive Biliary Surgery in the Treatment of Iatrogenic Bile Duct Injuries

Beata Jabłońska and Paweł Lampe
Medical University of Silesia in Katowice,
Department of Digestive Tract Surgery
Poland

1. Introduction

The aim of this chapter is to present different types of biliary reconstructions used in the surgical treatment of iatrogenic bile duct injuries (IBDI).

IBDI remain an important problem in gastrointestinal surgery. The most frequently, they are caused by laparoscopic cholecystectomy which is one of the commonest surgical procedure in the world. The early and proper diagnostics of IBDI is very important for surgeons and gastroenterologists, because unrecognized IBDI lead to serious complications such as biliary cirrhosis, hepatic failure and death. Choice of the proper treatment of IBDI is very important, because it may avoid these serious complications and improve quality of life in patients. Non-invasive, percutaneous radiological and endoscopic techniques are recommended as initial treatment of IBDI. When endoscopic treatment is not effective, surgical management is considered. The goal of surgical treatment is to reconstruct the proper bile flow to the alimentary tract. In order to achieve this goal, many techniques are used. There are contradictory reports on the effectiveness of bile duct reconstruction methods in the literature.

2. Historical perspectives of reconstructive biliary surgery

The first descriptions of the anatomy of the liver and bile ducts originate 2000 years BC in Babylon. The presence of gallbladder stones were found in mummy priestess who lived in the eleventh century BC. Historical records derived from ancient Mesopotamia, Greece, Egypt and Rome, also demonstrate the presence of biliary tract diseases in those days. The first surgical procedures within the bile ducts were simple and uncomplicated. In 1618, Fabricus removed gallstones from the gallbladder. In 1867, Bobbs performed cholecystostomy. Cholecystostomy procedures were also performed by: Sims in 1878, Kocher in 1878 and Tait in 1879. The first planned cholecystectomy, performed on July 15, 1882, by the Berlin surgeon Langenbuch (1846-1901), was a breakthrough in the development of biliary surgery. In 1890, Couvoissier the performed the first choledochotomy. Development of operations performed on the bile ducts caused the the problem of iatrogenic bile duct injuries. In 1891, Sprengel, first described the case of bile duct injury. With the rise of this problem, the first reports of surgical reconstruction of the injuried bile ducts have appeared. In 1892, Doyen, as first, described the biliary ductal end-to-end anastomosis. The idea of biliary-alimentary anastomoses appeared as early as the nineteenth century. Cholecystoenterostomy (anastomosis between the gallbladder and colon), made by Winiwater in 1881, was the he first recorded biliary-alimentary anastomosis. In 1905, Mayo made the first biliary reconstruction as the end-to-side anastomosis between the common bile duct anastomosis (CBD) and the duodenum called choledochoduodenostomy. In 1908, Monprofit described biliary-alimentary anastomosis with a loop of small intestine Roux-Y as a way to repair the biliary tract. In 1909, Dahl reported a similar case. In 1944, Manteuffel performed hepaticojejunostomy conncting intrahepatic biliary ducts with a small intestine. In 1948, Cole attempted to produce mucosal-intestinal anastomosis by moving a segment of small intestine mucosa by incision the proximal hepatic duct. However, in this method, the mucosal fragment had not got sufficient blood supply. This technique was modified in 1969 by Smith, who described it as a mucosal graft. In 1964, Gilbert and in 1969, Grassi used in the insertion of the small intestine pedunculated on biliary vessels in the biliary reconstruction. The role of the Berlin surgeon Kehr (1862-1916), as the creator of the most widely used today T biliary drain, should be also emphasized. The French surgeons, Couinaud in 1954 and in 1956, Hepp and Couinaud, described the hepatic hilum of the liver and long extrahepatic left hepatic duct, using it to perform a wide biliary-alimentary anastomosis, after the dissection of tissue within the hilum the liver to perform, in cases of intrahepatic bile duct injuries. In 1948, Longmire and Sanford also described a technique of isolating the left hepatic duct to use it for a biliary-intestinal anastomosis, consisting of partial resection of the left lobe of the liver. In 1957, this technique has been modified and used by Soupault and Couinaud to isolate the hepatic segment of the third hepatic segment in order to perform the biliary-intestinal anastomosis in the case of atypical sectoral biliary system. In 1994, Blumgart described the technique of the hilar and intrahepatic biliary-enteric anastomosis. In 1965, Thomford and Hallenbeck described the modification of an animal model of biliary-enteric anastomosis using Roux-Y loop, consisting of the jejunostomy (intestinal loop sutured into the abdominal shell) which allowed postoperative endoscopic control and dilatation of the anastomosis. In 1984, Hutson described the application of this technique in patients with postoperative stenosis within the biliary anastomosis. This method of reconstruction has not been widely accepted and incorporated into the standard surgical treatment of iatrogenic bile duct injuries (IBDI). In Poland, the modified biliary-enteric anastomosis with using Roux-Y loop sutured into the hole in the layer of musculo-fascial, was first described in 1997 by Jędrzejczyk et al. [8]. The increase in the IBDI incidence has been reported in the early 90's, which was connected with the introduction of laparoscopic cholecystectomy. The first laparoscopic cholecystectomy was performed in 1986 by Muhe.

3. Pathogenesis of bile duct injuries

Iatrogenic bile duct injury account for about 95% of all benign biliary strictures (BBS). "Benign biliary strictures" is a broad concept encompassing not only strictures caused by injuries, but also as a result of other causal factors [1, 11 12]. Causes of BBS can be divided into several groups and they are summarized in table 1.

There are two basic groups of surgical procedures, which may lead to IBDI. The first group are the operations performed on the bile ducts: an open cholecystectomy (OC) and

Congenital strictures: Biliary atresia and congenital cysts
Bile duct injuries:
Iatrogenic: postoperative, following endoscopic and percutaneous procedures
Following blunt or penetrating trauma of the abdomen
Inflammatory strictures:
Cholelithiasis and choledocholithiasis
Mirizzi's syndrome
Chronic pancretitis
Chronic ulcer or diverticulum of duodenum
Abscess or inflammation of liver or subhepatic region
Parasitic, viral infection
Toxic drugs
Recurrent pyogenic cholangitis
Primary sclerosing cholangitis
Radiation-induced strictures
Papillary stenosis

Table 1. Main causes of benign biliary strictures.

laparoscopic cholecystectomy (LC), choledochotomy, and previous biliary reconstruction. The second group includes the operations performed on other abdominal organs, such as gastric resection (Bilroth II partial resection), liver resection, liver transplantation, pancreatic resection (pancreatoduodenectomy, extended distal pancreatic resection and pancreatic cyst drainage), biliary-enteric and porto-caval anastomoses, and lymphadenectomy or other procedures within the hepatoduodenal ligament.Cholecystectomy is the most common cause of IBDI. Injuries caused during cholecystectomy represent 92.5% of IBDI.

Data regarding the exact prevalence of IBDI after OC and laparoscopic LC vary depending on the literature source. However, according to most authors IBDI occur 2-4 times more likely after laparoscopic cholecystectomy than after open cholecystectomy. IBDI number has increased in recent years, twice in connection with the introduction of laparoscopic cholecystectomy. Table 2 summarizes IBDI incidence following OC and LC.

Author	IBDI incidence following OC	IBDI incidence following LC
Mc Mahon 1995	0.2%	0.81%
Strasberg 1995	0.7%	0.5%
Shea 1996	0.19-0.29%	0.36-0.47%
Targarona 1998	0.6%	0.95%
Lillemoe 2000	0.3%	0.4-0.6%
Gazzaniga 2001	0.0-0.5%	0.07-0.95%
Savar 2004	0.18%	0.21%
Moore 2004	0.2%	0.4%
Misra 2004	0.1-0.3%	0.4-0.6%
Gentileschi 2004	0.0-0.7%	0.1-1.1%
Kaman 2006	0.3%	0.6%

BDI iatrogenic bile duct injuries; OC open cholecystectomy; LC laparoscopic cholecystectomy.

Table 2. Incidence of IBDI following cholecystectomy.

There are many factors that increase the IBDI risk during surgery. Coexisting chronic or exacerbated inflammation of the operated area, obese patient, the presence of abundant adipose tissue around the hepatoduodenal ligament, not sufficiently broad insight into the operative field, and bleeding increases the difficulty of surgery and promote bile duct injuries. The conditions in which laparoscopic cholecystectomy is performed, also affect the rate of IBDI formation. Adverse factors include older age, male gender and long duration of symptoms prior to surgery. Biliary anomalies and variability of the arteries are also the factors associated with increased IBDI risk. Unusually reputed hepatic duct may be mistakenly regarded as the cystic duct and ligated or cut. Excessive, more than is necessary, dissection around the hepatoduodenal ligament during cholecystectomy may lead to damage to the axial arteries running along the CBD. Vascular damage is the cause of postoperative biliary strictures due to ischemia . According to the literature, during the distal bile duct injury the axial artery damage usually occurs (incidence 10-15% of cases), while during high biliary injuries of the proximal bile duct damage to the branches of the proper hepatic artery occurs (incidence 40-60% of cases).

4. Clinical presentation of iatrogenic bile duct injuries

The most frequently observed clinical symptoms include jaundice, fever, chills, abdominal pain, pruritus. Clinical symptoms can be divided into two main groups. The first group are patients with the bile leakage in the early postoperative period due to the bile duct injury. In the presence of a drain in the peritoneal cavity, the injury indicates the appearance of bile in the drain. In patients without a catheter in the peritoneal cavity, bile leak into the abdominal cavity, leading to biloma or bile peritonitis. In these patients, jaundice is not observed because there is no cholestasis. In the second group of patients, usually in a remote time after surgery, there are primarily clinical symptoms resulting from cholestasis due to biliary obstruction. This is most commonly jaundice,

5. Diagnosis of iatrogenic bile duct injuries

5.1 Laboratory diagnosis

Laboratory tests and imaging are used in IBDI diagnostics. In the laboratory tests, cholestasis and liver function indicators, such as bilirubin, alkaline phosphatase (FA), gamma-glutamyl-transpeptidase (GGT), alanine transaminase (ALT) and aspartate transaminase (AST), are the most useful. In patients with biliary stenosis cholestasis parameters are increased: serum bilirubin, FA, GGT and 5'-nucleotidase and leucine aminoptidase (LAP) (less marked in the laboratory), and transaminase values usually remain normal (the liver is not damaged). Elevated transaminase levels indicate damage to liver parenchyma and the development of secondary biliary cirrhosis hypoalbuminemia and prolonged prothrombin time occur due to damaged liver synthetic function.

5.2 Radiological diagnosis

In IBDI diagnostics, imaging ultrasound (USG), abdominal computed tomography (CT) scan of the abdominal cavity, percutaneous cholangiography, endoscopic cholangiography and magnetic resonance imaging are performed. Abdominal ultrasound allows the visualization of intra-and extrahepatic bile ducts with the measurement of width and visibility of the biloma within the peritoneal cavity in the case of bile leakage. In doubtful cases, you can perform abdominal CT to accurately depict the reservoir of bile. Accurate assessment of biliary tree can be made using cholangiography. Percutaneous cholangiography (percutaneous transhepatic cholangiography, PTC) is useful to evaluate the bile ducts proximal to the injury. Endoscopic cholangiography (endoscopic retrograde cholangiopancreatography, ERCP) plays a very important role in the imaging of biliary tract injuries. During ERCP it is possible to supply minor injuries through the establishment of the prosthesis into the lumen of the damaged bile ducts. The advantage of magnetic resonance cholangiography (cholangio-MR) imaging is the high accuracy of the biliary tree and it is non-invasive. This investigation is primarily used to assess the biliary tract before the reconstructive surgery.

6. Classification of iatrogenic bile duct injuries

Different IBDI classifications are described in the literature. In our opinion, the Bismuth classification is the most useful in a clinical practice (described in figure 1). It is based on location of the injury in the biliary tract. This classification is very helpful in prognosis after repair, but does not involve the wide spectrum of possible biliary injuries. The another classification is the Strasberg scale which, in difference from the Bismuth scale, allows to distinguish small (bile leakage from the cystic duct) and serious injuries performed during laparoscopic cholecystectomy, but it does not play an important role in choice of surgical treatment method. The Mattox classification of IBDI takes into consideration a kind of injuring factor (contusion, laceration, perforation, transsection, distraction or interruption of the bile duct or the gallbladder). There are several classifications of IBDI performed during laparoscopic cholecystectomy (Steward and Way, Schmidt, Hannover) in the literature.

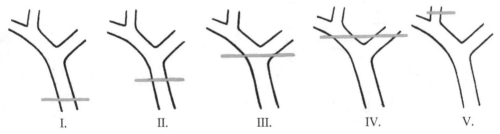

I.   II.   III.   IV.   V.

I. Common bile duct (CBD) and low common hepatic duct (CHD) > 2cm. from hepatic duct confluence. II. Proximal CHD < 2cm from confluence. III. Hilar injury with no residual CHD – confluence intact. IV. Destruction of confluence – right and left hepatic ducts separated. V. Involvement of aberrant right sectoral hepatic duct alone or with concomitant injury of CHD.

Fig. 1. Bismuth classification of IBDI.

7. Treatment of iatrogenic bile duct injuries

7.1 Non-invasive treatment of iatrogenic bile duct injuries

Non-invasive, percutaneous radiological end endoscopic techniques are recommended as initial treatment of IBDI. When these techniques are not effective, surgical management is considered.

Type	Injury type
A	Injury of small bile ducts in communication with the main biliary system, with leakage of bile from the Luschka's or cystic ducts.
B	Injury of the sectoral bile duct, with subsequent obstruction of the main biliary system.
C	Injury of the sectoral bile duct with bile leakage of bile from bile duct, without communication with the main biliary system.
D	Side extrahepatic bile duct injury.
E1	CBD or CHD stricture at a distance> 2 cm from the hepatic duct confluence.
E2	CHD stricture at a distance< 2 cm from the hepatic duct confluence.
E3	CHD stricture within the hepatic duct confluence.
E4	Stricture involving the right and left hepatic ducts separately.
E5	Complete closure of all the bile ducts, including sectoral bile ducts.

Table 3. Strasberg classification of IBDI.

Type	Injury type
I	Contusion of the gallbladder or hepatic triad.
II	Jagged or perforation of the gallbladder.
III	The total separation of the gallbladder from the liver.
IV	CBD or CHD partial <50% CBD or CHD laceration or CSF.
V	CBD or CHD transsection> 50% and injury of intrapancreatic or intraduodenal part of bile ducts.

Table 4. Mattox classification of IBDI.

Type	Injury type
I	Small incisions or incomplete intersections of CBD.
II	Stricture caused by thermal injury or clips.
III	Total transsection or excision of the or CBD, CHD or the right or left hepatic ducts.
IV	Resection of the right hepatic cord erroneously recognized as the cystic duct.

Table 5. Steward i Way classification of IBDI.

Type	Injury type
A	Leak from the cystic duct (A1) or an accessory hepatic duct within gallbladder fossa (A2).
B	Clip closure of CBD or CHD incomplete (B1) or complete (B2).
C	Side injury of CBD or CHD over a distance of up to 5 mm (C1) or more than 5 mm (C2).
D	Transsection of CBD or CHD without loss (D1) or loss (D2) of bile duct.
E	Stricture of CBD or CHD over a distance of up to 5 mm (E1),> 5 mm (E2) or the hepatic ducts confluence (E3) or only the right hepatic duct (E4).

Table 6. Schmidt classification of IBDI.

Type	Injury type
A	Peripheal bile leakage (in communication with main biliary system).
A1	Bile leakage from the cystic duct.
A2	Bile leakage from the gallbalder fossa.
B	CHD or CBD stricture without damage (eg caused by a clip).
B1	Incomplete.
B2	Complete.
C	Lateral CHD or CBD injury.
C1	Small spot injury (< 5 mm).
C2	Large injury (> 5 mm) below the hepatic ducts confluence.
C3	Large injury at the level of the hepatic ducts confluence.
C4	Large injury above the hepatic ducts confluence.
D	Total transsection of CHD Or CBD.
D1	Without ductal loss below the hepatic ducts confluence.
D2	With ductal loss below the hepatic ducts confluence.
D3	At the level of the hepatic ducts confluence.
D4	Above the hepatic ducts confluence. (with or without ductal loss).
E	CHD or CBD stricture.
E1	Short, circular (< 5 mm) CHD or CBD stricture.
E2	Longitudinal CBD stricture (>5 mm).
E3	Stricture at the level of the hepatic ducts confluence
E4	Stricture of the right hepatic duct / sectorral hepatic duct.
E5	The complete closure of all the bile ducts, including sectoral bile ducts.

Table 7. Hannover classification of IBDI.

7.1.1 Percutaneous dilatation under radiological control

The effectiveness of percutaneous diltatation of biliary strictures with transhepatic insertion of the stent under radiological control is 40-85%. The main treatment-related complications associated with the liver puncture include haemorrhage, bile leakage and cholangitis. The other less common complications include pneumothorax which is the result of damage to the pleura, biliary-pleural fistula and perforation of adjacent organs, including the colon. Percutaneous technique is less effective (52%) than surgical therapy (89%). Also frequently than post-surgical complications observed (35% and 25% of complications). It is also associated with the higher number of complications (35%) than surgery (25%). The most frequently, it is recommended in very difficult cases of very high, hilar biliary strictures or in the treatment of very small bile ducts in the diameter.

7.1.2 Endoscopic dilatation during ERCP

Endoscopic dilatation associated with insertion of biliary prosthesis during ERCP investigation is the most frequently used non-surgical method in the treatment of IBDI. The effectiveness of endoscopic (72%) and surgical (83%) treatment is comparable. Incidence of complications in both methods of treatment is also comparable (35% vs. 26%). The common complications of endoscopic techniques regarding placement of biliary prosthesis include cholangitis, pancreatitis, prosthesis occlusion, migration, dislodgement and perforation of the bile duct.

Endoscopic treatment is recommended as initial treatment of benign biliary strictures, biliary fistula in the presence and in patients not not qualified to surgical treatment.

7.2 Surgical treatment of iatrogenic bile duct injuries

7.2.1 Immediate repair of IBDI

In the case of intraoperative recognition of bile duct injury, it is recommended that intraoperative cholangiography or conversion from laparoscopic cholecystectomy to open, allowing a better insight into the operative field and immediate repair. The injury should be repaired by an experienced hepatobiliary surgeon. If it is impossible, a patient should be transferred to a referral hepatobiliary surgery center, after adequate drainage of a subhepatic region. If the cut bile duct is less than 2-3 mm in diameter, without communication with the main biliary system, it should be ligated in order to avoid postoperative bile leak leading to development of the biloma and abscess in the subhepatic region. Bile ducts with a diameter of 3-4 mm or more should be surgically repaired because they drain the larger area of the liver. Interruption of CHD or CBD continuity can be repaired by immediate tension-free end-to-end ductal anastomosis with or without a T tube, using absorbable sutures. Security of the immediately repaired bile duct with a T tube is controversial. If the bile duct loss is too long and immediate end-to-end biliary anastomosis is not possible without tension, hepaticojejunostomy Roux-Y is recommended.

7.2.2 Surgical reconstructions of iatrogenic bile duct injuries

Over 2/3 bile duct injuries are recognized at least a few days after surgery, during which the injury occurred. The surgical treatment of elective IBDI is made using different methods of biliary reconstructions. The main aim of surgical treatment is the reconstruction of proper flow of bile to the alimentary tract. The following operations are performed in biliary injuries surgical treatment: Roux-Y hepaticojejunostomy, end-to-end ductal biliary anastomosis with T drainage or endoprothesis conducted into the duodenum according to Górka, choledochoduodenostomy, Lahey hepaticojejunostomy, jejunal interposition hepaticoduodenostomy, Blumgart (Hepp) anastomosis, Heinecke-Mikulicz biliary plastic reconstruction and Smith mucosal graft.

Conditions of proper healing of each biliary anastomosis

- The anastomosed edges should be healthy, without inflammation, ischemia and fibrosis.
- The anastomosis should be tension-free and properly vascularized.
- It should be performed in a single layer with absorbable sutures.

7.2.2.1 Types of surgical reconstructions performed in IBDI

7.2.2.1.1 End-to-end ductal anastomosis (EE)

We recommend this method as the first, because end-to-end ductal anastomosis (EE) is the most physiological biliary reconstruction [1, 46, 48, 49]. In this type of reconstruction, extensive mobilization of the duodenum with the pancreatic head through the Kocher maneuver, excision of the bile duct stricture, and refreshment of the proximal and distal stumps should be performed. Anastomosis is performed in a single layer with interrupted absorbable PDS 4-0 or 5-0 sutures. This reconstruction is not recommended by most authors due to the higher number of anastomosis strictures in comparison with Roux-y hepaticojejunostomy (HJ). We recommend EE first, because in some patients, extensive mobilization of the duodenum with the pancreatic head by the Kocher maneuver allows to perform the tension-free anastomosis after the extensive length-loss of the bile duct. Excision of the bile duct stricture, dissection and refreshing of the proximal and distal stumps as far as the tissues are healthy and without inflammation, and the use of non-traumatic, monofilament-interrupted sutures 5-0 allows the achievement of good long-term results. Using of an internal Y tube conducting from the right and left hepatic ducts into the duodenum through EE and the papilla of Vater also allows the proper healing of this anastomosis. This reconstruction can be performed when the bile duct loss is from 0.5 to 4 cm. It allows the achievement of very good long-term results with effectiveness comparable with HJ. It is important that establishing a physiological bile pathway allows proper digestion and absorption, which causes a higher gain weight in patients following EE, which was noted in study performed in our department. Another essential advantage of EE is possibility of of endoscopic control after surgery.The lower number of early complications is observed after EE than HJ, which is associated with opening of the alimentary tract and the higher number of performed anastomoses (biliary-enteric and entero-enteric) in patients with HJ. The disadvantage is the higher incidence of recorded postoperative stenosis at the anastomosis due to poorer blood supply of the operated area. It can't be performed in patients with bile duct loss more than 4 cm. The diameter of both anastomosed ends should be comparable. If there is a difference between a diameter of anastomosed ends, the thinner end should be incised longitudinally in the anterior surface in order to extend it before creation of anastomosis. This repair should not be carried out in bile ducts that are too thin (diameter less than 4 mm). In our opinion a patient, whom we perform first or exceptionally second bile ducts repair, is a candidate for EE. Because of a number of advantages, EE is recommended as the first method of choice for patients with IBDI.

7.2.2.1.2 Roux-Y hepaticojejunostomy

Roux-Y hepaticojejunostomy (HJ) is the most frequently performed surgical reconstruction of IBDI. In this surgical technique, a proximal common hepatic duct is identified and prepared and the distal common bile duct is sutured. End-to-side or end-to-end HJ is performed in a single layer using interrupted absorbable polydioxanone (PDS 4-0 or 5-0) sutures. Most authors prefer HJ due to the lower number of postoperative anastomosis strictures. According to Terblanche et al, HJ is effective in 90% of cases [50]. However, after this reconstruction, bile flow into the alimentary tract is not physiological, because the duodenum and upper part of the jejunum are excluded from bile passage. Physiological conditions within the proximal gastrointestinal tract are changed as a result of duodenal exclusion from bile passage. An altered bile pathway is a cause of disturbances in the release of gastrointestinal hormones. There is a hypothesis that in patients with HJ, the bile bypass induces gastric hypersecretion leading to a pH change secondary to altered bile synthesis and release of gastrin. A higher number of duodenal ulcers is observed in patients with HJ, which may be associated with a loss of the neutralizing effect of the bile, including bicarbonates and the secondary gastric hypersecretion. Laboratory investigations revealed increased gastrin and glucagon-like immunoreactivity (GLI) plasma levels and decreased triglycerides, gastric inhibitory polypeptide (GIP), and insulin plasma levels in patients with HJ. An altered pathway of bile flow is also a cause of disturbance in fat metabolism in patients undergoing HJ. Moreover, the total surface of absorption in these patients is also decreased due to exclusion of the duodenum and upper jejunum from the food passage. In our department a significantly lower weight gain in patients undergoing HJ in comparison to patients following physiological end-to-end ductal anastomosis was reported [1, 49]. The another disadvantage of HJ is a lack of capability of control endoscopic examination and endoscopic dilatation of strictured biliary anastomosis. In order to resolve this problem, a longer jejunal loop (jejunostomy) is prepared and sutured to the abdominal subcutaneous tissue in the right subcostal region. Jejunostomy can be open or closed with possibility of opening in a case of biliary anastomosis stricture, which should be endoscopically dilated. Jejunostomy is asscociated with bile loss of about 40 ml/day in patients.

7.2.2.1.3 Choledochoduodenostomy (ChD)

Choledochoduodenostomy (ChD) is actually rarely performed operation recommended by some authors only in cases of injury within the distal portion of the common bile duct. It guarantees physiological bile flow into duodenum and anastomosis endoscopic control, and it is easier technically. It is recommended in some cases of distal strictures, when use of the jejunal loop due to numerous adhesions is impossible. It should be performed on the large common bile duct (>15 mm diameter) because the postoperative strictures are more frequent within the narrow duct. ChD should be created between the duodenum and the distal CBD in order to decrease a risk of so-called sump syndrome noted in 0.14-3.3% of cases in the literature. In patients following ChD, recurrent ascending cholangitis due to bile reflux is noted in 0-4%. A higher rate of bile duct cancer in patients with ChD in comparison of HJ (7.6 vs. 1.9%) was reported in the literature .

7.2.2.1.4 Jejunal interposition hepaticoduodenostomy (JIHD)

Jejunal interposition hepaticoduodenostomy, using 25-35 cm of the jejunal loop, is performed in some surgical centers including our department. This reconstruction includes three (biliary-enteric, enteric-duodenal and entero-enteric) anastomoses. Biliary-enteric anastomosis is performed in a single layer with interrupted absorbable sutures 5-0 and enteric-duodenal in a single layer with interrupted or continuous absorbable sutures 4-0. In our opinion, JIHD should be used only in patients in good general condition, without active inflammation within the peritoneal cavity, with protein level more than 6 g/dl and serum bilirubin level less than 20 mg/dl. Good condition of the duodenal wall is important factor for proper healing of hepaticoduodenostomy with jejunal interposition. The advantage of this reconstruction is physiological bile flow into the duodenum, which prevents duodenal ulcer caused by changes in the neurohormonal axis within the upper alimentary tract. This method of reconstruction is recommended mainly in patients with concomitant duodenal ulcer The disadvantage is a higher number of early complications due to presence of three anastomoses.

7.2.2.1.5 Reconstructions of hilar bile duct injuries

The repair of hilar IBDI requires special surgical techniques. In the past, so-called "mucosal graft technique" described by Smith in the 1960s was performed. This reconstruction involves creating a mucosal dome of jejunum (by removing a seromuscular patch) near the end of Roux-Y loop through which a straight rubber tube is brought via hepatic ducts and through liver parenchyma. This technique is based on the hypothesis that jejunal mucosa grafts to the biliary epithelium and mucosa-to-mucosa anastomosis is created. Short-term results were good, but in long-term results a high number of anastomosis strictures was observed. Therefore, currently, not Smith but Blumgart-Hepp technique is used in reconstruction of hilar IBDI. In this technique, dorsal surface of the left hepatic duct parallel to the quadrate hepatic lobe. Dissection and opening of the left hepatic duct longitudinally allows to create a wide anastomosis of 1-3 cm in diameter.

Other methods of IBDI reconstruction, such as Lahey hepaticojejunostomy, jejunal Heinecke-Mikulicz biliary plastic operation Kirtley operation and others are performed sporadically.

7.2.2.2 Types of surgical biliary drainage used in IBDI reconstructions

7.2.2.2.1 External T-drainage

External T-drainage - using a typical Kehr tube with insertion of its short branches into the bile duct and conducting of its long branch through the abdominal wall outside.

7.2.2.2.2 External Y-drainage

External Y-drainage - insertion of short branches of the Kehr tube into both right and left hepatic ducts, splinting of the anastomosis and conducting of its long branch through the jejunal loop and abdominal wall outside.

7.2.2.3 Internal Y-drainage

Internal Y-drainage - insertion of short branches of the Kehr tube into both right and left hepatic ducts, splinting of the anastomosis and conducting of its long branch into the duodenum by the papilla of Vater.

7.2.2.4 Rodney-Smith drainage

Rodney Smith drainage - using two straight rubber tubes splinting the biliary-enteric anastomosis that are brought via hepatic ducts and through liver parenchyma and conducted through the abdominal wall outside. This drainage type is used in high intrahilar biliary-enteric anastomosis. In the past, it was used in Smith "mucosal graft technique".

7.2.2.5 No drainage

Drainage using is still controversial. The advantage of biliary drainage is limitation of the inflammation and fibrosis occurring after the surgical procedure. In some authors' opinion, the presence of the biliary tube prevents anastomosis stricture. The disadvantage of biliary drainage is a higher risk of postoperative complications. There are recommendations (according to Mercado et al) to use transanastomotic stents when there is a thin bile duct less than 4 mm in diameter, and when there is inflammation within the ductal anastomosed edges that makes proper healing of the anastomosis questionable.

8. Treatment of iatrogenic bile duct injuries – Assesment of results in the surgical treatment of iatrogenic bile duct injuries

8.1 Short-term results and early complications

The early postoperative morbidity rate is 20-30% and mortality rate 0-2%. The most frequent early complication is wound infection (8-17.7%). Other complications are the following: bile collection, intra-abdominal abscess, biliary-enteric anastomosis dehiscence, biliary fistula, cholangitis, peritonitis, eventration, pneumonia, circulatory insufficiency, intra-abdominal bleeding, sepsis, infection of the urinary tract, pneumothorax, acute pancreatitis, thrombosis and embolic complications, diarrhea, ileus and multi-organ insufficiency.

8.2 Long-term results and quality of life

8.2.1 Follow-up after surgical reconstructions

8.2.1.1 Duration of follow-up

IBDI remain a serious clinical problem and a challenge for even the most experienced surgical centers of reference. According to literature, the effectiveness of surgical treatment of IBDI is 70-90%. The recurrent strictures after biliary reconstruction occur in 10-30% of cases. About 80% of postoperative recurrence of biliary strictures are observed during the first five years following reconstruction. Two-thirds (65%) of recurrent biliary strictures develop within 2-3 years after the reconstruction, 80% within 5 years, and 90% within 7 years. Recurrent strictures 10 years after the surgical procedure are also described in the literature. Therefore, the objective assessment of long-term results of surgical treatment plays an important role in the observation period (follow-up) (FU). According to most authors, patients following biliary reconstruction should be observed at least 3 years; according to some authors even 5 to 10 years. Satisfactory length of follow-up, which is necessary in order to assess the long-term results of the repair procedure, is 2 to 5 years. Some authors recommend 10 or 20 years of observation. The criteria of success of surgery include: the absence of clinical symptoms such as biliary jaundice or cholangitis and absence of recurrent stenosis after surgery requiring endoscopic or surgical correction.

The early proper biliary reconstruction is very important, because duration of biliary obstruction is the most important risk factor of biliary cirrhosis. According to literature, prolonged time from injury to repair and portal hypertension are important parameters correlating with secondary biliary cirrhosis. So, early biliary repair can prevent liver fibrosis. According to the literature, biliary cirrhosis occurs in two thirds of patients without effective biliary repair. Portal hypertension is noted in 15-25% of patients with biliary cirrhosis due to IBDI. Reoperations within inflammation, fibrosis and a higher risk of intra-operative bleeding due to portal hypertension with collateral circulation and intraperitoneal adhesions are very difficult and associated with increased mortality rate. Therefore, early and proper biliary reconstruction increases survival rate and decreases morbidity and mortality rates in patients with IBDI.

8.2.1.2 Follow-up classifications

Different classifications are used for an objective assessment of the effectiveness of biliary repair. The Terblanche scale taking into account clinical parameters is the most frequently used classification [50, 72]. Other less frequently used classifications are the following: the McDonald, Brummelkamp Lygidakis, Cardenas and Munoz, and Nielubowicz scales.

I	**Excellent result.** No biliary symptoms with normal liver function.
II	**Good result.** Transitory symptoms, currently no symptoms and normal liver function.
III	**Fair result.** Clearly related symptoms requiring medical therapy and/or deteriorating liver function.
IV	**Poor result.** Recurrent stricture requiring correction or related death.

Table 8. Terblanche classification.

A	No clinical symptoms from the biliary tract, proper laboratory liver funtion parameters tests.
B	No clinical signs, laboratory liver function parameters tests slightly elevated liver function parameters, or periodically occurring episodes of pain or fever.
C	Pain, cholangitis with the presence of fever with jaundice and abnormalities in laboratory tests.
D	Condition requiring surgical or endoscopic correction.

Table 9. McDonald classification.

I	Without pain, normal liver function tests.
II	Minor clinical symptoms due to periodic cholangitis resolved after antibiotic therapy, occurring 2-3 times a year, not requiring hospitalization. Proper liver function tests, except of increased serum bilirubin and alkaline phosphatase, with rapid normalization after symptoms resolution.
III	Severe recurrent cholangitis, occuring in more 3 times a year,, lasting over a week and requiring hospitalization. Laboratory tests showing a tendency do increased ALT and AST and transit but rapid increased serum bilirubin and alkaline phosphatase.

Table 10. Lygidakis i Brummelkamp classification.

I	Asymtomatic course.
II	Minor clinical symtoms.
III	Recurrent cholangitis.

Table 11. Muñoz-Cardenas classification.

Very good result	Without clinical symptoms.
Good result	Cholangitis 1-2 a year without jaundice, and without debilitating normal life and work of the patient.
Poor result	Often repeated bouts of cholangitis with jaundice, showing recurrence of stenosis.

Table 12. Nielubowicz classification.

9. Conclusion

The early and proper treatment of IBDI is very important, because it can prevent serious complications and improve quality of life in patients. Non-invasive methods are used as initial treatment. When it is not effective, surgical management should be considered. Surgical treatement includes different types of reconstructions.

10. References

[1] Ahrendt S.; & Pitt H. (2001). Surgical Therapy of Iatrogenic Lesions of Biliary Tract. Word J Surg, Vol. 25, pp. 1360-1365.

[2] Barker E.M.; & Winkler M. (1984). Permanent-access hepaticojejunostomy. Br J Surg, Vol. 71, pp. 188-191.

[3] Beal J.M. (1984). Historical perspective of gallstone disease. Surg Gynecol Obstet, Vol. 158, pp. 181-189.

[4] Bektas H.; Schrem H.; Winny M.; & Klempnauer J. (2007). Surgical treatment and outcome of iatrogenic bile duct lesions after cholecystectomy and the impact od different clinical classification systems. Br J Surg 2007, Vol. 94, No. 9, pp. 1119-1127.

[5] Bismuth H.; & Franco D. (1978). Long term results of Roux-en-Y hepaticojejunostomy. Surg Gyn Obstet, Vol. 146, No. 2, pp. 161-167.

[6] Bismuth H.; & Majno P.E. (2001). Biliary strictures: classification based on the principles of surgical treatment. Word J Surg, Vol. 25, pp. 1241-1244.

[7] Blumgart L.H. (1994). Hilar and intrahepatic biliary enteric anastomosis. Surg Clin North Am;, Vol. 74, pp. 731-740

[8] Bolton J.S.; Braasch J.W.; & Rossi R.L. (1980). Management of benign biliary stricture. Surg Clin North Am, Vol. 60, pp. 313-332.

[9] Braasch J.W. (1994). Historical perspectives of biliary tract injuries . Surg Clin North Am, Vol 74, No. 4 pp. 731-740.

[10] Buell J.F.; Cronin D.C.; Funaki B.; & al. (2002). Devastating and Fatal Compilactions Associated With Combined Vascular and Bile Injuries During Cholecystectomy. Ann Surg, Vol. 137, pp. 703-710.

[11] Chaudhary A.; Chandra A.; Negi S.; & Sachdev A. (2002). Reoperative Surgery for Postcholecystectomy Bile Duct Injuries. Dig Surg, Vol. 19, pp. 22-27.

[12] Coleman J.A.; & Yeo Ch.J. (2000). Postoperative Bile Duct Strictures: Management and Outcome In the 1990s. Ann Surg, Vol. 232, No. 3, pp. 430-441.

[13] Connor S.; & Garden O.J. (2006). Bile duct injury in the era of laparoscopic cholecystectomy. Br J Surg, Vol. 93, pp. 158-168.

[14] Davids P.; Tanka A.; Rauws E, Gulik T.; Leeuwen D.; Wit L.; Verbeek P,.; Huibregtse K.; Heyde N.; & Tytgat G. (1993). Benign Biliary Strictures. Surgery or Endoscopy? Ann Surg, Vol. 217, No. 3, pp. 237-243.

[15] Flum D.R.; Cheadle A.; Prela C.; Dellinger E.P.; & Chan L. (2003). Bile Duct Injury During Cholecystectomy and Survival in Medicare Beneficiares. JAMA 2003, Vol. 290, No. 16, pp. 2168-2173.

[16] Gazzaniga G.M.; Filauro M.; & Mori L. (2001). Surgical treatment of Iatrogenic Lesions of the Proximal Common Bile Duct. Word J Surg, Vol. 25, pp. 1254-1259.

[17] Gentileschi P.; Di Paola M.; Catarci M.; & al. (2004). Bile duct injuries during laparoscopic cholecystectomy. A 1994-2001 audit on 13,718 operations in the area of Rome. Surg Endosc, Vol. 18, pp. 232-236.

[18] Górka Z.; & Rudnicki M. (1991). Zespolenie przewodowo-czczo-dwunastnicze w operacjach odtwórczych dróg żółciowych. Pol Przegl Chir, Vol. 63, pp. 1003-1008.

[19] Górka Z.; Ziaja K.; Nowak J.; Lampe P.; & Wojtyczka A. (1992). 195 operacji kalectwa żółciowego. Pol Przegl Chir, Vol. 64:, pp. 969-976.

[20] Górka Z.; Ziaja K.; Wojtyczka A.; Kabat J.; & Nowak J. (1992). End-to-end anastomosis as a method of choice in surgical treatment of selected cases of biliary handicap. Pol J Surg, Vol. 64, pp. 977-979

[21] Gouma D.J.; & Obertop H. (2002). Management of Bile Duct Injuries: Treatment and Long-Term Results. Dig Surg; Vol. 19, pp. 117-122.

[22] Hall J.G.; & Pappas TN. (2004). Current Management of Biliary Strictures. J Gastrointest Surg, Vol. 8, No. 8, pp. 1098-1110.

[23] Hardy K.J. (1993). Carl Langenbuch and the lasarus Hospital: events and circumstanses surrounding the first cholecystectomyAust N Z J Surg, Vol. 63, No. 1, pp. 56-64.

[24] Imamura M.; Takahashi M.; Sasaki I.; Yamauchi H.; & Sato T. (1988). Effects of the Pathway of Bile Flow on the Digestion of FAT and the Release of Gastrointestinal Hormones. Am J Gastroenterol, Vol. 83, pp. 386-392.

[25] Jabłońska B.; Lampe P.; Olakowski M.; Lekstan A.; & Górka Z. (2008). Surgical treatment of iatrogenic biliary injuries – early complications. Przegl Chir, Vol. 80, No. 6, pp. 299-305.

[26] Jabłońska B.; Lampe P.; Olakowski M.; Górka Z.; Lekstan A.; & Gruszka T. (2009). Hepaticojejunostomy vs. end-to-end biliary reconstructions in the treatment of iatrogenic bile duct injuries. J Gastrointest Surg, Vol. 13, No.6, pp. 1084-1093.

[27] Jabłońska B.; & Lampe P. (2009). Iatrogenic bile duct injuries – etiology, diagnosis and management. WorldJ Gastroenterol, Vol. 15, No. 33, pp. 4097-4104.

[28] Jabłońska B.; Lampe P.; Olakowski M.; Lekstan A.; & Górka Z. (2010). Long-term Results in the Surgical Treatment of Iatrogenic Bile Duct Injuries. Pol J Surg, Vol. 82, No. 6, pp. 354-361.

[29] Jarnagin W.R,.; & Blumgart LH (1999). Operative Repair of Bile Duct Injuries Involving the Hepatic Duct Confluence. Arch Sur, Vol. 134, pp. 769-775.

[30] Jarnagin W.R.; & Blumgart L.H. (2002). Benign biliary strictures. [In:] Blumgart LH, Fong Y, ed. Surgery of the liver and biliary tract. WB Saunders Company, Philadelphia 2002: pp. 895-929.

[31] Jędrzejczyk W.; Juźków H.; & Jackowski M. (1997). Modyfikacja techniki operacyjnej w kalectwie dróg żółciowych – nadzieje i obawy. Pol Przegl Chir, Vol. 69, No. 3, pp. 297-300.

[32] Kaman L.; Sanyal S.; Behera A.; Singh R.; & Katariya R.N. (2006). Comparision of major bile duct injuries following laparoscopic cholecystectomy and open cholecystectomy. ANZ J Surg, Vol. 76, pp. 788-791.

[33] Koffron A.; Ferrario M.; Parsons W.; Nemcek A.; Saker M.; & Abecassis M. (2001). Failed primary management of iatrogenic biliary injury: Incidence and significance of concomitant hepatic arterial disruption. Surgery, Vol. 130, pp. 722-731.

[34] Kosiński B.; Umiński M.; J& agielski G. (1995). Kalectwo dróg żółciowych. Pol Przegl Chir, Vol. 67, No. 2, pp. 141-144.

[35] Kozicki I.; & Bielecki K. (1997). Hepaticojejunostomy in Benign Biliary Stricture – Influence of Careful Postoperative Observations on Long-Term Results. Dig Surg, Vol. 14, pp. 527-533.

[36] Kozicki I.; & Bielecki K.; the late Kowalski A.; & Krolicki L. (1994). Repeated reconstruction for recurrent benign bile duct stricture. Br J Surg, Vol. 81, pp. 677-679.

[37] Kozicki I.; Bielecki K.; & Lembas L. (2000). Leczenie śródwnękowych urazów dróg żółciowych po cholecystektomii laparoskopowej. Pol Przegl Chir, Vol. 72, No. 11, pp. 1049-1060.

[38] Krawczyk M.; & Patkowski W. (2001). Taktyka postępowania w jatrogennym uszkodzeniu dróg żółciowych. Pol Przegl Chir, Vol. 73, No. 1, pp. 4-16.

[39] Lillemoe K.D.; Melton G.B.; Cameron J.L.; Pitt H.A.; Campbell K.A.; Talamini M.A.; Sauter P.A.; Coleman J.; & Yeo C.J. (2000). Postoperative Bile Duct Strictures: Management and Outcome in the 1990s. Ann Surg, Vol.232, No. 3, pp. 430-441.

[40] Lygidakis N.J.; & Brummelkamp W.H. (1986). Surgical management of proximal benign biliary strictures. Acta Chir Scand, Vol. 152, pp. 367-371.

[41] Mattox K.L.; Feliciano D.V.; & Moore E.E.(1996). Trauma. 3rd Ed. Stamford, CT: Applenton&Lange, 1996: 515-519.

[42] Mc Mahon A.J.; Fullarton G.; Barter J.N.; & O'Dwyer P.J. (1995). Bile duct injury and bile leakage In laparosopic cholecystectomy. Br J Surg; Vol. 82, pp. 307-313.

[43] McDonald M.L.; Farnell M.B.; Nagorney D.M.; Ilstrup D.M.; & Kutch J.M. (1995). Benign biliary strictures: repair and outcome with contemporary approach. Surgery, Vol. 118, pp. 582-591.

[44] Mercado M.A.; Chan C.; Orozco H.; Cano-Gutiérrez G.; Chaparro J.M.; Galindo E.; Vilatobá M..; & Samaniego-Arvizu G. (2002) To stent or not to stent bilioenteric anastomosis after iatrogenic injury: A Dilemma not answered? Surgery, Vol. 137:, pp. 60-63.

[45] Mercado M.A.; Chan C.; Orozco H.; Tielve M.; & Hinojosa C.A. (2003). Acute bile duct injury. The need for a high repair. Surg Endosc, Vol. 17, pp. 1351-1355.

[46] Misra S.; Melton G.B.; Geschwind J.F.; Venbrux A.C.; Cameron J.L.; & Lillemoe K.D. (2004). Percutaneous Management of Bile Duct Strictures and Injuries Associated with Laparoscopic Cholecystectomy: A Decade of Experience. J Am Coll Surg, Vol. 198, pp. 218-226.

[47] Moore D.F.; Feurer I..D.; Holzman M.D.; & al. (2004). Long-term Detrimental Effect of Bile Injury on Health-Related Quality of Life. Arch Surg, Vol. 139, pp. 476-482.

[48] Muňoz R.; & Cardenas S. (1990). Thirty Years' Experience with Biliary Tract Reconstruction by Hepaticoenterostomy and Transhepatic T Tube. Am J Surg, Vol. 159, pp. 405-410.

[49] Murr M.M.; Gigot J.F.; Nagorney D.M.; Harmsen W.S.; Ilstrup D.M.; & Farnell MB. (1999). Long-term Results of Biliary Reconstruction After Laparoscopic Bile Duct injuries. Arch Surg, Vol. 134, No. 6, pp. 604-610

[50] Negi S.S,.; Sakhuja P.; Malhotra V.; & al. (2004). Factors Predicting Advanced Hepatic Fibrosis in Patients With Postcholecystectomy Bile Duct Strictures. Arch Surg, Vol. 139, pp. 299-303.

[51] Nielsen M.K.; Jensen S.L.; Malstrom J.; & Niwlsen O.V. (1980). Gastryn and gastric acid secretion in hepaticojejunostomy Roux-en-Y. Surg Gyn Obstet, Vol. 150, pp. 61-64.

[52] Nielubowicz J.; Olszewski K.; & Szostek M. (1973). Operacje odtwórcze w kalctwie dróg żółciowych. Pol Przegl Chir, Vol. XLV, No. 12, pp. 1389-1395.

[53] Pellegrini C.A.; Thomas M.J.; & Way L.W. (1984). Recurrent biliary stricture: patterns of recurrence and outcome of surgical therapy. Am J Surg, No. 147, pp. 175-180.

[54] Perakath B.; Sitaram V.; Mathew G.; & al.(2003). Postcholecystectomy benign biliary stricture with portal hypertension: is a portosystemic shunt before hepaticojejunostomy necessary? Ann R Coll Surg Engl, Vol. 85, pp. 317-320.

[55] Pitt H.A.; Kaufman H.S.; Coleman J.; White R.I.; & Cameron JL. (1989). Benign postoperative biliare strictures. Operate or dilate? Ann Surg, Vol. 210, pp. 417-425.

[56] Pitt H.A.; Miyamoto T.; Parapatis S.K.; Tompkins R.K.; & Longmire W.P .Jr. (1982). Factors influencing outcome in patients with postoperative biliary strictures. Am J Surg, Vol. 144, pp. 14-21.

[57] Reynolds W. Jr. 2001The first laparoscopic cholecystectomy. JSLS. Jan-Mar;5(1):89-94.

[58] Robinson T.N,.; Stiegmann G.V.; Durham J.D.; Johnson S.I.; Wachs M.E.; Serra A.D.; & Kumpe D.A. (2001). Management of major bile duct injury associated with laparoscopic cholecystectomy. Surg Endosc, Vol. 15, pp. 1381-1385.

[59] Rossi R.L.; & Tsao J.I. (1994). Biliary reconstruction. Surg Clin North Am, Vol. 74, No. 4, pp. 825-841.

[60] Rudnicki M.; McFadden D.W.; Sheriff S. & Ischer J.E. (1992). Roux-en-Y jejunal Bypass abolishes postprandial neuropeptide Y release. J Surg Res, Vol. 53, pp. 7-11.

[61] Savar A.; Carmody I.; Hiatt J.R.; & Busuttil R.W. (2004). Laparoscopic Bile Duct Injuries: Management at a Tertiary Liver Center. Am Surg, Vol. 70, pp. 906-909.

[62] Schmidt S.C.; Langrehr J.M.; Hintze R.E.; & Neuhaus P. (2005). Long-term results and risk factors influencing outcome of major bile duct injuries following cholecystectomy. Br J Surg, Vol. 92, pp. 76-82.

[63] Schmidt S.C.; Settmacher U.; Langrehr J.M.; & Neuhaus P. (2004). Management and outcome of patients with combined bile duct and hepatic arterial injuries after laparoscopic cholecystectomy. Surgery, No. 135, pp. 613-618.

[64] Shamiyeh A.; & Wayand W. (2004). Laparoscopic cholecystectomy: early and late complications and their treatment. Langenbecks Arch Surg, No. 389, Vo.3, pp. 164-171.

[65] Shea J.A.; Healey M.J.; Jesse A.; & al. (1996). Mortality and Complications Associated with Laparoscopic Cholecystectomy: A Meta-Analysis. Ann Surg, Vo. 224, No. 5, pp. 609-620.

[66] Sicklick J.K.; Camp M.S.; Lillemoe K.D.; & al. (2005). Surgical Management of Bile Duct Injuries Sustained During Laparoscopic Cholecystectomy. Perioperative Results in 200 Patients. Ann Surg, Vol. 241, No. 5, pp. 786-795.

[67] Sicklick J.K.; Camp M.S.; Lillemoe K.D.; Melton G.B.; Yeo C.J.; Campbell K.A.; Talamini M.A.; Pitt H.A.; Coleman J.; Sauter P.A,.; & Cameron J.L. (2005). Surgical Management of Bile Duct Injuries Sustained During Laparoscopic Cholecystectomy. Perioperative Results in 200 Patients. Ann Surg, Vol. 241, pp. 786-795.

[68] Sikora S.S.; Pottakkat B.; Srikanth G.; Kumar A.; Saxena R.; & Kapoor V.K. (2006). Postcholecystectomy Benign Biliary Strictures – Long-Term Results. Dig Surg, Vol. 23, pp. 304-312.

[69] Sikora S.S.; Srikanth G.; Agrawal V.; & al. (2008). Liver histology in benign biliary stricture: fibrosis to cirrhosis... and reversal? J Gastroenterol Hepatol, Vol. 23, No. 12, pp. 1879-84.

[70] Smith R. (1964). Hepaticojejunostomy with transhepatic intubation: a technique for very high strictures of the hepatic ducts. Br J Surg, Vol. 51, pp. 186-194.

[71] Steward L.; & Way L.W. (1995). Bile Duct Injuries During Laparoscopic Cholecystectomy. Factors That Influence the Results of Treatment. Arch Surg, Vol. 130, pp. 1123-1128.

[72] Strasberg S.M.; Hertz M.; & Soper N.J. (1995). An analysis of the problem of biliary injury during laparoscopic cholecystectomy. J Am Coll Surg, Vol. 189, pp. 101-125.

[73] Targarona E.M.; Marco C.; Balague C.; & al. (1998). How, when and why bile duct injury occurs. A comparision between open and laparoscopic cholecystectomy. Surg Endosc, Vol. 12, No. 4, pp. 322-326.

[74] Terblanche J.; Worthley C.; & Krige J. (1990). High or low hepaticojejunostomy for bile duct strictures? Surgery, Vol. 108, pp. 828-834.

[75] Tocchi A.; Costa G.; Lepre L.; Lotta G.; Mazzoni G.; & Sita A. (1996). The Long-Term Outcome of Hepaticojejunostomy In the Treatment of Benign Bile Duct Strictures. Ann Surg, Vol. 224, No. 2, pp. 162-167.

[76] Tocchi A.; Mazzoni G.; Liotta G.; Costa G.; Lepre L.; Miccini M.; Masi E.; Lamazza M.A.; & Fiori E. (2000). Management of Benign Biliary Strictures. Arch Surg, Vol. 135, No. 2, pp. 153-157.

[77] Tocchi A.; Mazzoni G.; Lotta G.; Lepre L.; Cassini D.; & Miccini M. (2001). Late Development of Bile Duct Cancer in Patients Who Had Biliary-Enteric Drainage for Benign Disease: A Follow-Up Study of More Than 1,000 Patients. Ann Surg, Vol. 234, No. 2, pp. 210-214 .

[78] Tsalis K.G.; Christoforidis E.C.; Dimitriadis C.A.; Kalfadis S.C.; Botsios D.S.; & Dadoukis J.D. (2003). Management of bile duct injury during and after laparoscopic cholecystectomy. Surd Endosc, Vol. 17, pp. 31-37.

[79] van Gulik T.M. (1986). Langenbuch's cholecystectomy, once a remarkably controversial operation. Neth J Surg, Vol. 38, No. 5, p. 138-141.

[80] Waage A.; & Nilsson M. (2006). Iatrogenic Bile Duct Injury. A Population-Based Study of 152 776 Cholecystectomies in the Swedish Inpatient Registry. Arch Surg, Vol. 141, pp. 1207-1213.

[81] Warren K.W.; & Jefferson M. (1973). Prevention and Repair of Strictures of the Extrahepatic Bile Ducts. Surg Clin North Am, No. 53, Vol. 5, pp. 1169-1190.

[82] Wexler M.J.; & Smith R. (1975). Jejunal mucosal graft: a sutureless technic for repair of high bile duct strictures. Am J Surg, Vol. 129, pp. 204-211.

[83] Wudel L.J.; Wright J.K.; Pinson C.W.; Herline A.; Debelak J.; Seidel S.; Revis K.; & Chapman W. (2001). Bile Duct Injury Following Laparoscopic Cholecystectomy: A Cause for Continued Concern. The Amer Surg, Vol. 67, No. 6, pp. 557-564.

[84] Yeo Ch.J.; Lillemoe K.D.; Ahrendt S.; & Pitt A.P. (2002). Operative Management of Strictures and Benign Obstructive Disorders of the Bile Duct. [In:] Zuidema GD, Yeo ChJ, ed. Shackelford's Surgery of the Alimentary Tract. Vol III. 5th edition. WB Saunders Company, Philadelphia 2002: pp. 247-261.

14

Selected Algorithms of Computational Intelligence in Gastric Cancer Decision Making

Elisabeth Rakus-Andersson
Blekinge Institute of Technology
Sweden

1. Introduction

Due to the latest research (Engelbrecht, 2007; Rutkowski, 2008) the subject of Computational Intelligence has been divided into five main regions, namely, neural networks, evolutionary algorithms, swarm intelligence, immunological systems and fuzzy systems.

Our attention has been attracted by the possibilities of medical applications provided by immunological computation algorithms. Immunological computation systems are based on immune reactions of the living organisms in order to defend the bodies from pathological substances. Especially, the mechanisms of the T-cell reactions to detect strangers have been converted into artificial numerical algorithms.

Immunological systems have been developed in scientific books and reports appearing during the two last decades (de Castro & Timmis, 2002; Dasgupta & Nino, 2008; Engelbrecht, 2007; Forrest et al., 1997). The basic negative selection algorithm NS was invented by Stefanie Forrest (Forrest et al., 1997) to give rise to some technical applications. We can note such applications of NS as computer virus detection (Antunes & Correia, 2011; Harmer et al., 2002; Zhang & Zhao, 2010), reduction of noise effect (Igawa & Ohashi, 2010), communication of autonomous agents (Ishida, 2004) or identification of time varying systems (Wakizono et al., 2006). Even a trial of connection between a computer and biological systems has been proved by means of immunological computation (Cohen, 2006).

Hybrids made between different fields can provide researchers with richer results; therefore associations between immunological systems and neural networks (Gao et al., 2008) have been developed as well.

In the current chapter we propose another hybrid between the NS algorithm and chosen solutions coming from fuzzy systems (Rakus-Andersson, 2007, 2009, 2010a, 2010b, 2011; Rakus-Andersson & Jain, 2009). This hybrid constitutes the own model of adapting the NS algorithm to the operation decisions "operate" contra "do not operate" in gastric cancer surgery. The choice between two possibilities to treat patients is identified with the partition of a decision region in self and non-self, which is similar to the action of the NS algorithm. The partition is accomplished on the basis of patient data strings/vectors that contain codes of states concerning some essential biological markers. To be able to identify the strings that characterize the "operate" decision we add the own method of computing the patients' characteristics as real values. The evaluation of the patients' characteristics is supported by inserting importance weights assigned to powerful biological indices taking place in the operation decision process. To compute the weights of importance the Saaty algorithm (Saaty, 1978) is adopted.

We introduce the medical task to solve in Section 2. In order to establish the code systems for clinical data the fuzzification of biological markers is discussed in Section 3. In Section 4 we analyze the way of determining the patient characteristics, which should connect the mix of different codes in one value. The adaptation of the NS algorithm to surgery assumptions is made in Section 5. Finally, in Section 6 we test clinical data to prove the action of the model introduced in the paper as an applicable novelty.

2. The description of the medical objective in gastric cancer surgery

Gastric cancer patients are mostly cured by operating on them. Different types of surgery are taken into account. Two of them, namely, the partial resection surgery contra the radical surgery are considered by surgeons when evaluating biological markers in the context of their deviations from normal values (Do-Kyong Kim et al., 2009; de Mello et al., 1983).

Nevertheless, a surgeon often must decide if any operation on a patient is possible. The choice between the status "operate" and "do not operate" will constitute the main problem to solve by engaging different algorithms with their origins in Computational Intelligence. The selection will be made on the basis of three biological markers listed as $X = age$, $Y = CRP\text{-}value$ (C reactive proteins), and $Z = body\ weight$ (Do-Kyong Kim et al., 2009; de Mello et al., 1983). These are considered as the most important indices in gastric cancer surgery decision making.

As a leading method, which should provide us with decisions "operate" against "do not operate", we adapt the NS (Negative Selection) algorithm of immunological computation. To comprehend better some associations between the body immunological system and artificially invented algorithms based on the body protection system let us recall the most essential definitions of immunity.

Immunity refers to the condition, in which the organism can resist diseases. A broader definition of immunity is a reaction to foreign substances (pathogens). The biological immune system (BIS) has the ability to detect foreign substances and to respond them. One of the main capabilities of the immune system is to distinguish own body cells from foreign substances, which is called self/non-self discrimination (Dasgupta & Nino, 2008; Engelbrecht, 2007; Forrest et al., 1997).

This particular ability is assigned to a special kind of lymphocytes called T-cells produced in the bone marrow. The T-cells can differentiate own body cells from pathogenic cells; therefore they play the role of detectors. Both own cells belonging to the self region and foreign pathogen cells forming non-self domain have their special characteristics given in the form of vectors of coded or measured properties.

Let us adapt the meaning of distribution into self and non-self in the medical application sketched as follows. To make a decision concerning an individual patient we assign the immunological region of self to "operate", whereas the non-self field will be identified with "do not operate" (Rakus-Andersson, 2011).

To be able to use the self/non-self discrimination, accomplished by the NS algorithm, we need to create vectors of coded patient data. The own fuzzy technique will be involved to divide reference sets of X, Y and Z into subintervals assisting growth levels of these biological indices. To the subintervals, in turn, the codes are added. We will arrange a code vector assisting the patient's features after examining his/her values of X, Y and Z.

When implementing the NS algorithm we assume that vectors characteristic of self region are available as input data. We do not intend to test too many casual vectors to decide their similarity with self vectors since we want to use the NS algorithm in the effective way. We thus try to generate the strongest population of strings being representatives of the self region.

In order to select this population we provide another own algorithm that converts the code vector to a real value. This value will be recognized as "characteristics of the patient".

3. Fuzzification of X, Y and Z in the creation of code vectors

Before studying the technique of making the self/non-self discrimination to state if the patient can be operated or not we should first be able to compare different strings $v = (x = age, y = CRP, z = body\ weight)$, $x \in X$, $y \in Y$, $z \in Z$, to decide their grades of affinity (coverage). We thus should design sets of codes for each biological parameter.

The markers *age*, *CRP*, and *body weight* are measurable features. Hence, we intend to determine the collections of codes assisting intervals, which correspond to the markers' levels. We want to accomplish a process of fuzzification of the measurable markers in order not to decide lengths of the level intervals intuitively (Rakus-Andersson, 2009, 2010a, 2010b, Rakus-Andersson & Jain, 2009).

A fuzzy set, say, A in the universe X is a collection of elements followed by the membership degrees that are computed by means of the membership function $\mu_A : X \rightarrow [0,1]$. Therefore A is denoted as $A = \{(x, \mu_A(x)), x \in X\}$. A is called normal if at least one element in the set A is assigned to the membership degree equal to 1. The support of A is a non-fuzzy set that consists of elements accompanied by membership degrees greater than 0.

The three quantitative markers X, Y and Z will be then differentiated into levels expressed by lists of terms. The terms from the lists are represented by fuzzy sets (Rakus-Andesson, 2007, 2010b), restricted by the membership functions lying over the domains $[x_{min}, x_{max}]$, $[y_{min}, y_{max}]$ and $[z_{min}, z_{max}]$ respectively.

In conformity with the physician's suggestions we introduce five levels of X, Y and Z as the collections

$$X = "age" = \{ X_1 = "very\ young", X_2 = "young", X_3 = "middle\text{-}aged", X_4 = "old", X_5 = "very\ old"\}$$

$$Y = "CRP\text{-}value" = \{Y_1 = "very\ low", Y_2 = "low", Y_3 = "medium", Y_4 = "high", Y_5 = "very\ high"\}$$

and

$$Z = "body\ weight" = \{Z_1 = "very\ underweighted", Z_2 = "underweighted", Z_3 = "normal", Z_4 = "over\ weighted", Z_5 = "very\ over\ weighted"\}.$$

To accomplish a formal mathematical design of level restrictions let us study the special own technique of their implementations (Rakus-Andersson, 2007, 2010b). In general, we suggest that the linguistic list of terms is converted to a sampling of fuzzy sets $L_1,...,L_m$, where m is an odd positive integer. Each term is represented by the corresponding fuzzy set, whose restriction is supposed to be created as the common formula depending on the lth value, where $l = 1,...,m$. We assume that supports of restrictions $\mu_{L_l}(w)$, $l = 1,...,m$, will cover parts of the reference set $L = [\min(L_1),\max(L_m)]$, $w \in L$. We introduce $E = |L|$ as the length of L.

We divide all expressions L_l in three groups, namely, a family of "*leftmost*" sets $L_1,..., L_{\frac{m-1}{2}}$, the set $L_{\frac{m+1}{2}}$ "*in the middle*" and a collection of "*rightmost*" sets $L_{\frac{m+3}{2}},...,L_m$. To design the membership functions of L_l the s-class function

$$s(w,\alpha,\beta,\gamma) = \begin{cases} 0 & \text{for} \quad w \le \alpha, \\ 2\left(\frac{w-\alpha}{\gamma-\alpha}\right)^2 & \text{for} \quad \alpha \le w \le \beta, \\ 1-2\left(\frac{w-\gamma}{\gamma-\alpha}\right)^2 & \text{for} \quad \beta \le w \le \gamma, \\ 1 & \text{for} \quad w \ge \gamma, \end{cases} \tag{1}$$

will be adopted. The point $(a, 0)$ starts the graph of the s-function, whereas the point $(\gamma, 1)$ terminates this graph. The parameter β is found as the arithmetic mean of a and γ. In $w = \beta$ the s-function reaches the value of 0.5.

When designing parameters of each class function we want to consider the possibility to obtain the equal lengths of these parts of L_l's supports, which assist membership values greater than or equal to 0.5. The parts are regarded as the important representatives of fuzzy sets as they possess the largest index of the relationship to the set. We thus determine the breadth of each L_l to be $\frac{E}{m}$ on the membership level equal to 0.5.

Let us first design the parameters of the membership function "*in the middle*". The function of $L_{\frac{m+1}{2}}$ is constructed as a π-function

$$\pi(w) = \begin{cases} s(w,\alpha_1,\beta_1,\gamma_1 = \alpha_2) & \text{for} \quad w \le \gamma_1 = \alpha_2, \\ 1-s(w,\alpha_2 = \gamma_1,\beta_2,\gamma_2) & \text{for} \quad w \ge \gamma_1 = \alpha_2. \end{cases} \tag{2}$$

We suppose that $L_{\frac{m+1}{2}}$ will be a normal fuzzy set in $\gamma_1 = \alpha_2 = \frac{E}{2}$.

In order to guarantee the breadth $\frac{E}{m}$ on the membership level 0.5, function $L_{\frac{m+1}{2}}$ should take $\beta_1 = \frac{E}{2} - \frac{E}{2m} = \frac{E(m-1)}{2m}$ and $\beta_2 = \frac{E}{2} + \frac{E}{2m} = \frac{E(m+1)}{2m}$. Since $L_{\frac{m+1}{2}}$ is expected to preserve the uniform and symmetric shape then $\alpha_1 = \frac{E}{2} - 2\frac{E}{2m} = \frac{E(m-2)}{2m}$ and $\alpha_2 = \frac{E}{2} + 2\frac{E}{2m} = \frac{E(m+2)}{2m}$. We state $L_{\frac{m+1}{2}}$'s formula as

$$\mu_{L_{\frac{m+1}{2}}}(w) = \begin{cases} 0 & \text{for } w \leq \frac{E(m-2)}{2m}, \\ 2\left(\frac{w-\frac{E(m-2)}{2m}}{\frac{E}{m}}\right)^2 & \text{for } \frac{E(m-2)}{2m} \leq w \leq \frac{E(m-1)}{2m}, \\ 1-2\left(\frac{w-\frac{E}{2}}{\frac{E}{m}}\right)^2 & \text{for } \frac{E(m-1)}{2m} \leq w \leq \frac{E}{2}, \\ 1-2\left(\frac{w-\frac{E}{2}}{\frac{E}{m}}\right)^2 & \text{for } \frac{E}{2} \leq w \leq \frac{E(m+1)}{2m}, \\ 2\left(\frac{w-\frac{E(m+2)}{2m}}{\frac{E}{m}}\right)^2 & \text{for } \frac{E(m+1)}{2m} \leq w \leq \frac{E(m+2)}{2m}, \\ 0 & \text{for } w \geq \frac{E(m+2)}{2m}. \end{cases} \tag{3}$$

For the "*leftmost*" family $L_1,..., L_{\frac{m-1}{2}}$ we make suggestions that the top segments of functions lying on the membership level 1 will have the same lengths. Moreover, the last "*left*" function $L_{\frac{m-1}{2}}$ should have the intersection point with "*in the middle*" function on the membership level 0.5. Each upper segment of L_t, $t = 1,..., \frac{m-1}{2}$, will be thus equal to $\frac{\frac{E}{2}}{\frac{m-1}{2}+1} = \frac{E}{m+1}$. Particularly, $\alpha_{L_{\frac{m-1}{2}}} = \frac{E(m-1)}{2(m+1)}$ after multiplying the length of the distinct upper segment by the number of the last left function. We have already found $\beta_1 = \frac{E(m-1)}{2m}$ of the "*in the middle*" function $L_{\frac{m+1}{2}}$. Due to the previously made assumption the functions $L_{\frac{m-1}{2}}$ and $L_{\frac{m+1}{2}}$ should intersect each other in point $\left(\frac{E(m-1)}{2m}, 0.5\right)$; therefore $\beta_{L_{\frac{m-1}{2}}} = \frac{E(m-1)}{2m}$. The difference between $\alpha_{L_{\frac{m-1}{2}}}$ and $\beta_{L_{\frac{m-1}{2}}}$ is evaluated to be $\frac{E(m-1)}{2m(m+1)}$. To find a uniform slope of $L_{\frac{m-1}{2}}$ we determine $\gamma_{L_{\frac{m-1}{2}}} = \beta_{L_{\frac{m-1}{2}}} + \frac{E(m-1)}{2m(m+1)} = \frac{E(m-1)(m+2)}{2m(m+1)}$.

Since the beginning of $L_{\frac{m-1}{2}}$ is planned to be placed in $(\min(L_1), 1)$ then $\mu_{L_{\frac{m-1}{2}}}(w) = 1 - s\left(w, \frac{E(m-1)}{2(m+1)}, \frac{E(m-1)}{2m}, \frac{E(m-1)(m+2)}{2m(m+1)}\right)$. The membership function of $L_{\frac{m-1}{2}}$ is thus expanded as

$$\mu_{L_{\frac{m-1}{2}}}(w) = \begin{cases} 1 & \text{for } w \leq \frac{E(m-1)}{2(m+1)}, \\ 1-2\left(\frac{w-\frac{E(m-1)}{2(m+1)}}{\frac{E(m-1)}{m(m+1)}}\right)^2 & \text{for } \frac{E(m-1)}{2(m+1)} \leq w \leq \frac{E(m-1)}{2m}, \\ 2\left(\frac{w-\frac{E(m-1)(m+2)}{2m(m+1)}}{\frac{E(m-1)}{m(m+1)}}\right)^2 & \text{for } \frac{E(m-1)}{2m} \leq w \leq \frac{E(m-1)(m+2)}{2m(m+1)}, \\ 0 & \text{for } w \geq \frac{E(m-1)(m+2)}{2m(m+1)}. \end{cases} \tag{4}$$

All constraints characteristic of the "*leftmost*" family of fuzzy sets will be given after inserting parameter $\delta(t) = \frac{2}{m-1} \cdot t$, $t = 1,\ldots,\frac{m-1}{2}$, in (4) to form it as (Rakus-Andersson, 2007)

$$
\mu_{L_t}(w) = \begin{cases}
1 & \text{for } w \leq \frac{E(m-1)}{2(m+1)}\delta(t), \\[2ex]
1 - 2\left(\dfrac{w - \frac{E(m-1)}{2(m+1)}\delta(t)}{\frac{E(m-1)}{m(m+1)}\delta(t)}\right)^2 & \text{for } \frac{E(m-1)}{2(m+1)}\delta(t) \leq w \leq \frac{E(m-1)}{2m}\delta(t), \\[2ex]
2\left(\dfrac{w - \frac{E(m-1)(m+2)}{2m(m+1)}\delta(t)}{\frac{E(m-1)}{m(m+1)}\delta(t)}\right)^2 & \text{for } \frac{E(m-1)}{2m}\delta(t) \leq w \leq \frac{E(m-1)(m+2)}{2m(m+1)}\delta(t), \\[2ex]
0 & \text{for } w \geq \frac{E(m-1)(m+2)}{2m(m+1)}\delta(t).
\end{cases}
\tag{5}
$$

Parameter $\delta(t)$ takes the value of 1 for $t = \frac{m-1}{2}$, which means that $\delta(\frac{m-1}{2})$ in (5) has no influence on the shape of the last left function. However, the introduction of $\delta(t)$ in (5) induces the narrowing effects in the supports of the other left function shapes. To preserve the same lengths of upper segments corresponding to membership 1 and middle segments attached to membership 0.5 we adjust $\delta(t)$, assisting the left function L_t, to be equal to $\frac{1}{\frac{m-1}{2}}$ multiplied by the function number t.

In order to start the implementation of the "*rightmost*" family functions let us note that the first right function $\mu_{L_{\frac{m+3}{2}}}(w)$ should possess $\mu_{L_{\frac{m-1}{2}}}(w)$'s inverted shape. We generate the membership function of $L_{\frac{m+3}{2}}$ by

$$
\mu_{L_{\frac{m+3}{2}}}(w) = \begin{cases}
0 & \text{for } w \leq E - \frac{E(m-1)(m+2)}{2m(m+1)}, \\[2ex]
2\left(\dfrac{w - \left(E - \frac{E(m-1)(m+2)}{2m(m+1)}\right)}{\frac{E(m-1)}{m(m+1)}}\right)^2 & \text{for } E - \frac{E(m-1)(m+2)}{2m(m+1)} \leq w \leq E - \frac{E(m-1)}{2m}, \\[2ex]
1 - 2\left(\dfrac{w - \left(E - \frac{E(m-1)}{2(m+1)}\right)}{\frac{E(m-1)}{m(m+1)}}\right)^2 & \text{for } E - \frac{E(m-1)}{2m} \leq w \leq E - \frac{E(m-1)}{2(m+1)}, \\[2ex]
1 & \text{for } w \geq E - \frac{E(m-1)}{2(m+1)}.
\end{cases}
\tag{6}
$$

The function of $L_{\frac{m+3}{2}}$ is symmetrically inverted to the function of $L_{\frac{m-1}{2}}$ over interval $[\min(L_1),\max(L_m)]$.

Hence, the membership function $\mu_{L_{\frac{m-1}{2}}}(w) = 1 - s\left(w, \frac{E(m-1)}{2(m+1)}, \frac{E(m-1)}{2m}, \frac{E(m-1)(m+2)}{2m(m+1)}\right)$ will be changed into $\mu_{L_{\frac{m+3}{2}}}(w) = s\left(w, E - \frac{E(m-1)(m+2)}{2m(m+1)}, E - \frac{E(m-1)}{2m}, E - \frac{E(m-1)}{2(m+1)}\right)$.

To generate the "*rightmost*" family of sets $L_{\frac{m+3}{2}},\ldots,L_m$ we need to create a new parameter $\varepsilon(t) = 1 - \frac{2}{m-1}(t-1)$, $t = 1,\ldots,\frac{m-1}{2}$, which will be inserted in (6). The construction of $\varepsilon(t)$, when comparing to the creation of $\varepsilon(t)$, is authorized by the fact that $t = 1$ should be followed by $\varepsilon(1) = 1$, whereas $t = \frac{m-1}{2}$ is helped by $\varepsilon(\frac{m-1}{2}) = \frac{2}{m-1}$. Formula (7) constitutes a common base for deriving membership functions

$$\mu_{L_{\frac{m+3}{2}+t-1}}(w) =$$

$$
\begin{cases}
0 & \text{for } w \le E - \frac{E(m-1)(m+2)}{2m(m+1)}\varepsilon(t), \\[2ex]
2\left(\frac{w-\left(E-\frac{E(m-1)(m+2)}{2m(m+1)}\varepsilon(t)\right)}{\frac{E(m-1)}{m(m+1)}\varepsilon(t)}\right)^2 & \text{for } E - \frac{E(m-1)(m+2)}{2m(m+1)}\varepsilon(t) \le w \le E - \frac{E(m-1)}{2m}\varepsilon(t), \\[2ex]
1-2\left(\frac{w-\left(E-\frac{E(m-1)}{2(m+1)}\varepsilon(t)\right)}{\frac{E(m-1)}{m(m+1)}\varepsilon(t)}\right)^2 & \text{for } E - \frac{E(m-1)}{2m}\varepsilon(t) \le w \le E - \frac{E(m-1)}{2(m+1)}\varepsilon(t), \\[2ex]
1 & \text{for } w \ge E - \frac{E(m-1)}{2(m+1)}\varepsilon(t).
\end{cases}
\tag{7}
$$

The functions of fuzzy sets $L_1,...,L_m$ intend to maintain the same distances on the membership level 0.5. This property allows assigning to $L_1,...,L_m$ the relevant parts of their supports possessing the same length. The relevant parts of fuzzy sets consist of the sets' elements that reveal the membership degree values greater than or equal to 0.5. When forming the supports of the same length, in turn, we warrant the partition of $[\min(L_1),\max(L_m)]$ in equal subintervals standing for L_l levels, $l = 1,...,m$. Apart from that, the "leftmost" and "rightmost" functions also keep the same distances on the membership level 1. This feature provides us with a harmonious arrangement of function shapes.

All steps of the discussed algorithm, which initiates three sets of membership functions corresponding to a list of terms, can be sampled in the block scheme. We need to follow the steps of the scheme together with formulas (3), (5) and (7) to write the excerpt of a computer program. We emphasize that the only data, used in the algorithm, are the length of the reference set and the number of functions. We do not need to specify the sets' borders in the process of the program initialization, as most of programmers do, since the borders are computed automatically by formulas (3), (5) and (7). The steps of the algorithm flow chart are sampled in Fig. 1.

The procedure discussed above has started introduction of membership functions typical of levels of X, Y and Z which, in turn, represent *age*, *CRP* and *body weight*.

For five levels of $X = [0, 100]$, $L = X$, $w = x$, $m = 5$, $E = 100$, the leftmost family is revealed by

$$
\mu_{X_t}(x) = \begin{cases}
1 & \text{for } x \le 33.33(0.5t), \\[2ex]
1-2\left(\frac{x-33.33(0.5t)}{13.33(0.5t)}\right)^2 & \text{for } 33.33(0.5t) \le x \le 40(0.5t), \\[2ex]
2\left(\frac{x-46.66(0.5t)}{13.33(0.5t)}\right)^2 & \text{for } 40(0.5t) \le x \le 46.66(0.5t), \\[2ex]
0 & \text{for } x \ge 46.66(0.5t),
\end{cases}
\tag{8}
$$

for $t = 1, 2$ due to (5).

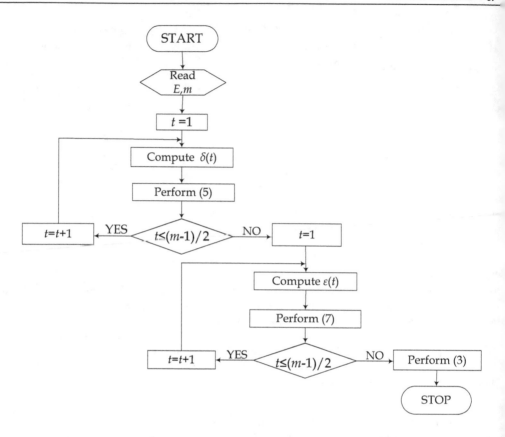

Fig. 1. The flow chart of the $L_1,\ldots,L_m$ implementation

The rightmost family of X-levels, composed with conformity with (7), is stated as

$$\mu_{X_{4+t-1}}(x) =$$
$$\begin{cases} 0 \text{ for } x \leq 100 - 46.66(1 - 0.5(t-1)), \\ 2\left(\frac{x-(100-46.66(1-0.5(t-1)))}{13.33(1-0.5(t-1))}\right)^2 \\ \quad \text{for } 100 - 46.66(1 - 0.5(t-1)) \leq x \leq 100 - 40(1 - 0.5(t-1)), \\ 1 - 2\left(\frac{x-(100-33.33(1-0.5(t-1)))}{13.33(1-0.5(t-1))}\right)^2 \\ \quad \text{for } 100 - 40(1 - 0.5(t-1)) \leq x \leq 100 - 33.33(1 - 0.5(t-1)), \\ 1 \text{ for } x \geq 100 - 33.33(1 - 0.5(t-1)), \end{cases} \qquad (9)$$

for $t = 1, 2$.

The "*in the middle*" X-level "*middle-aged*" has, in accord with (3), the constraint

$$\mu_{X_3}(x) = \begin{cases} 0 & \text{for} \quad x \le 30, \\ 2\left(\frac{x-30}{20}\right)^2 & \text{for} \quad 30 \le x \le 40, \\ 1 - 2\left(\frac{x-50}{20}\right)^2 & \text{for} \quad 40 \le x \le 50, \\ 1 - 2\left(\frac{x-50}{20}\right)^2 & \text{for} \quad 50 \le x \le 60, \\ 2\left(\frac{x-70}{20}\right)^2 & \text{for} \quad 60 \le x \le 70, \\ 0 & \text{for} \quad x \ge 70. \end{cases} \tag{10}$$

All levels of X are sketched in Fig. 2.

The parts of X_1-X_5 supports should be consisted of elements, which have the strongest connections with the X_1-X_5 fuzzy sets. Therefore we only select the elements having the membership degrees greater than or equal to 0.5.

To make the partition of X in subintervals representing levels X_1-X_5 we return to formulas (8), (9) and (10). Due to (8), to find the subinterval of X assisting X_1 when $t = 1$, we concatenate the intervals $x \le 33.33(0.5 \cdot 1)$ and $33.33(0.5 \cdot 1) \le x \le 40(0.5 \cdot 1)$, leading to [0, 20].

We have chosen these intervals, which contain elements of X_1 furnished with membership degrees greater than or equal to 0.5. For $t = 2$, set in two first intervals of (8), we aggregate $x \le 33.33(0.5 \cdot 2)$ and $33.33(0.5 \cdot 2) \le x \le 40(0.5 \cdot 2)$ in [0, 40]. This generates the interval [0, 40]-[0, 20] = [20, 40] typical of X_2. By (10) we find [40, 60] = [40, 50] + [50, 60] as an essential part of X_3. The insertion of $t = 2$ in (9) produces a joint of

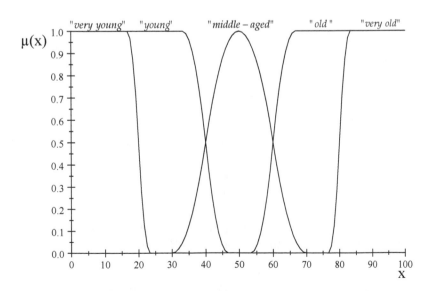

Fig. 2. The fuzzy sets X_1-X_5

$100 - 40(1 - 0.5(2 - 1)) \le x \le 100 - 33.33(1 - 0.5(2 - 1))$ and $x \ge 100 - 33.33(1 - 0.5(2 - 1))$ to be a common interval [80, 100] regarded as the domain of X_5. By setting $t = 1$ in the last intervals of (9) we get the field [60, 100]. It means that X_4 will be given by [60, 80] = [60, 100]–[80, 100]. We are furnished with the same intervals after accomplishing the close analysis of Fig. 2 on the membership level 0.5.

Let us now initiate the associations among the terms of X, characteristic intervals of these terms and assigned to them codes due to the scheme

name of X-level	representative interval	code
X_1	0–20	0
X_2	20–40	1
X_3	40–60	2
X_4	60–80	3
X_5	80–100	4

We emphasize the role of an elegant mathematical design of X's membership functions, which allows making the partition of the X-domain in equal intervals. Definitely, we obtain the same results when dividing the length of X by the number of levels to get a length of one part but the effects computed by means of membership functions only confirm this intuitive calculation. Moreover we can modify the arbitrary lengths of X-subintervals by making changes in the formulas of $\delta(t)$ and $\varepsilon(t)$.

By applying the same technique to $Y = [0, 60]$, $L = Y$, $w = y$, $m = 5$, $E = 60$ we generate the code pattern

name of Y-level	representative interval	code
Y_1	0–12	0
Y_2	12–24	1
Y_3	24–36	2
Y_4	36–48	3
Y_5	48–60	4

Lastly, if $Z = [40, 120]$ for men, $L = Z$, $w = z$, $m = 5$, $E = 80$ then

name of Y-level	representative interval	code
Z_1	40–56	0
Z_2	56–72	1
Z_3	72–88	2
Z_4	88–104	3
Z_5	104–120	4

If we collect clinical data, concerning a patient examined then we will be now capable to create code vectors taking place in the discrimination NS algorithm.

Example 1

An eighty one-year-old man, whose CRP is 17 and weight is 91, will be given by the vector $v = (4, 1, 3)$.

In order to measure the affinity (coverage) of two code vectors v_1 and v_2 of the same length over the same alphabet we are furnished with the r-contiguous bit matching rule, which provides us with a true match(v_1, v_2) if v_1 and v_2 agree in r contiguous locations.

Example 2

For $v_1 = (3, 1, 3)$ and $v_2 = (3, 1, 2)$, when $r = 2$, match(v_1, v_2) is true.

4. The selection of the most representative data vectors for the decision "operate"

We have already mentioned that we need the "operate" types of patient data vectors as the entries of the NS discrimination algorithm. We thus want to prepare typical data strings for the decision "operate" in advance.

Let us first treat the vector $v = (x, y, z)$ as the string of integers $v = (x\ y\ z)$, where x, y and z can take the code values 0, 1, 2, 3, 4. We form the function $f(x\ y\ z) = x + y + z$ to measure the common code value of the data vector. To make the selection of "operate" type vectors even more accurate let us assign the weights of power-importance to the biological indices considered in the operation decision. In the gastric cancer operation decision we first concentrate our attention on the changes of CRP- values, which points out CRP as the most decisive factor. The analysis of CRP is followed by the judgment of age and, finally, we check the values of body weights. Hence, we state the ranking of the symptom importance as $CRP \succ age \succ body\ weight$, provided that $\succ$ means "more important than".

A procedure for obtaining a ratio scale of importance for a group of m elements (in the considered case – biological markers) was developed by Saaty (Saaty, 1978). Assume that we have m objects (symptoms) and we want to construct a scale, rating these objects as to their importance with respect to the decision. We ask a decision-maker to compare the objects in paired comparison. If we compare object j with object k, j, $k = 1,...,m$, then we will assign the values b_{jk} and b_{kj} as follows

1. $b_{kj} = \dfrac{1}{b_{jk}}$.

2. If objective j is more important than objective k then b_{jk} gets assigned a number according to the following scheme:

Intensity of importance expressed by the value of b_{jk}	Definition
1	Equal importance of x_j and x_k
3	Weak importance of x_j over x_k
5	Strong importance of x_j over x_k
7	Demonstrated importance of x_j over x_k
9	Absolute importance of x_j over x_k
2, 4, 6, 8	Intermediate values

If object k is more important than object j, we assign the value of b_{kj}.

Having obtained the above judgments an $m \times m$ importance matrix $B = \left(b_{jk}\right)_{j,k=1}^{m}$ is constructed. The importance weights are decided as components of this eigenvector that corresponds to the largest in magnitude eigenvalue of the matrix B.

Example 3

For priorities $Y = CRP \succ X = age \succ Z = body\ weight$ we determine the contents of B as

$$B = \begin{array}{c} \\ X \\ Y \\ Z \end{array} \begin{array}{ccc} X & Y & Z \\ \left[\begin{array}{ccc} 1 & \frac{1}{3} & 3 \\ 3 & 1 & 5 \\ \frac{1}{3} & \frac{1}{5} & 1 \end{array}\right] \end{array}$$

The largest eigenvalue ($\lambda = 3.033$) of B has the associated eigenvector $V = (0.37, 0.92, 0.15)$. V is composed of coordinates that are interpreted as the importance weights w_1, w_2, w_3 sought for X, Y, Z.

Let us rearrange the form of function f by adding the weights of importance to the vector code values. The new pattern of f is designed as $f(x\ y\ z) = w_1x + w_2y + w_3z$. The function value yields the patient's characteristics given by a combination of codes stated for different symptoms.

Example 4

The patient vector $v = (3, 1, 2)$ has the characteristics $f(312) = 0.37 \cdot 3 + 0.92 \cdot 1 + 0.15 \cdot 2 = 2.33$.

Due to the physician's expertise we assume that we can operate patients who are characterized by codes of age equal to 1, 2 and 3, codes of CRP recognized as 0, 1 and 2 and codes of body weight determined as 1, 2 and 3. The minimal patient characteristics to be operated is thus $f(101) = 0.37 \cdot 1 + 0.92 \cdot 0 + 0.15 \cdot 1 = 0.52$, whereas the maximal data characteristics, classifying the patient for the operation is given by $f(323) = 0.37 \cdot 3 + 0.92 \cdot 2 + 0.15 \cdot 3 = 3.4$. We conclude that the patient who is capable to be operated should have the characteristics $f(x\ y\ z)$ included in the interval [0.52, 3.4]. It is worth emphasizing that the decisions are made with respect to the decisive power of biological markers age, CRP and $body\ weight$.

Example 5

We test $v = (4, 2, 4)$. As $f(424) = 0.37 \cdot 4 + 0.92 \cdot 2 + 0.15 \cdot 4 = 3.92$, which lies beyond the boundaries of the "operate" interval, then the patient with data $v = (4, 2, 4)$ should not be operated. For vectors $v_1 = (3, 2, 2)$, $v_2 = (2, 0, 2)$, $v_3 = (3, 1, 3)$, $v_4 = (3, 1, 2)$ the decision will be made as "operate".

The flow chart, sketched in Fig. 3, will show the selection of vectors typical of the decision "operate".

The vectors v_1, v_2, v_3 and v_4 will be included in the experimental population of representative data strings for the positive decision of the operation. We intend to use them in the next part of the chapter, when discussing the action of the NS algorithm adapted to the operation model.

5. The negative selection algorithm

After coding the patient data and selecting the initial data, which are given into account for the decision "operate", we can make a choice between two alternatives concerning the cure

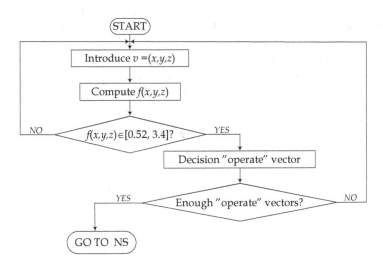

Fig. 3. The flow chart of the selection of "operate" type vectors

of gastric cancer patients. We intend to adapt the technique of an immunological algorithm based on the T cell behaviour. We use the negative selection algorithm NS proposed by Forrest (Forrest et al., 1997).

The goal of NS is to cover the non-self space with a set of detectors. For the sake of the surgery aim, already outlined in Section 2, the algorithm should lead to discrimination of the statements "operate" and "do not operate" provided that vectors characteristic of type "operate" are available. This assumption is motivated by the surgeon's intention to cure the patient from his/her cancer disease by making surgery if the patient's state allows accomplishing it. The patient data reports, which register his/her parameters in the case of operating, are clearly interpretable. However, the physician can have some doubts when he denies an operation for the patient. Therefore we have used the strings confirming the "operate" decision as the more convincing vectors in the entrance of NS.

We distinguish two steps in the surgery NS algorithm prepared on the basis of the general NS (Dasgupta & Nino, 2008; Engelbrecht, 2007; Forrest et al., 1997):

1. Generation of detectors, which should possess the property vectors corresponding to the decision "do not operate" on a patient. These strings are not recognized as obviously as the strings of "operate"; that is why we get some help from the algorithm in generating their patterns.
2. Selection of the surgery settlements "operate" or "do not operate" for any patient data vector due to the matching criterion concerning detectors.

In the first step a set of detectors is generated. To accomplish this task we use as an input a collection of vectors found by the method of preparing "operate" strings, which have been discussed in Section 4. Candidate detectors that match any of the "operate" type vector samples are eliminated whereas unmatched ones are kept. We adopt the r-contiguous bit matching rule for the patient data vectors as a measure of "the distance" between the "operate" type and the "do not operate" decision.

In the second step of NS the stored detectors, generated in the first stage, are used to check whether new incoming samples of patient data vectors correspond to the "operate" type or to the "do not operate" type. If an input sample, characterizing a patient, matches any detector then the patient should not be operated. When we cannot find a match between detectors and the incoming patient data vector it will mean that the decision about the surgery should be made. Figure 4 collects all steps of the surgery NS algorithm in the flow chart.

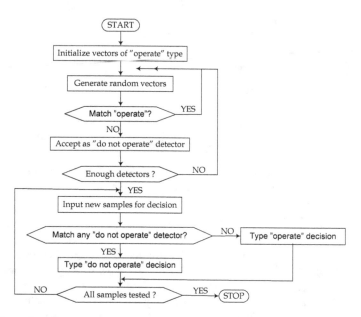

Fig. 4. The flow chart of the surgery NS algorithm

6. The surgery decision based on the NS algorithm

We wish now to follow the steps of the surgery NS algorithm to study its action in practical decision cases concerning the operation decision.

Let us thus go through the following example.

Step 1. *Initialization*

As the input data we introduce the set $V = \{v_1, v_2, v_3, v_4\}$, which consists of four patient data vectors characteristic of the "operate" type. The length of each vector is decided to be three in conformity with previously made suggestions. In Section 4 we have already initialized

$v_1 = (3, 2, 2),$
$v_2 = (2, 0, 2),$

$v_3 = (3, 1, 3)$,
$v_4 = (3, 1, 2)$.

The vectors emerge the clinical data concerning elderly patients whose the CRP- values are not very high. The patients' weights are not radically deviated from normal standards either. Hence, they have been operated in conformity with the surgeon's determination.

We now wish to generate the set D of four detectors d_1, d_2, d_3, d_4 that should not match any of v_j, $j = 1,...,4$. At the beginning of the procedure D is an empty set.

To measure the match grade between v_j and candidates to be detectors we state, e.g., $r = 2$ in the r-contiguous bit matching rule.

Step 2. *Introduction of random candidates to act as detectors*

We present $d = (3, 1, 1)$ and check matches between d and each v_j, $j = 1,...,4$, as

match$((3, 2, 2), (3, 1, 1))$ is false,
match$((2, 0, 2), (3, 1, 1))$ is false,
match$((3, 1, 3), (3, 1, 1))$ is true,
match$((3, 1, 2), (3, 1, 1))$ is true.

Since d matches v_3 and v_4 then it cannot be classified as a detector.

We prove the next candidate $d = (4, 3, 1)$ to make matches between d and each v_j, $j = 1,...,4$, in the form of

match$((3, 2, 2), (4, 3, 1))$ is false,
match$((2, 0, 2), (4, 3, 1))$ is false,
match$((3, 1, 3), (4, 3, 1))$ is false,
match$((3, 1, 2), (4, 3, 1))$ is false.

All matches are false, which means that $d_1 = d$ is the first detector placed in D. The set of detectors now contains one element $d_1 = (4, 3, 1)$. We repeat the procedure until we determine four detectors in set D. D is finally formed as

$D = \{(4, 3, 1), (2, 3, 4), (4, 4, 1), (3, 4, 0)\}$.

Step 3. *Operation decision making*

In the second phase of the algorithm we test data strings to organize them in either the "operate" type or in the "do not operate" type decisions. If the data vector matches any detector from D then the decision is made as "do not operate" (the non-self region). Otherwise, for all false matches between the data vector and d_k, $k = 1,...,4$, we accept the operation (the self region).

We introduce $v = (3, 2, 3)$. The matches to detectors are determined as

match$((4, 3, 1), (3, 2, 3))$ is false,
match$((2, 3, 4), (3, 2, 3))$ is false,
match$((4, 4, 1), (3, 2, 3))$ is false,
match$((3, 4, 0), (3, 2, 3))$ is false.

As all matches to detectors are false we conclude the performance of surgery (decision "operate").

Another test vector $v = (3, 4, 1)$ is inserted into the checking system. The match results are shown as

match$((4, 3, 1), (3, 4, 1))$ is false,
match$((2, 3, 4), (3, 4, 1))$ is false,
match$((4, 4, 1), (3, 4, 1))$ is true,
match$((3, 4, 0), (3, 4, 1))$ is true.

Vector v converges to two detectors, which means the decision to be referred to "do not operate".

By setting $r = 2$ in the contiguous bit matching rule we have preserved a margin of imprecision in decision making, since we do not demand all contiguous vector codes to be equal. This gives a certain chance of operating for the patients whose mix of biological indices cannot be precisely judged. For $r = 3$ the decision will be quite strict.

The method of making medical decisions by means of immunological systems is an applicable novelty. The example has a more didactic and experimental meaning than a real medical investigation. If we really want to use the method for making decisions in the surgery discipline we should, at first, extend the length of data strings by introducing more biological markers. A very dense set of initial vectors from "self" ("operate") ought to be chosen by the algorithm belonging to Section 4. Nevertheless, the proposal of combining fuzzy systems and weighted characteristics of vectors with the NS algorithm to create the hybrid can start a new applied domain in medicine.

7. Conclusion

In the process of creation of a new medical application model we have inserted some elements of fuzzy systems into the negative selection immunological algorithm. This hybrid, attached to two disciplines of Computational Intelligence, has found a practical application in surgery decision making. As self and non-self constitute two regions of the NS partition of objects then we could identify these regions with decisions "operate" against "do not operate" in the case of curing gastric cancer patients. The action of the modified NS could help us to determine the surgery or its lack for individual patients with respect to their clinical data entry vectors.

To make the action of the NS algorithm more efficient we have complemented the method by preparing the population of the most representative vectors standing for the "operate" type. The vectors have been converted to real values giving the common characteristics of a patient. In that characteristics the weights of importance, assigned to biological markers, will play the essential role in the final judgment of the vectors' influence on the decision "operate".

We wish to add that the excerpts from fuzzy systems, involved in NS, come from own research, which has been concentrated on the creation of compact parametric formulas. These formulas concern the generation of a family of membership functions without predetermining their borders in advance.

All parts of the methodology have been prepared in the form of numerical algorithms given by flow charts. This allows composing a common computer program to test large samples of vectors in a real clinical application.

We emphasize that the proposal is a novel contribution in medical applications and should be still tested on larger samples of data. We can expect that, in future investigations, an introduction of the neural artificial perceptron model instead of the NS algorithm will provide us with similar results concerning surgery decisions. As an extension of the model we also wish to adapt the real-value negative selection algorithm in order to insert measured values of biological markers in data vectors instead of codes. This procedure should improve the reliability of a decision. Having results from more models we can select the most efficient one to work on its further development.

8. Acknowledgment

The author thanks the Blekinge Research Board in Sweden for the grant funding the current research. The author is also grateful to Associate Professor Henrik Forssell for supporting these investigations with medical advice and data.

9. References

Antunes, M. & Correia, M.E. (2011). Tunable Immune Detectors for Behavior-Based Network Intrusion Detection, *Artificial Immune Systems: 10th International Conference, ICARIS 2011*, Cambridge, UK, pp. 334–347, LNCS, vol. 6825, Springer, ISBN 978-3-642-22370-9

De Castro, L.N. & Timmis, J. (2002). *Artificial Immune Systems*, Springer, ISBN 978-1-85233-594-6, Berlin Heidelberg

Cohen, I.R. (2006). Immune System Computation and the Immunological Homunculus, LNCS, vol. 4199, pp. 49–52, ISBN 978-3-540-45772-5

Dasgupta, D. & Nino, F. (2008). *Immunological Computation: Theory and Applications*, Auerbach Publishers Inc., ISBN 978-1-420-06545-9, London

Do-Kyong Kim, Sung Yong Oh, Hyuk-Chan Kwon, Suee Lee, Kyung A Kwon, Byung Geun Kim, Seong-Geun Kim, Sung-Hyun Kim, Jin Seok Jang, Min Chan Kim, Kyeong Hee Kim, Jin-Yeong Han & Hyo-Jin Kim (2009). Clinical Significances of Preoperative Serum Interleukin-6 and C-reactive Protein Level in Operable Gastric Cancer, *BMC Cancer* 9, pp. 155–156, ISSN 1471-2407

Engelbrecht, A.P. (2007). *Computational Intelligence*, Wiley & Sons Ltd., ISBN 978-0-470-03561-0, Chichester

Forrest, S., Hofmeyr, A.S. & Somayaji, A. (1997). Computer Immunology, *Communications of the ACM*, vol. 40, nr 10, pp. 88–96, ISSN 1017-4656

Gao, X.Z., Ovaska, S.I., Wang, X. & Chow, M.Y. (2008). A Neural Networks-based Negative Selection Algorithm in Fault Diagnosis, *Neural Computing & Applications*, vol. 17, nr 1, pp. 91–98, ISSN 1433-3058

Harmer, P.K., Williams, P.D., Gunsch, G.H. & Lamont, G.B. (2002). An Artificial Immune System Architecture for Computer Security Applications, *IEEE Transactions on Evolutionary Computation*, vol. 6, nr 3, pp. 252–280, ISSN 1089-778X

Igawa, K. & Ohashi, H. (2009). A Negative Selection Algorithm for Classification and Reduction of the Noise Effect, *Journal of Applied Soft Computing*, vol. 9, nr 1, pp. 431–438, ISSN 1568-4946

Ishida, Y. (2004). *Immunity-Based Systems: A Design Perspective*, Springer, ISBN 3-540-00896-9, Berlin Heidelberg New York

de Mello, J., Struthers, L., Turner, R., Cooper, E.H. & Giles, G.R. (1983). Multivariate Analyses as Aids to Diagnosis and Assessment of Prognosis in Gastrointestinal Cancer, *Br. J. Cancer*, nr 48, pp. 341–348, ISSN 0007-0920

Rakus-Andersson, E. (2007). *Fuzzy and Rough Techniques in Medical Diagnosis and Medication*, Springer, ISBN 978-3-540-49707-3, Berlin Heidelberg

Rakus-Andersson, E. & Jain, L. (2009). Computational Intelligence in Medical Decisions Making, *Recent Advances in Decision Making*, Springer, Berlin Heidelberg, pp. 145–159, ISBN 978-3-642-02186-2

Rakus-Andersson, E. (2009). Approximate Reasoning in Surgical Decisions, *Proceedings of the International Fuzzy Systems Association World Congress – IFSA 2009*, Instituto Superior Technico, pp. 225–230, ISBN 978-989-95079-6-8

Rakus-Andersson, E. (2010a). One-dimensional Model of Approximate Reasoning in Surgical Considerations, *Developments in Fuzzy Sets, Intuitionistic Fuzzy Sets, Generalized Nets and Related Topics*, vol. II, System Research Institute of Polish Academy of Sciences, pp. 233–246, ISBN 139788389475305

Rakus-Andersson, E. (2010b). Adjusted s-parametric Functions in the Creation of Symmetric Constraints, *Proceedings of the 10th International Conference on Intelligent Systems Design and Applications - ISDA 2010*, Cairo, Egypt, pp. 451–456, ISBN 978-1-4244-8135-4

Rakus-Andersson, E. (2011). Hybridization of Immunological Computation and Fuzzy Systems in Surgery Decision Making, *Proceedings of the 15th Conference on Knowledge Expert Systems – KES 2011*, Kaiserslauntern, Germany, LNCS/LNAI, vol. 6884, Springer, Berlin Heidelberg, pp. 399–408, ISBN 978-3-642-23865-9

Rutkowski, L. (2008). *Computational Intelligence: Methods and Techniques*, ISBN 978-3-540-76287-4, Springer, Berlin Heidelberg

Saaty, T.L. (1978). Exploring the Interface between Hierarchies, Multiplied Objectives and Fuzzy Sets, *Fuzzy Sets and Systems* 1, pp. 57–58, ISSN 0165-0114

Wakizono, M., Hatanaka, T. & Uosaki, K. (2006). Time Varying System Identification with Immune Based Evolutionary Computation, *Proceedings of SICE-ICASE, 2006*, Busan, Korea, pp. 5608–5613, ISBN 89-950038-4-7

Zhang, Q. & Zhao, H. (2010). The Research of Generation Algorithm of Detectors in a New Negative Selection Algorithm, *Proceedings of the International Conference on Technology Management and Innovation 2010*, paper 78, ISBN 13-978-0-791-85961-2

Permissions

The contributors of this book come from diverse backgrounds, making this book a truly international effort. This book will bring forth new frontiers with its revolutionizing research information and detailed analysis of the nascent developments around the world.

We would like to thank Tomasz Brzozowski, for lending his expertise to make the book truly unique. He has played a crucial role in the development of this book. Without his invaluable contribution this book wouldn't have been possible. He has made vital efforts to compile up to date information on the varied aspects of this subject to make this book a valuable addition to the collection of many professionals and students.

This book was conceptualized with the vision of imparting up-to-date information and advanced data in this field. To ensure the same, a matchless editorial board was set up. Every individual on the board went through rigorous rounds of assessment to prove their worth. After which they invested a large part of their time researching and compiling the most relevant data for our readers. Conferences and sessions were held from time to time between the editorial board and the contributing authors to present the data in the most comprehensible form. The editorial team has worked tirelessly to provide valuable and valid information to help people across the globe.

Every chapter published in this book has been scrutinized by our experts. Their significance has been extensively debated. The topics covered herein carry significant findings which will fuel the growth of the discipline. They may even be implemented as practical applications or may be referred to as a beginning point for another development. Chapters in this book were first published by InTech; hereby published with permission under the Creative Commons Attribution License or equivalent.

The editorial board has been involved in producing this book since its inception. They have spent rigorous hours researching and exploring the diverse topics which have resulted in the successful publishing of this book. They have passed on their knowledge of decades through this book. To expedite this challenging task, the publisher supported the team at every step. A small team of assistant editors was also appointed to further simplify the editing procedure and attain best results for the readers.

Our editorial team has been hand-picked from every corner of the world. Their multi-ethnicity adds dynamic inputs to the discussions which result in innovative outcomes. These outcomes are then further discussed with the researchers and contributors who give their valuable feedback and opinion regarding the same. The feedback is then collaborated with the researches and they are edited in a comprehensive manner to aid the understanding of the subject.

Apart from the editorial board, the designing team has also invested a significant amount of their time in understanding the subject and creating the most relevant covers. They scrutinized every image to scout for the most suitable representation of the subject and create an appropriate cover for the book.

The publishing team has been involved in this book since its early stages. They were actively engaged in every process, be it collecting the data, connecting with the contributors or procuring relevant information. The team has been an ardent support to the editorial, designing and production team. Their endless efforts to recruit the best for this project, has resulted in the accomplishment of this book. They are a veteran in the field of academics and their pool of knowledge is as vast as their experience in printing. Their expertise and guidance has proved useful at every step. Their uncompromising quality standards have made this book an exceptional effort. Their encouragement from time to time has been an inspiration for everyone.

The publisher and the editorial board hope that this book will prove to be a valuable piece of knowledge for researchers, students, practitioners and scholars across the globe.

List of Contributors

Bhavani Prasad Kota and Basil D. Roufogalis
University of Sydney, Australia

Aik Wei Teoh
Ferngrove Pharmaceuticals, Australia

Saoussen Turki and Héla Kallel
Unité de Biofermentation, Institut Pasteur de Tunis, Tunisia

Neeraj Prasad
Royal Albert Edward Infirmary, Wigan, University of Salford, United Kingdom

In-Hyun Lee, Jung Wan Hong, Yura Jang, Yeong Taek Park and Hesson Chung
Korea Institute of Science and Technology and Daehwa Pharmaceutical, Korea

Soňa Gancarčíková
University of Veterinary Medicine and Pharmacy, Košice, Slovakia

Rani Sophia and Waseem Ahmad Bashir
Yeovil Hospital NHS Foundation Trust, Yeovil, Somerset, United Kingdom

S. Burmeister, P.C. Bornman, J.E.J. Krige and S.R. Thomson
University of Cape Town, South Africa

Antonio Marte, Lucia Pintozzi and Pio Parmeggiani
Pediatric Surgery, 2nd University of Naples, Naples, Italy

Gianpaolo Marte
General Surgery, 2nd University of Naples, Naples, Italy

Yoko Uchiyama-Tanaka
Yoko Clinic, Japan

Nam Q. Nguyen
Department of Gastroenterology, Royal Adelaide Hospital, North Terrace, Adelaide, SA, Australia

Om Parkash, Adil Aub and Saeed Hamid
Aga Khan University, Karachi, Pakistan

A. Lorenzo Hernández and E. Ramirez
University Autonoma of Madrid, Spain

Jf. Sánchez Muñoz-Torrero
University of Extremadura, Spain

Beata Jabłońska and Paweł Lampe
Medical University of Silesia in Katowice, Department of Digestive Tract Surgery, Poland

Elisabeth Rakus-Andersson
Blekinge Institute of Technology, Sweden

Printed in the USA
CPSIA information can be obtained
at www.ICGtesting.com
LVHW051033190224
772231LV00003B/23